An Introduction to the Medical History of Ethiopia

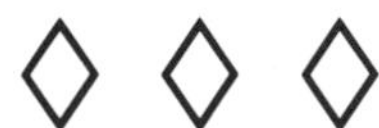

Richard Pankhurst

with a Postscript by Asrat Waldeyes

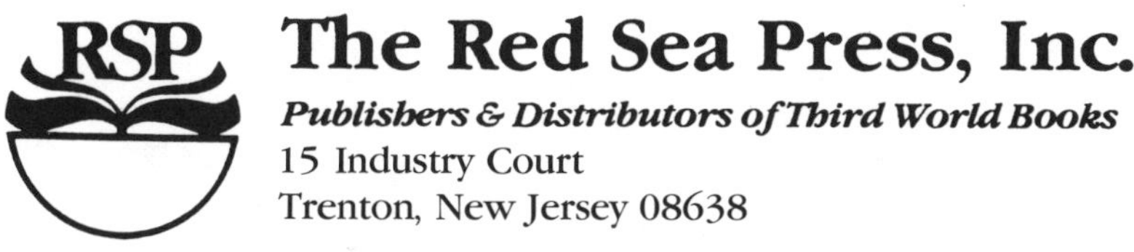

The Red Sea Press, Inc.
Publishers & Distributors of Third World Books
15 Industry Court
Trenton, New Jersey 08638

Red Sea Press
15 Industry Court
Trenton, NJ 08638

Cover design by Ife Nii Owoo

Typeset by TypeHouse of Pennington, Inc.

Book design by Francesca Kindron

Library of Congress Catalog Card Number: 90-816622

ISBN: 0-932415-44-x   cloth
       0-932415-45-8   paper

Contents

For Rita

Part I

Epidemics, Diseases and Traditional Approaches to Medicine

I

Introduction: Some Factors Affecting Health

Climatic Factors

Ethiopia on many counts was geographically well situated. Normally, the climate of the highlands with its bright sunshine yet gentle heat is salubrious and invigorating, and two annual rainy seasons do much to cleanse the country of infection. The value of these rains impressed observers such as the Englishman Charles Rey, who, writing of Addis Ababa in the 1920s, observed that after seven or eight months one looked forward to "the coming fierce downpours, to bring freshness to the air and cleanliness to the town." His compatriot Christine Sandford agreed that the weather did much to compensate for lack of medical facilities. "It was," she wrote, "only the wonderful climate of the highlands," with their "dry air, brilliant sunshine, yet temperate heat," followed by the "cleansing torrents of the rainy season," that "checked the spread of infection and made epidemics very uncommon." On a more personal note, she commented:

> The author brought up a family of six children in Addis Ababa and its vicinity without any infectious illness among them in over fifteen years, with the exception of one case of whooping cough, and occasional conjunctivitis, which, after a little experience, was avoided altogether.

The highlands suffered, however, from sudden drops in temperature, particularly at night, as well as from considerable humidity during rains. Cold nights following upon warm or hot days were probably responsible for the high incidence of pneumonia, pleurisy, bronchitis, catarrh and other diseases of the respiratory organs. Heavy rainfall was likewise conducive to the colds, influenza, and bronchitis that were sometimes prevalent during the rains.

The lowlands, on the other hand, tended to be infested with mosquitoes and thus were subject to malaria. This disease was widespread in areas of low elevation, particularly during the rains, and was especially prevalent in narrow, densely wooded, and damp river valleys and swampy plains near rivers and lakes, as well as in the coastal area.

The extent of malaria has been attested by innumerable observers. Early in the nineteenth century the British traveler Henry Salt observed that the high incidence of the disease in the Massawa area was responsible for the Ethiopians' "great dread and horror of the coast," while King Sahla Sellasé of Shawa, speaking of the lowlands of Adal, remarked, "The water of the *qwolla* (i.e., low country) is putrid, and the air hot and unwholesome." The French travelers Ferret and Galinier, writing of Tegré and Lake Tana, likewise observed: "Toward the end of the rainy season the humid atmosphere and the soil, which is soaked and productive of a pernicious miasma, turn the country into a fatal region." Walter Plowden, a British consul of the 1850s, wrote that fevers were common around Lake Tana, while his contemporary Henry Stern complained that they "overspread" the lowlands "for more than six months in the year." Similar testimony was provided by eye-witnesses in other regions. Lejean stated that the disease was prevalent in the Sheré lowlands, Hayes in the Blue Nile–Lake Tana area, Marcel Cohen in the Awash Valley, Traversi around Lake Zway, Hugh Le Roux in the environs of Harar, Macfie in Ogaden, Hodson in the neighborhood of Lake Margherita and the Omo, Bartleet around Gambela, and Boyes on the Kenya frontier. Traders visiting the lowlands, according to Dr. Mérab, a Georgian pharmacist in early twentieth-century Addis Ababa, were also often badly affected.

Most of the lowlands, particularly to the east and south, historically consisted of arid scrub-lands, some giving way to deserts. These regions, because of the sand and dust in the air, and the glare of the cloudless sky, often suffered from a higher than average incidence of eye disease. The prevalence of eye infections among the Danakil was noticed by several nineteenth-century observers, among them Johnston, Krapf, Munzinger, and Soleillet, and was also reported in the Harar area by Richard Burton and Franz Pedar, in Ogaden by Jennings, and in Borana by Maud. The high incidence of eye complaints in the eastern provinces is likewise evident from the statistics of the Russian Red Cross mission of 1896, which indicate that such cases accounted for 30% of its consultations in Harar as compared with only 12% in Addis Ababa.

Agricultural Factors: Abundance and Scarcity

Ethiopia traditionally enjoyed abundant agriculture. In 1520 the Portuguese priest Francisco Alvares, traveling through the May Tzada region of Tegré, exclaimed: "It seems to me that in the whole world there is not so populous a country or one so abundant in crops." Further to the south in the

Farso area, near modern May Chaw, he saw "thick maize fields as high as large cane." The inhabitants told him that

> They gathered so much crops of all kinds, that were it not for the worm, there would have been abundance for ten years. And because I was amazed they said to me: "Honoured guest, do not be amazed, because in the years that we harvest little we gather for three years' plenty in the country; and if it were not for the multitudes of locusts and hail, which sometimes do great damage, we should not sow the half of what we sow because so much remains that it cannot be believed; so it is sowing wheat, or barley, lentils, pulse or any seed. We sow so much with the hope that even if each of the said plagues should come some would be spoiled but some would remain, and if all were spoiled the year before, our produce is in such manner abundant that we have no scarcity."

Livestock resources were also immense, as seen from the description by Alvares of "infinite herds." Writing again of the Farso region he declared: "Those of our company guessed them at fifty thousand cows. I do not say a larger number, and yet the multitude cannot be believed." Such abundance probably ensured an adequate consumption of food in normal years by the population at large.

Droughts and crop failures, outbreaks of cattle disease, plagues of locusts, the ravages of war, and looting by soldiers, however, led to frequent acute famines. These, as recorded in the Ethiopian royal chronicles and travel literature, are known to have occurred in the following years: 1540, 1543, 1567, 1611, 1623, 1625, 1633, 1635, 1636, 1647, 1650, 1653, 1678, 1700, 1702, 1721, 1722, 1747, 1748, 1752, 1783, 1789, 1797, 1800, 1828, 1829, 1835, 1836, 1837, 1864, 1868, 1876, 1888, 1889, 1890, 1891, 1892, 1905, 1913, 1914, 1928, and 1929.

These famines were invariably accompanied by a drastic deterioration of public health, often followed by serious epidemics. This correlation between famine and epidemics was based on four main factors: 1) the starving and debilitated populations had little resistance to disease; 2) famine victims often resorted to eating impure food, such as carcasses of decaying animals; 3) people dying during famines were frequently left unburied, thus themselves becoming a source of infection; 4) famished persons wandering around the country in search of food served as carriers of disease.

The earliest documented instance of this relationship between famine and disease is in the first half of the ninth century when, according to the *Ethiopian Synaxarium*, a harvest failure and consequent famine were followed by an outbreak of plague. The chronology of many of the epidemics which followed cannot be established, but a number, as we shall see, were demonstrably related to famines. The Great Famine of 1888-1892, which is better documented than any earlier outbreak, was, for example, clearly followed by a lamentable deterioration of hygienic and sanitary conditions.

Contemporary observers left a terrible tale of woe. The Ethiopian author Afawarq Gabra Iyasus recorded that the "people, dying of hunger, began to collapse or lie down on the roads, in the woods, around the enclosures of churches and the houses of dignitaries." Vanderheym, a French traveler, stated that it was not unusual for hyenas and jackals to leave Addis Ababa at daybreak without having consumed all the unburied corpses, while Martini, the governor of the Italian colony of Eritrea, told of "abandoned corpses" and "walking skeletons," as well as of "young boys searching in the excrement of camels to find a grain of durra." The missionary Clemente da Terzorio, describing the situation at Harar, wrote of large numbers of flies, which after sucking the putrefying matter of corpses, alighted on the living. Under such circumstances it is hardly surprising that there were large-scale epidemics of cholera, smallpox, typhus, dysentery, and influenza.

Societal and Personal Factors

Fasting

Ethiopian Christians were often physically debilitated by their strict observance of periods of fast and abstinence, which in many cases were followed by excessive feasting. There were a minimum of 158 and a maximum of 208 days of abstinence per year, or an average of 183 days out of 365, approximately half the total. On days of abstinence the population refrained from consuming any animal food (i.e., meat, milk, butter, cheese, or eggs). This limitation was considered by some to also include fish, which in any event was virtually impossible for most people to obtain. During fasts it was forbidden to eat or drink until noon (except on Saturdays and Sundays) and in Holy Week this prohibition was often extended to mid-afternoon or even sunset.

Abstinence from animal food was prescribed on the following occasions:

1. Every Wednesday and Friday, except during the 50-day period from the end of Lent to the feast of *Bala Hamsa*, or Feast of Fifty, and on a Wednesday or Friday if it coincided with Christmas or the Epiphany.
2. The long period of *Hudadé*, or Lent. This comprised 40 days in which mornings of total fasting were followed by afternoons and evenings of abstinence from animal food. Since Saturdays and Sundays in Lent were days of abstinence, but not of morning fasting, they were excluded from the reckoning. The total period of Lent thus extended for eight weeks, the last of which, Holy Week, was accompanied by fasting until at least 1:00 P.M. Lent comprised 40 days of morning fasting and abstinence from animal food, together with an additional 16 days of abstinence, or a total of 56 days. This great fast, according to Harry Hyatt, was observed with "greater vigour" than any other, and was practically a test of Christianity, for anyone violating it was traditionally "considered almost a pagan."
3. A period of at least 40 days preceding Christmas. This was sometimes reckoned as 40 days from Hedar 18 to the *gahad*, or Eve, of Christmas on

Tahsas 28, though many persons increased it to 43 days beginning on Heder 15, so that the 40 days should be exclusive of the one-day fasts of the Blessed Virgin, Incarnation, and Message of Gabriel.

4. A period of from 10 to 40 days, depending on the date of Easter, known as *Somé Hawaryat*, or Fast of the Apostles, to commemorate St. Peter and St. Paul. This period normally began eight days after *Bala Hamsa* and continued until Hamlé 5. In Tegré, however, it was often considered to begin on *Bala Hamsa*, and was hence eight days longer.

5. One day on the Eve of the Epiphany.

In addition to these fasts, which were kept almost universally, there were three others observed by the most religious segments of the population. These were the 40-day fast of Qwasquam from Maskaram 26 to Hedar 6, the 15-day fast of Nineveh, which lasted from Monday to Wednesday two weeks before the beginning of Lent. Monks, nuns, and the most pious clergy were commanded to observe several additional fasts.

Children under the age of thirteen were often said to be exempt from fasting, but this relaxation was in many cases applied only to those of much more tender age.

Fasting was virtually universal among the Christian population. Almost the only historical figure known to have departed from the custom was Emperor Téwodros, who, according to chronicler Walda Maryam and the British envoy Hormuzd Rassam, did so towards the end of his reign. He allowed his soldiers and followers a similar indulgence, which, however, they mainly refused to follow. Fasting was therefore still almost unanimously practiced on the eve of the Italian war, though pupils at the Boy Scout School were reported by the Hungarian journalist Ladislas Farago to have broken from this tradition.

In view of the paucity of information on the diet of former times the medical consequences of traditional fasting and abstinence are difficult to assess. It is, however, significant that at the end of the fifteenth century the Muslim invader Mahfud always launched his attacks against the highlands in Lent, when, according to James Bruce, the Christian soldiers had "become so weak" on account of the fast that they were "unable to bear any fatigue."

Diet

Certain aspects of the traditional diet had a direct effect on health. The practice of eating raw meat, which was first reported by Alvares in the early sixteenth century, led to a high incidence of tapeworm. Testimony to the extent of infestation is provided by several early nineteenth-century foreign travelers, among them the German Eduard Rüppell, the Frenchman Combes and Tamisier, and the Englishman Plowden, all of whom describe the complaint as virtually "universal," while the latter's compatriot De Cosson believed that it affected "all the natives and two out of three travellers."

Ascarides and other types of internal worm were also common, particularly among children, as noted by both Plowden and Mérab.

Another characteristic of the traditional diet was the large content of both *barbaré*, or red pepper, and fat, which, in the absence of vinegar, preserves, or sweetened drinks such as coffee or tea, led, Dr. Mérab believed, to a high incidence of gastritis and other complaints of the stomach. Such disorders, he thought, might also have been accentuated by excessive doses of *kosso* (*Hagenia abyssinica*) and other strong purges taken in the treatment of tapeworm, as well as in Addis Ababa by excessive drinking of the Greek-distilled *araqi*.

The absence of sugar, though possibly detrimental to digestion, was undoubtedly advantageous for the preservation of the teeth. Madame Dabbert, a pre–World War II Addis Ababa dentist who also practiced at Dire Dawa and Jibuti, says that at the latter port she had many more patients than in the interior of Ethiopia. The inhabitants of the coast, she explains, ate many sweet things and drank sweetened tea and coffee, whereas most Ethiopians scarcely consumed any sugar at all. Even the nobility drank coffee with salt rather than sugar. Sweet cakes which delighted the Arabs, Somalis, and Indians were unknown. The inhabitants of Jibuti, being much more involved in trade, purchased sweets for their children, while youngsters in Ethiopia made do with roasted grain which was much better for their teeth.

Deficiency in diet and drinking water were responsible in certain limited areas for a considerable amount of goiter and pellagra. The former was prevalent in some mountain valleys of Shawa, Gojjam, Walaga and Wallo, as well as on the snow-capped heights of Samén where Rüppell called it a national disease. It was later described by the twentieth century Italian physician Dr. Calo as fairly widespread in the Gondar area, while his com-patriot Dr. Lanzoni recalled that it was also "very common" among women in Goré whose throats sometimes swelled almost to the size of their heads. Pellagra was likewise serious in the Goré area where the population lived largely on maize, which did not ripen properly owing to excessive rain for four months of the year, and also suffered from an acute scarcity of salt. Excellent results were obtained, Lanzoni claimed, by Ras Nadaw, who, on his advice, caused many people to change from a diet of maize to one of sorghum.

Drunkenness

Drunkenness, which was largely an urban phenomenon, seems to have become serious towards the end of the nineteenth century when *araqi* produced locally by Greeks became available in large quantities. During the construction of the church of Maryam at Entotto, Empress Taytu was "much grieved," according to Gabra Sellasé's chronicle, to find that the building workers were often drunk, and De Coppet, the French editor of the chronicle, comments that it was only since the opening of European distilleries that alcoholism "made progress in Ethiopia, above all in Addis Ababa."

The growth of drunkenness was facilitated by the opening in early twentieth century Addis Ababa of numerous drinking houses. Their number increased, according to Dr. Mérab, from 50 in 1908 to 100 in 1913, and might have reached a thousand or more by 1922. Commenting on this expansion he says that he had never seen anyone the worse for drinking the traditional Ethiopian drinks *taj* (or mead) and *talla* (or beer), but the *araqi* sold in these houses was often harmful and led for example to atrophied cirrhosis. Drunkenness in the city, he believed, was very common among Shanqellas, Gimiras, and Walamos, and fairly widespread among people of Amhara, Gojjam, Shawa, and Tegré, but remarkably rare among Guragés. Drunkenness, confirmed the post-World War II Ethiopian writer, Maaza Lamma, became a problem only after the establishment of Addis Ababa, when those who consumed *araqi* became poor while those who sold it became rich. Many of the roads, he complained, became noisy with disputes and "the peace of the town was absolutely destroyed."

Personal Hygiene and Sanitation

Standards of personal hygiene varied greatly but, as foreign travelers' reports suggest, were often low. Large sections of the population suffered from impure water and poor sanitary conditions, particularly in the larger towns and military camps where typhus and typhoid fever consequently were not uncommon.

Cleanliness in old-time Ethiopia inevitably left much to be desired. Washing, when practicable, was not unpopular. Henry Salt remarked that Ethiopians were "very fond of bathing," and that they did so whenever they had an opportunity, such as in a running stream. A century later his compatriot R.E. Cheesman observed that, on halting by a river, Ethiopians never missed an opportunity to take off their clothes and wash themselves. Most villages and homesteads, however, for strategic and other reasons, were situated on or near the tops of hills, at a considerable distance from rivers and lakes. Water, therefore, tended to be scarce, so that most people were compelled by circumstance to be dirty. Mansfield Parkyns, after three years' residence in Tegré, observed that there were "many who beyond washing their hands before meals, and their feet after a journey, never troubled the water from one year's end to another," while De Cosson noted that "most people" displayed "utter disregard" for cleanliness. The German Gerhard Rohlfs roundly declared that "no one" washed, while the Englishman A.B. Wylde observed that "the lower class Abyssinian," though "A 1 at godliness," knew "nothing about cleanliness," and the "higher class" was "but little cleaner." This judgement was accepted by Mérab who claimed that Christians sometimes considered undue washing a Muslim practice. There was, however, he noted, a considerable amount of washing twice a year—on New Year's Day and at Epiphany, when large numbers of people would immerse themselves in nearby rivers or lakes. On the other hand, Muslims, who washed for religious reasons, were reported to be relatively clean, and the same was said of the Falashas, or Judaic Ethiopians.

Traditional dress, as worn by most inhabitants of the plateau, was made of cotton, and, being comparatively easy to wash, was healthier than clothing of either wool or skin. The washing of clothes in streams and rivers was integral to the culture, particularly before feast days. Washing clothes, which was usually (but not exclusively) a man's occupation, was carried out with the aid of the pulverized seeds of the *endod* plant (*Phytolacca dodecandra*). This washing agent did not make clothes very white, observed De Cosson, but did produce "a sufficiently good lather" to clean them.

Clothing was, however, by no means always clean. The people of Bagémder, claimed Stern, had "a strong prejudice" against clean clothes, while according to the Roman Catholic missionary Francesco da Offejo, the costumes of the Eritrean plateau started off white but gradually took on the color almost of soot. At the time of the Italian invasion, Guragés of Addis Ababa told the British journalist George Steer that they "never" washed their clothes, for it not only cost money but made them wear out "before their time."

Traditional housing, moreover, was often unhealthy. As Johnston noted of mid-nineteenth-century Shawa, domestic animals in many cases spent the night in the same apartment as their owners. Half a century later Wylde observed, "Lower class and poorer people have but one room. . . . Here all the family sleep, and all the household goods are stored. . . . The rest of the room is taken up by the animals, and a mixed crowed it is." Early twentieth-century observers, such as Francesco da Offejo and the Duchesne-Fournet mission, confirm that humans and their livestock frequently co-habited cheek by jowl.

Houses were "generally very dirty," Wylde asserted, and abounded with fleas and lice. Most dwellings thus swarmed with "vermin of all sorts and of the worst kinds," and, as he knew to his cost, "domestic and personal insects" were to be got "either in the king's palace or in the peasants' huts." After spending a night in a typical dwelling he commented: "I shall never forget the next morning! What our bodies looked like, lumps, bumps and knobs over every part!" A similar picture of the Harar area was drawn by the late nineteenth century Russian doctor Schusev, while in the north-west of the country a British physician, Dr. Hayes, observed that almost the entire population, Muslim as well as Christian, was "infested . . . with body lice."

Conditions were, however, by no means uniform. The houses of kings and some of the nobles were, according to Wylde, often "thoroughly clean," and the Duchesne-Fournet mission agreed that dwellings belonging to persons of higher rank were better looked after than those of the common people. Persons who had traveled abroad, or had been the servants of Europeans, in Wylde's opinion, also tended to have a higher than average standard of cleanliness. They kept their houses "fairly clean," wore "properly washed" clothing, undressed before going to bed, cleaned their face and hands daily, and took a bath in hot water every day. This was "a scale of decency," he claims, which compared well with that of continental Europe. Most traditional houses were, however, dark, and, having neither windows nor chimneys, suffered from a smoky atmosphere, which, Salt believed, probably injured the inhabitants' eyes—a view which was supported by later observers, including Dr. Mérab.

Sanitation and Water Supplies

Sanitation in former times was rudimentary. In rural areas with a scattered population this was of little consequence, but in the larger villages and towns it presented a major health hazard. Harris, while often an unjust critic, was not wholly exaggerating when he observed that the population of Ethiopian settlements, in "the absence of drains and sewers," from time to time lived in a "miasma of decomposing matter and stagnant water."

Water supplies were often impure. Dead livestock, according to the early twentieth-century German traveler Rosen, was seldom removed from streams and rivers which served for the washing and drinking of man and beast alike. Diseased mules frequently died in or near the water to which they were taken to drink and the people were "too lazy or indifferent to bury the pestilentially-smelling corpses or even to pull them out of the water." No less unfortunate was the practice at Sheik Husein in Ogaden, reported by Donaldson Smith, whereby the Somalis buried their dead around the edge of the pond from which they drank.

Such poor sanitation, together with poor hygiene and the absence in many areas of pure water, led to a high incidence of disease, and in particular to serious epidemics and dysentery.

Traditional Town Life

The principal Ethiopian towns, such as Adwa, Gondar, Ankobar, and Harar, like old-time urban settlements in other parts of the world, were crowded and as the unflattering accounts of many foreign observers claim, often suffered from unsanitary conditions.

Adwa in former days was a particularly unhealthy place. "The streets," wrote Hewett, a British diplomat, in 1884,

> are very narrow and revoltingly filthy. They are in no place broad enough for two mules to walk abreast, while in many places two foot-passengers cannot do so. They appear to be the recognized depot for all the offal, dead cattle and domestic cattle; any beast of burden which falls dead in the street is suffered to remain there until devoured by dogs, hyenas and vultures. All these substances in an active state of putrefaction, together with large quantities of human excreta, render a walk through town a thing not willingly repeated.

A similar picture was drawn by Wylde who observed that the streets, as a rule, were "disgracefully dirty, and all the refuse of the houses, including bones of slaughtered animals," were "thrown out of doors and left to the mercy of dogs, vultures and hyenas."

Gondar, apart from the imperial quarter, was perhaps scarcely better. Its crooked, steep, and narrow streets, noted the mid-nineteenth century German traveler Theodor von Heuglin, were "in the highest degree dirty." The city was also chronically short of drinking water, for although there were several springs at the foot of the nearby hills, most dried up during the dry season when it was necessary to rely on river water.

Ankobar likewise suffered from abominable sanitary conditions. It too had "narrow tortuous roads full of stones" which made it difficult to walk even on foot, while its "nauseating smell," rendered any stay "disagreeable," according to the French traveler Aubry.

Harar was even more unhealthy. A city of rough stone houses with very few trees, its streets were "narrow" lanes "strewed with gigantic rubbish heaps," Burton noted in 1855. The Egyptians, during their occupation of 1875–1885, attempted to introduce piped water but the project was soon abandoned. The sanitary situation in the early twentieth century was therefore strikingly similar to that in Burton's day. The British traveler A.E. Pease wrote, "It is of all the filthy towns I ever saw, the dirtiest. Its rock-hewn gutters and open sewers choked with manure heaps and decaying carcases." His compatriot John Boyes likewise recalled that he had described Harar as "the rottenest place" it had been his "misfortune to enter," and commented, "The language may not be very elegant, but it correctly describes my impression. Every inch of ground. . . . had been built upon without regard for health. . . . There was not the remotest attempt at sanitation, and the streets were running with filth and refuse of all kinds exuding a noisome stench. Such a place," he concluded, "might be a veritable city of plague, but fortunately it was often visited by torrential rains, which washed away the filth and did the cleaning which the inhabitants neglected to do for themselves."

Little provision for refuse disposal was made in any town. Some street cleaning was, however, carried out in early twentieth century Harar by women who collected dirt in baskets, and tipped it outside the walls, but "beyond this fraction of prophylaxis," noted Jennings, an English visitor, there was "no such thing as sanitation."

Town cleaning was in fact left virtually entirely to nature. The rainy season was thus of considerable sanitary importance, for household refuse would then be "swept away," as Harris reported, by "descending torrents."

Hyenas and other scavengers also played a useful role in the removal of animal carcasses. At Adwa for example Wylde remarked:

The hyenas are the best municipal workers in the place, and I have been down a street in the afternoon and seen a dead bullock or a dead mule on the ground and passed the next morning and found only a few bones. What the town would do without these scavengers I don't know. As it is they have hard jaw-work to keep pace with the supply of filth thrown out by the inhabitants.

Animal scavengers were no less important in other cities, including Harar, where, in Vivian's words, "all the scavenging" was done by "kindly hyenas and accommodating jackals," who crept into the town after dusk and at dawn scurried out through the holes in the walls.

A virtually unchanged pattern of town life was described a few generations later, at the time of the Italian invasion, by the British journalist Harmsworth in the following melodramatic terms:

> Harar has no sanitary system. . . . the householders, instead of placing their refuse in the dustbin to be collected in the morning, throw their rubbish in a heap outside their front doors. After dusk the scavengers appear, their green eyes shining with a sinister light through the blackness, and in the morning the streets are clean.

Despite the activities of scavengers, however, sanitary conditions often remained poor, as evident from the abundance of flies. Liano observed that although in many towns flies were plentiful, it was impossible to find one with a larger number than Harar.

Such unhealthy conditions led inevitably to a high incidence of disease: most towns suffered, as we shall see, from periodic epidemics of smallpox, cholera, typhus, and dysentery.

Army Camps and Battlefields

Traditional army camps, because of their size and absence of sanitation, were also often unhealthy. They were described by Rohlfs as both unsanitary and smelly, and led Wylde to observe: "The remains of an English camp is never a very cheerful sight, but that of an Abyssinian camp is still less."

Battlefields tended to be equally unsalubrious, for the killed were often left unburied. After the battle of Chalanqo between Menilek and the Amir of Harar in 1887, the Italian traveler Robecchi-Bricchetti found many skeletons lying about the site. Wylde, who visited Adwa shortly after the famous battle of 1896, likewise noted:

> Here were the remains of unburied humanity, dirt, filth and corruption at every step, and, although there had been heavy rains which had washed away part of the fragments, and the grass was growing luxuriantly, still a sickly smell of decaying flesh pervaded the atmosphere, and every few yards I had to put my handkerchief to my nose and go on as fast as possible. I asked Schimper if he called it healthy and a fit place to come to, and he replied, "Oh, this is nothing to what it was ten days ago; it was not sweet then."

The principal churchyard was "very foul-smelling," for the bodies buried there had "only a slight covering of earth over them, and many of the extremities were protruding, while in one of the deserted gate-houses several corpses remained without any attempt at interment." Wylde described his visits to the battlefield as perhaps the "most disagreeable task he had ever performed in his life," for each position was "more foul smelling and disgusting" than the next:

> A burying party of Italian engineers had been allowed . . . to come and inter the dead, but the condition of the corpses prevented them from being moved, and a few loose stones were their only covering which, instead of facilitating decomposition, only retarded it; not half of the bodies had been attended to, and in some places, putrescent masses held together by ragged clothes marked the details of the fight. . . . I used to be sick half-a-dozen times a day. . . . my Abyssinian guides used to tie their cloths around their nostrils and mouths and ask me if I had not seen enough.

Concluding his gruesome description, Wylde declared: "Bird and animal life was absent, even they could not face the horrible Golgotha, and the hyenas had long ago left the district to procure something more tempting. . . . There are some things in one's life that can never be forgotten, and this is one of them that I shall carry with me as long as I live."

As a result of such unsanitary conditions, soldiers and camp followers, like town-dwellers, often suffered from major epidemics, particularly of cholera, typhus, and dysentery.

Warfare

Throughout her long history, Ethiopia was seriously impoverished both by civil wars and by foreign invasions. Warfare, and the movement of soldiers throughout the country, seem also to have contributed to the spread of venereal diseases, for the warriors tended to travel without their spouses, and were, according to Rüppell, in the habit of taking wives wherever they went. Itinerant traders followed a similar practice, and therefore in many cases suffered from syphilis as well as malaria contracted in the lowlands.

II

Early Unidentified Epidemics

Ethiopia, as we shall see, has suffered over the centuries from innumerable epidemics, primarily of smallpox, cholera, typhus, dysentery, and influenza. The precise character of most early outbreaks, however, cannot be established, for the records of the time—many of which relate miracles alleged to have occurred in such times of distress—neither mention diseases by name nor provide sufficient detail to allow identification. Nevertheless, many of the unidentified "pestilences" of the past, to judge from the evidence available, were just as serious as later, medically diagnosed outbreaks. Several, as we shall see, followed in the wake of famine, and in some cases led to migration from the more affected areas.

The First Recorded Epidemics

The first two "pestilences" (i.e., epidemics) on record—both of them in the *Mashafa Senkesar*, or *Ethiopian Synaxarium*—each came in the wake of famine. The first is mentioned in the section to be read on the 23rd day of the month of Teqemt (i.e., in October), which recalls the life of Abba Joseph, the fifty-second patriarch of Alexandria, who held office from A.D. 831 to 849. The story is told that Abba Yohannes, the *abun* (or head) of the Ethiopian church, was at that time expelled from Ethiopia, and returned to Egypt. His expulsion so angered the Lord, it is claimed, that it resulted in a famine and plague which caused the then emperor to write a terrified letter to the patriarch. The letter stated that because certain people had gone astray, "great tribulation" had "come upon our land, and all our men are dying of the plague, and our beasts and cattle have perished, and God hath restrained the heavens so that they cannot rain upon our land." On receiving this message the patriarch is said to have appointed "brave men" to return with Abba Yohannes to

Ethiopia, whereupon, the *Synaxarium* claimed, "the plague ceased, and rain fell from heaven."

The second epidemic, which seems to have occurred three centuries later, is mentioned in the passage of the *Synaxarium* for the tenth of Miyazya (i.e., in April), which commemorates the life of Saint Gabriel, the seventieth patriarch of Alexandria, who held office from A.D. 1131 to 1145. The text states that the then Ethiopian emperor wished to appoint additional bishops, but the ruler of Egypt opposed this on the ground that it would make the Ethiopians "wax bold." He therefore, ordered the patriarch to "send a letter and curse the King of Ethiopia." The prelate complied, and, the *Synaxarium* adds:

> When that letter reached the King of Ethiopia. . . . famine and plague broke out in the land, and the rain would not fall on the fields, and great tribulation came upon the people.

The emperor thereupon "turned to God and repented," after which the Almighty "removed His anger; and the rain descended upon them, and God removed the famine and the plague and the people rejoiced with great joy."

Reference to another early epidemic is found in a Harari Arabic manuscript recording that a major pestilence struck the Harar area in A.H. 660 (i.e., A.D. 1261–1262). This was the first such event that can be dated with any certainty.

Early Hagiographical Accounts: Twelfth to Fourteenth Centuries

Epidemics figure extensively in several hagiographical accounts of early times. Most biographies of St. Takla Haymanot, a holy man thought to have lived in Shawa in the twelfth or thirteenth century, claim that when he grew old he was forewarned of his coming demise. According to one such account, the Lord spoke to him, saying, "Thou hath finished they contending, and there is nothing left for thee except to die. And behold, thou shalt die through the pain of pestilence, an evil death, and I will reckon it as if thou hadst been crucified, and will regard it as the blood of the martyrs who were before thee. And not thyself only, but also thy sons who shall die through sickness of pestilence. . . . I will number with the martyrs."

The holy man, it is said, informed his followers of his impending death, and "on the same day the sickness of pestilence came to them, and it seized those monks whose names he had declared." Though the community was apparently small, consisting perhaps of only a few dozen, no less than fourteen men are said to have perished. The text presents the pestilence in personalized terms. Mention is thus made of an "army of the pestilence," with whose leaders the saint held discourse.

Another biography of Takla Haymanot declares that when a "terrible epidemic" decimated the monks a frightful demon emanating from the disease appeared, whereupon the holy man turned to her, saying, "God will uproot you," at which she turned pale, and died. The plague, we are told, "lasted a long while, and many of the monks passed from life to death."

Such tales, preserved in the biography of one of the principal saints of the Ethiopian church, had their counterparts in many later writings.

The *Acts* of St. Anoréwos, a monk believed to have lived at the time of Emperor Amda Seyon (1314–1344), tells of several epidemics. On one occasion, allegedly as a divine punishment on the king, white flies appeared, biting horses and men, as a result of which many animals and people died. A later pestilence is said to have been called forth by Anoréwos as a punishment for a witch called Budi, but was brought to an end by the good man's prayers. Another epidemic (influenza?) affected the saint himself in the throat, but was cured by the will of God. There is also mention of a fourth plague in which "many people" perished and the rest fled, only one of the holy man's disciples remaining in the area.

Another fourteenth-century outbreak of disease is described in the *Acts* of Abuna Aron, who lived in Dabra Darit in Bagémder during the reign of Emperor Sayfa Ared (1344–1372). A plague "moved down the whole of Ethiopia," and was so serious that one thousand of Aron's disciples succumbed and his church was filled with corpses. The men and women who survived closed their houses and fled. Even after the saint's own death, it was reported to the subsequent *abun*, Abba Salama, that the bodies of the dead were piled on the grave of Aron and that the church was so filled with corpses that it was impossible to set foot inside it. Thereupon the *abun* ordered the old church closed and a new place of worship built to hold Aron's remains.

The pestilence referred to above may well have been one mentioned in the *Acts* of Filipos, a monk who lived at Dabra Libanos during the reigns of both Amda Seyon and Sayfa Ared. The narrative states that fifty-three monks died, besides an unspecified number of women and children.

This same epidemic may also be that referred to in the *Acts* of Zéna Maryam, a nun of Enfraz near Lake Tana who lived in the second half of the fourteenth century. An outbreak, from which her mother died, is said to have occurred in her childhood. Her family, weeping bitter tears, buried her, whereupon "all the servants and neighbours fled from fear of the plague." Zéna Maryam left home with her brothers and found refuge in a cave. She cut down branches and built a fence as a defense against wild animals. She prayed to the Holy Trinity not to desert them, but the plague struck down one of her elder brothers. He was eaten alive by wild animals and his sister found and buried his remains. One by one all her brothers perished; Zéna Maryam alone was spared, it is claimed, by the clemency of the Lord.

The magnitude of one of the plagues of this obscure period is apparent from the *Acts* of Yohannes, a monk of Dabra Bizan who lived from 1369 to 1448. This account relates that a famine, supposedly caused by the wickedness of the monks, was followed by an epidemic that had been foreseen by Yohannes in a revelation. All the monks suffered and many old people and children died, but the holy man comforted the survivors by reminding them of the trials and tribulations of biblical times.

The importance attached to such calamities is likewise seen in the *Acts* of Marqorewos, a fifteenth century monk of Tegré whose followers did not forget his precepts "even in time of epidemics."

The Fifteenth Century

The epidemics of the fifteenth century, though still largely undiagnosable, are on the whole better documented than those of earlier times.

Two of the earliest outbreaks of this period can be dated with some certainty. The first was reported by the Arab historian Maqrisi to have occurred in A.H. 839 (i.e., A.D. 1435-1436), a year or so after the accession of Emperor Zara Ya'qob (1434-1468), and was described as "a pestilence ranging far and wide destroying the inhabitants of Abyssinia. The *Hati* (i.e., emperor) fell to it, and so many people that the whole country is said to be depopulated." The ruler referred to was probably not Zara Ya'qob, who lived on for over thirty years, but rather one of his immediate predecessors, Endreyas, Takla Maryam, Sarwé Iyasus, or Amda Iyasus, all of whom had unusually short reigns, together totaling only four years.

The reign of Zara Ya'qob nevertheless witnessed a serious epidemic which, to deduce from his chronicle, probably occurred between 1454 and 1468. It is recorded that the monarch was at his newly established capital, Dabra Berhan, when there was "a great pestilence which killed so large a number of people that no one remained to bury the dead." Zara Ya'qob therefore ordered the construction of a new church, called Béta Qirqos, in the hope that this would cause God to remove the disease from Dabra Berhan, in accordance with the promise that "the plague will not come to the spot where a temple will be built." The chronicler claimed that his master's "faith and confidence" was successful, for it "turned away the illness from the enclosure of his palace just as he had hoped."

Zara Ya'qob insisted that the corpses should be properly buried. "When the plague decimated the country," the chronicle states, he "ordered all the inhabitants to come together to bury the dead." He told them to assemble for this purpose with sticks and branches, and to sprinkle holy water. These groups of men he termed "Congregations of the Evangelist," and the branches, "Sticks of Moses." To reinforce his orders he commanded the *shums* (or lesser chiefs) to pillage the houses and seize the goods of anyone who failed to inter the dead.

This epidemic seems to be alluded to in other texts of the period. The *Acts* of Batérgéla Maryam, one of Zara Ya'qob's sons, related that "there arose a murderous plague so great that it was impossible to describe." The young man went at that time into an area infected by the disease, but the Virgin Mary saved him by causing his father to recall him home. Thus, it is claimed,

Batérgéla Maryam was preserved, though two of his brothers fell victim to the disease.

The same epidemic seems also to be mentioned in the *Acts* of Krestos Samra, a Shawan nun who founded a hermitage on the island of Gwangut in Lake Tana. She is quoted as stating that the plague came upon "all the confines of the world" and remained for three years. "Many people" perished, and their houses were "filled with tears and lamentations." The epidemic is spoken of as a kind of army, and the text claims that the holy woman was able to converse with one of its soldiers.

Reference to this same pestilence is likewise found in the *Acts* of St. Feré Mika'él and St. Zara Abreham, who lived in the land of Warab during the reign of Zara Ya'qob. Feré Mika'él, it is said, prayed for "all the people, men, women and children, far and near," but he, his brother, and two nephews all died of the plague.

Ethiopian preoccupation with such pestilence is apparent in an early fifteenth century manuscript of the *Miracles of the Blessed Virgin Mary*, which tells of three successive epidemics, the last and most serious of which "killed many people, including women and children," causing everyone to mourn in anticipation of their own death.

The Sixteenth Century

At least five major epidemics are known to have occurred during the sixteenth century.

The first, which was the earliest to be recorded by a European observer, was described by Francisco Alvares, chaplain of the Portuguese diplomatic mission of the 1520s. He recalls that while his party was at the monastery of Dabra Bizan in May 1520, "the people fell sick, both the Portuguese and our slaves; few or none remained who were not affected, and many were in danger of death." Patients, in accordance with contemporary medical practice, were "often bled and purged." Those not so treated were attacked by the disease "with all its force." Among those who died was Murad, an Armenian envoy in Ethiopian service, as well as one of the Portuguese servants.

This outbreak may well have been that referred to in the *Life* of Enbakom, abbot of Dabra Libanos, which mentions an epidemic in which the good man buried no less than 400 monks in one year.

The second recorded pestilence occurred half a century later. It is mentioned in a Harari Arabic manuscript which records that there was a severe famine in A.H. 975 (i.e., A.D. 1567–1568) followed by a plague in which the then ruler of Harar, Amir Nur, perished.

A third epidemic was reported towards the end of the reign of Sarsa Dengel (1563–1597), whose chronicle states that it broke out in the King's camp and "many men" died. This outbreak, or another of the period, is referred to in the *Acts* of Batra Maryam, founder of a church at Zagé by Lake Tana.

A fourth plague, according to the same text, broke out in Damot, where the holy man and his disciples all fell ill but were cured by his prayers.

A famine, however, later broke out in the same country, allegedly because the people were "wicked" and did not know the Lord. "Many" fell ill as a consequence and were "near to death," but were saved by Batra Maryam calling them to prayer, as a result of which his fame spread throughout the land.

The Seventeenth Century

Though the medically more detailed records of the seventeenth century provide the first diagnoses of epidemics, several of the outbreaks chronicled remain unidentified.

The first, according to the chronicles, occurred in the fifth year of the reign of Susenyos (i.e., in A.D. 1611), and was so severe that it was called *manan tita*, literally "Who did it leave?" It is said that "many people" died, particularly in Dambeya. One of the chronicles comments that this outbreak was too severe to describe.

An eyewitness account of a somewhat later epidemic was provided by a Jesuit missionary, Aloysius de Azevedo, who reported that in 1616 there was "a great pestilence" that was especially severe in Tegré, where it carried off entire villages—although, he claims, it did not touch any Catholics, thus proving God's "paternal care" for them.

This outbreak was followed a couple of years later by another which is mentioned both in Susneyos' chronicle and by the Jesuits. The former source states that many people succumbed, including Kantiba Za Giyorgis, the governor of Dambeya, and that the monarch grieved greatly for them. The disease then carried off many nobles at the king's camp at Gorgora by Lake Tana. The victims included one of the principal church officials, 'Aqabé Sa'at Abba Egwalé, the governor of the coastal province, Bahr Nagash Del Ba Iyasus, and two other prominent courtiers, Dajazmach Kefla Wahed and Abétahun Yolyos. So many people perished that no one could count the dead. Their kinsmen buried them anywhere they could, without looking for any church. The number of bodies was so great that the monarch found it necessary to abandon his camp by the lake and move to higher ground.

Azevedo, whose report confirms much of the above account, observed in October 1618 that the country was suffering from a plague that killed three important personalities, and that the monarch was obliged to transfer his headquarters to the cooler (i.e., healthier) region of Danqaz. Even there mortality was high. The victims included several Portuguese to whom the Jesuits gave the sacraments, a notable deed, Azevedo claims, as the local clergy were refusing to visit the dying for fear of the disease which "spread and killed like the plague." In the majority of cases people were not properly interred, but were merely dragged into some cave. Catholics, however, were buried with pomp according to the Roman rite. Ever anxious to assert that his coreligionists enjoyed divine protection, the missionary declared that when one of the Ethiopian converts died, the latter's Orthodox brother would claim that he had perished as a result of his conversion, but adds with satisfaction that the unconverted brother, his wife, and several relatives were struck down by the disease a few days later.

Despite such fanciful assertions of divine partiality, the account of the monarch's flight from infection seems well corroborated. This practice, which had occurred on many previous occasions, caused Hiob Ludolf, the renowned German scholar, to comment of the Ethiopians:

> If a Pestilence chances to break out, they leave their Houses and Villages, and retire with their Herds to the Mountains, putting all their Security in flying from the Contagion.

By the time of the founding of Gondar in 1636 the more important epidemics recorded in the chronicles seem to be identifiable. Several undiagnosed outbreaks are, however, also mentioned. During the latter years of the seventeenth century there is thus report of an illness called *labalb* which raged at Gondar and elsewhere in 1683, another known as *féra* which killed many of King Ya'qob's soldiers in 1685, an unidentified disease which was particularly acute at Aksum in 1693, and a "very serious plague" caclled *tanaka* which erupted during the following rainy season.

The early decades of the eighteenth century likewise witnessed at least two unidentified epidemics; a pestilence called *gudru* which struck the country during the rainy season of 1701, and a "fierce" plague which appeared during the rains of 1709. One last unidentified outbreak, possibly of typhus, which took place in 1772, is mentioned by the Scottish traveler James Bruce who states that it affected the camp of a rebel called Téwodros.

III

Smallpox and Variolation

Epidemics

Smallpox, the most serious epidemic from which Ethiopia suffered in the past, seems to have existed in the region for at least a millennium and a half. According to Arab tradition, the disease was brought to Arabia from Ethiopia by Aksumite soldiers around A.D. 370 and some historians believe that another epidemic broke out among the Aksumite troops in Arabia two centuries later, in 570 or 571.

Further outbreaks probably occurred in the Middle Ages, and may account for at least some of the unidentified epidemics mentioned, as we have seen, in the often tantalizingly brief records of that time.

Smallpox is known in Amharic as *kufagn*, a word first listed in Ludolf's Amharic-Latin dictionary of 1698, but was also spoken of as *fantata*, a term also used, as we shall see, for syphilis.

The first definitive account of smallpox in Ethiopia was provided by the Scottish traveler and historian, James Bruce, who reported that it reached epidemic proportions during the reign of Iyasu I (1682–1706), when it raged among the Gallas, or Oromos, "with such violence that whole provinces . . . became half desert." Subsequent chronicles tell of a violent attack of *kufagn* in 1718 in which many nobles died, and an outbreak in the middle of 1768 that carried off many persons in the capital, Gondar, and other areas as far as the frontiers of the realm. The later stages of this epidemic were described by Bruce, who himself treated some of its victims. He claimed that the outbreak had started at the coast, killing over one thousand people at the ports of Massawa and Arkiko. From there it advanced to Adwa in the autumn of 1769, and spread rapidly inland, reaching Gondar in the spring of the following year. The disease appeared "much more serious and fatal" than in England (where smallpox epidemics were still common), and Bruce was led to believe that it had resulted in considerable depopulation, particularly among the Saho and other people near Massawa and the Shanqellas in the west where it had "greatly reduced their numbers" and "extinguished to a man whole tribes of them."

Nineteenth-century travelers, who were both more numerous and more informative than those of earlier times, have revealed that at least half a dozen further smallpox epidemics occurred during that period, namely, in 1811–1812, in 1838 or 1839, in 1854, in 1878, in 1886, and in 1889–1890, or an average of once every generation.

The first of these outbreaks was graphically reported by Nathaniel Pearce, a British resident in Tegré, who described the disease as "the most destructive complaint" known in the country. Writing on September 13, 1811, during a period of civil war, he noted, "The small-pox . . . committed such ravages throughout the country, that all thoughts of war were abandoned. As the malady increased it became more like a plague than the small-pox, and in a great many towns and villages the people lost all their children, and numbers of grown-up persons, who had not had the disease before, died also." Appalled by the ferocity of the outbreak, Pearce added:

> At Axum the mortality among the people was so great as to occasion the loss of the cattle also, there not being a man or boy left in some families to open their pens and turn them out to grass. Thirty cows were found dead in one fold. At Adowa, the ravages of the disease were not so severe, as a great number of its inhabitants had previously had the disorder the last time it appeared amongst them; but all the other places in Amhara, Tigré, Enderta, and the adjoining districts, Samen, Lasta, Begemder, Gondar, shared the same fate . . . the smallpox carried off the people in all quarters, so that a great part of the country was left in a state of complete desolation.

Four months later, on January 4, 1812, he recorded that "the smallpox still raged like a plague" with the result that "throughout the country nothing was heard but lamentations." One refugee, alarmed at the extent of infection in Tegré, fled to Gojjam only to find that the disease was raging there too; he therefore went to one of the islands on Lake Tana, but, finding it there as well, was forced to abandon his efforts to escape the epidemic.

The gravity of the situation is confirmed by letters written by Ras Walda Sellasé, the ruler of Tegré, to the British traveler Henry Salt. These epistles contain such passages as the following: "The smallpox is a greater enemy of the country than the locust," "the smallpox has ravaged the land . . . affliction is heaped upon us," and "the smallpox fills the country with fear."

The occurrence of one or more smallpox outbreaks in the late 1830s or early 1840s is indicated in the writings of several foreign travelers, such as W.C. Harris, who declared that the disease "frequently" devastated the land; while Captain Haines, the British consul for the Somali coast, wrote in

December, 1845, that it was "still prevalent among the villages of the interior," though reported to be "on the decrease." Not long afterwards, in 1856, the orientalist Richard Burton described smallpox as "the most dangerous disease" known in the country. Some time earlier it had raged with great violence in the Harar area, killing many of the peasantry who demanded—and received—blood money from the local Amir.

A decade or so later Walter Plowden, the British consul in the north of the country, stated that smallpox was infrequent, but that when it did appear it carried off the population "in thousands." Shortly afterwards, in 1861, a Frenchman Alfred Courbon observed that mortality among the infected was high—50% in the case of children, and no less than 80% in that of adults. There were, he added, few Ethiopians without smallpox scars.

A major epidemic broke out during the latter years of the reign of Emperor Téwodros II (1855–1868). Blanc, one of his captives, noted that smallpox "now and then" made "fearful ravages," while another prisoner, Rosenthal, stated that the disease had killed "thousands" in the Magdala area. A contemporary chronicle told of a further outbreak in Addigrat shortly afterwards, in 1868.

The incidence of the disease was comparable in the south of the country where, according to Plowden, it broke out every ten years and considerably reduced the population. This statement is borne out by the great fear of the disease which the Italian missionary Massaia encountered in Jimma, Kaffa, and adjacent lands. Smallpox, he asserted, was also more or less endemic in Lagamara and Gudru.

An outbreak in 1878, which was mentioned by the Italian traveler Cecchi, was particularly serious in Shawa; at the town of Lecché, for instance, which had a population of 15,000, as many as 20 or 30 people were dying every day.

Perhaps the most serious late nineteenth-century epidemic occurred in 1886 (several years before the outbreak of the Great Famine) and, according to Dr. Mérab, lasted until 1898, when a major vaccination campaign was inaugurated. The Italian writer Alamanni stated that the disease first appeared in Massawa and made its way via Aylet and Asmara to Adwa where out of a population of 7,000 no less than 500 people died, including 300 children under the age of 14. The infection quickly spread inland, to Asmara, Gojjam, and Shawa, where, the contemporary French traveler Paul Soleillet stated, at least a quarter of the population bore smallpox scars. Menilek himself was no stranger to the disease, which, according to Powell-Cotton, had "pitted" his face. Hodson, a later British consul, suggested that the population of Arussi to the south was much depleted. This epidemic also affected western Eritrea, where, the German linguist Enno Littmann reported, the Mansa Bét Abraha tribe referred to 1886 as "the year of the smallpox," having lost "about seven hundred people, old and young."

A further wave of smallpox occurred at the height of the Great Famine of 1888-1892, when Emperor Menilek's Swiss advisor, Alfred Ilg, estimated that the army returning from Tegré at the beginning of 1890 lost 15% of its numbers as a result of smallpox, dysentery, typhus, and bronchitis.

Perhaps the last major smallpox epidemic broke out in 1904–1905, when the disease spread over a wide area of the country, as reported by Drake-Brockman at Bulhar in British Somaliland, by Dr. Rosen at Dire Dawa and, subsequently, by the American missionary Bergsma at Dambidolo.

The continued significance of smallpox in early twentieth-century Ethiopia is apparent from Mérab's statement that around the time of World War I about a fifth of the population of Shawa were still pock-marked, and that slaves who had survived smallpox—and were therefore thought to be proof against it— were considered twice as valuable as those liable to contract it.

Though no further large-scale epidemics were reported after this time, presumably because of the introduction of vaccination, smallpox continued to be endemic for several decades. Dr. Brielli, an Italian physician, reported in 1913 that there were frequent attacks of smallpox in the Dasé area; British consular reports for 1899-1900 and 1911-1912 stated that the disease was always prevalent in Harar; and the Swiss ethnographer Dr. Montandon noted in 1910–1911 that smallpox still resulted in a high death rate in most parts of the country. The situation was scarcely better in Eritrea, where, according to a British report for 1919, "smallpox frequently appears, especially along the caravan roads out of Abyssinia."

The prevalence of smallpox in pre–World War II Ethiopia was subsequently noted by the Phelps-Stokes mission, which reported that cases of the disease were "fairly frequent," while Rey remarked that they were "still very numerous" even in Addis Ababa, where Fan C. Dunckley described them as "common."

Traditional Methods of Treatment

Variolation

The most widespread traditional method of combating smallpox was variolation, which was practiced in most, if not all, parts of the country. Pearce, the first observer to describe the custom, noted that in early nineteenth-century Tegré,

> upon the approach of the disorder, the people of the country and villages collect their children and those who have not had it into one gang, for the purpose of having them inoculated. Everyone carries a piece of salt, or a measure of corn: they then march together to the neighboring town, or wherever the disorder may have made its appearance. Here they pick out a person, who is thickest covered with sores, and procure a skilful person or Dofter (i.e., *dabtara*, or lay priest) who takes a quantity of matter from him into an egg-shell, and then by turns he cuts a small cross with a razor on the arm, puts in it a little of the matter, and afterwards binds it up with a piece of rag. The salt and other articles which they carry are given to the Dofter, and he divides it with the person from whom the matter is taken. After this operation they all return home, singing and shouting praises to God, in a joyful

manner, and beseeching him to preserve them from death during the time of their disease.

Variolation was also described by several other observers. Harris, who wrote of Shawa, indicated that it was a social occasion, for "many hundred persons assemble, and a layman, chosen for the rectitude of his life . . . proceeds with a razor," while Dr. Petit of the French scientific mission of 1839-42 stated that chiefs in the northern provinces often ordered compulsory inoculation and that he had seen this done throughout Tegré by command of its ruler, Dajazmach Webé.

As for the operation itself, Harris and Mérab both noted that it was the practice to dilute the pus with either honey or butter, presumably to make it go further. Petit related further that the patient's skin would be folded at the lower front part of the forearm, four fingers' breadth above the wrist, after which an incision was made there with a razor. The virus was thereupon introduced by means of a so-called "magic stick" and the wound was then bandaged. Kirk, a physician who visited Shawa in the 1840s, said that care was taken to obtain the pus from free men and not from slaves, a statement confirmed by Harris as follows: "a free boy of pure blood is selected from among the number of the infected, and carefully secluded until the pustules are ripe." Courbon added that variolation was not usually carried out on children below the ages of 15 or 18 years, and was seldom repeated on persons already inoculated.

Observers varied in their assessment of the custom. Krapf, a well-informed missionary, complained that variolation was frequently undertaken too late, when the epidemic had reached considerable proportions, while other writers emphasized that use was made of an active smallpox virus which often actually spread the disease. It was also asserted that the practice led to the diffusion of other diseases. W.C. Harris described traditional inoculation as a "clumsy operation" from which death was "often the consequence," while Dr. Blanc agreed that it resulted in "considerable" mortality. Dr. Wurtz, a French physician sent by his government to treat the epidemic of 1897, gave the following examples: a rich Ethiopian had his eight maids inoculated, all of whom died of smallpox, while the French trader Savouré claimed that each of his nine servants had developed syphilis as a result of innoculation with vaccine derived from a person suffering from the venereal disease.

Two early twentieth-century observers, Dr. Mérab and Dr. Lincoln de Castro (the latter a physician attached to the Italian legation), were more optimistic. Mérab believed inoculation was usually well done, and confirmed earlier accounts that, as far as possible, pus for vaccine was drawn from persons in otherwise good health, especially from those who were not suffering from veneral disease. Chances of successful immunization, he believed, were actually higher than in the case of the European vaccination. De Castro agreed that variolation gave indisputable immunity, though the operation, he conceded, was sometimes badly carried out, in which case the patient was often infected.

Isolation

Several other methods of avoiding or preventing infection were employed. One of the simplest consisted in flight, a practice which, as we have seen, was noted by Ludolf, who had observed that on the outbreak of a pestilence people often retired to the mountains "putting all their security in flying from the contagion."

Attempts were also made to prevent the spread of infection by prohibiting or controlling the movement of persons. According to Krapf, when smallpox broke out at the Shawan capital, Ankokar, King Sahla Sellasé (1813-1847) would retire to the village of Mahal Wanz where no one was admitted to his presence. Merchants and travelers were forbidden from entering the realm by a kind of "cordon militaire." During the epidemic of 1856, claimed Burton, the peasants around Harar likewise prevented anyone from traveling to or from the city. Subsequently, the Italian traveler Naretti related that, on entering Ethiopia from Massawa during the outbreak of 1878, he received a letter from Emperor Yohannes ordering him to halt his journey because of an epidemic, almost certainly of smallpox. This order was later countermanded, presumably because normal conditions returned. Still, at the time of the epidemic of 1886, a British report stated, Emperor Yohannes prohibited fornication on account of "increased chance" which it gave for the spread of smallpox. Some years later, in 1897, Dr. Wurtz reported that many Addis Ababa children had been sent out of the capital to avoid the epidemic then raging, and were living under canvas in the nearby mountains. At Addisgé, a small village in Shawa, a woman of noble family who had left home and was camping with her maids near a stream posted guards nearby with instructions to allow no one to approach who had not first completely washed his body and clothes.

A Draconian Practice: Purification by Fire

A draconian method of dealing with a smallpox epidemic is alluded to by several writers. Bruce in the eighteenth century claimed that the Gallas of the Macha area lived in such terror of the disease, that when it broke out in a household, the neighbors, knowing it would spread to the whole area if unchecked, surrounded the house in the night and set fire to it. They then thrust the inamates back into the burning dwelling at spear point even though they were their neighbors or relatives. The Scotsman's comment was that though this might seem "a barbarity scarcely credible" it would be considered "quite otherwise" if one saw the "dreadful visitation" of the disease. Pearce, half a century or so later, told a similar story about the "pagan Gallas," and declared that, "horrible as it might appear, they considered this practice a very prudent mode of proceeding," and reproached the Christians for not doing the same, declaring that "infinite numbers of their brethren were thus preserved by the sacrifice of the few."

This practice, which the Italian missionary Massaia also learned of in Gudru, had its parallel among the Somalis. Burton in the middle of the nineteenth century and Bardey a generation or so later both record that Somali tribesmen on the outbreak of smallpox would often decamp, leaving the victims to be devoured by the hyenas who thus constituted a kind of sanitary squad. Though this custom later died out, doubtless because of its ruthlessness, it is not without interest that the Somalis were reported in the 1930s as practicing rigid isolation of smallpox victims, as well as burning houses and personal effects to prevent the spread of infection.

Sudorific Treatment

Sudorific treatment was widely practiced. Bruce, the first to report it, stated that an infected person would be confined to his room without the smallest breath of air, and would be given hot drinks, extra bed clothing, and a fire, the door being securely closed to keep the room in darkness. Pearce, who witnessed a similar treatment in early nineteenth-century Tegré, commented that the patient would be placed on ashes or river sand and kept in his house, which would be closed to both air and light, with visitors rigidly excluded.

The Somalis had a similar custom. In the mid-nineteenth century Burton stated that a patient, "if a man of note," would be "placed on the sand," which presumably was hot, "and fed with rice and millet bread till he recovers or dies." Half a century later, Puccioni reported the Somalis' use of fumigation, which was effected by placing aromatics under the bed of the patient, who would then be buried under the sun-warmed sand with only his head uncovered.

A different practice was reported by Petit who observed that smallpox patients in Tegré were told to eat and drink plentifully, and were obliged to consume a glass of melted butter every morning for eight days (Blanc suggests that linseed oil was sometimes taken instead of butter). If the cure was successful, patients had to wash themselves for twelve days in a river, after which their heads were shaved and they were considered unclean for some time before again being allowed to associate with other people.

Magic and Superstition

Several cures for smallpox involved a certain degree of magic. According to Bruce, a popular practice in eighteenth-century Gondar, devised by a monk of Waldebba, consisted of inscribing a tin plate with magical characters which were then washed off with a medicinal liquor and given to the patient to drink. An element of superstition was also involved in the above-mentoned sudorific treatment in Tegré, in as much as male animals and birds were not allowed in the vicinity of the patient, due to the belief, noted by Pearce, that sexual intercourse, even by livestock, would cause the Devil to bring the "shadow of death" upon the patient and kill him. Discussing this superstition, Pearce commented, "I have often asked them what they mean by the shadow, and how the shadow would come to a house or hut where everything was closed, and not a hole or crevice but was stopped up. They said that all connections (i.e., sexual intercourse) . . . done while the Almighty was angry with them would increase their illness and vex God so much as not to show mercy upon them at all."

IV

Cholera: The *Naftagna Fangal*

Cholera, the second of the major epidemics, differed from smallpox in that it was not endemic, but tended to enter Ethiopia from abroad, often from India or elsewhere in the East. The disease resembled smallpox, however, in that it resulted in a high rate of mortality, and inspired considerable terror.

Though cholera may have been responsible for some of the early epidemics (discussed in chapter II), its diagnosis cannot be firmly established until the early seventeenth century. The first such epidemic occurred after a famine early in the reign of Fasiladas (1632–1667). The epidemic was mentioned by the Jesuit Manoel de Almeida, who stated that after the expulsion of his Order, in 1633, "a horrible plague invaded nearly the whole region," so that the emperor was obliged to "change the seat of his palace to another place." Almeida, who depicted this plague as a curse of God, declared that it entered the country

> through Dambeya and soon assailed the camp and court at Danqaz with such fierceness that it was necessary to move the site to Libo. There the attacks continued in such a manner that they did not spare the imperial tents; within them the pestilence killed some of the emperor's pages, and forced him to go running away and moving to various places, wandering like another Cain. From Danqaz the disease passed to Wagara, to the mountains of Samén and to the famous Lamalmo, and forced the guards who collect the taxes, and cloth, in that pass to flee.

The epidemic did not stop at the elevated lands of Lamalmo, but "descended to Tegré," where it obliged the inhabitants to "leave many lands depopulated."

The above account is corroborated by that of another Jesuit, Diego de Mattos, who reported in 1643–1645 that his companions had learned that pestilence was "raging around the mountain of Lamalmo and had entered the province of Tegré."

This epidemic is also mentioned in the Ethiopian chronicles, which record that in the second year of the Emperor's reign (1634-1635) there was an outbreak of *fangal*, the word later used invariably for cholera. This statement would seem to establish the identity of the disease, and leads us to suppose that the outbreak was an extension of a major international epidemic of cholera first reported in Java in 1629.

An echo of this outbreak is found in the *Treatise* of Zara Ya'qob and Walda Heywat, a work of disputed authorship, which, following long established practice, blames the disaster on the wickedness of man, and declares that "famine struck, and after famine, the plague; many died, others were stricken by terror." The calamity, we are told, consisted of "two years of famine and plague."

The Early Nineteenth Century

Ethiopia suffered from at least five cholera epidemics in the nineteenth and early twentienth centuries.

The first occurred in the 1830s when the disease spread in many countries of the East. The medical historian Hirsch later observed that this attack was "probably the continuation of a pestilential progress from Egypt through Tripoli and Tunis, the wider ramifications of which may be seen in the epidemics that prevailed at the same time in Abyssinia, on the East Coast of Africa from Somaliland to Zanzibar, and in the Sudan." The chronology in Ethiopia, where at least two distinct outbreaks seem to have taken place, is obscure, however, for the travelers of the period—most of whom learned of the event at second hand—gave conflicting dates. Johnston gave 1830-1831; Harris, 1833; Kirk, 1834 and 1835; d'Abbadie, 1835; and Krapf, Wolff, and Gobat, 1836. All, however, agreed as to the epidemic's magnitude. Kirk, whose account is the most detailed, believed that there were in fact two outbreaks. The first, which took place in 1834, led to "great mortality" in Shawa. Explaining the geographical coverage of the disease, he observed:

> Its course is said to have been from north to south, first appearing on the frontiers of the Wollo country, and passing to the districts inhabited by the Galla tribes to the south and southwest, from whence most probably it penetrated to the unknown regions of central Africa. The more elevated regions of Shoa remained nearly free from the disease, a few isolated cases only appearing at Ankober and Angolalla. In character it appears to have resembled the Asiatic cholera, and to have been marked by vomiting, purging and spasm, the cases usually terminating fatally in twenty-four hours.

The second outbreak occurred in the following year, after a drought and a "severe famine." This epidemic was characterized by severe pain in the abdomen and frequent purging of blood, to which the sufferer usually succumbed in from eight to ten days. There was once again "great mortality" throughout Shawa, and Ankobar was "half depopulated." Johnston, a British ship's surgeon, explained that this outbreak was particularly serious as it came after two successive crop failures had reduced the population to "the greatest extremity" with the result that at Ankobar "nearly two thirds" of the poverty-stricken inhabitants perished of cholera, which was locally known as *agwert*. The epidemic's intensity also owed much to the capital's poor sanitary conditions. The disease, reported Harris, "spread with fearful virulence in the foul city" so that "one half of the whole population were speedily swept away."

The northern provinces were also serious affected. In the summer of 1835 no less than forty-four members of a caravan journeying inland from Massawa died between dawn and dusk, and, though a number of sufferers were taken back to the port, all perished, according to d'Abbadie. Daily mortality at Gondar in May of the following year was said by Gobat to have "averaged from thirty-six to forty in a population of about three thousand," which suggests that 700 to 800 persons, or about a quarter of the inhabitants, perished. The epidemic, Wolff reported, was still raging at Adwa four weeks later. The population of Wallo and Lasta, Krapf noted, was likewise "considerably thinned." In one fertile area, observed d'Abbadie, all cultivation was discontinued; the inhabitants abandoned the place, which consequently was almost entirely depopulated. The incidence of the disease, however, varied greatly from region to region. It was considerably greater towards the coast, and, though serious at Dabra Tabor where many soldiers and poor people were quartered, had entered neither Gojjam nor the lands south of the Blue Nile.

Early nineteenth-century Ethiopian society, as d'Abbadie insisted, was fully aware of the contagious character of the disease. So was King Sahla Sellasé, who, according to Harris, "sought strict seclusion in the remote palace at Machel-wans, where he would see no person until the plague was stayed; and those of his terror-stricken subjects who survived fled for a season from a hill which was declared by the superstitious priesthood to have been blasted by a curse from heaven." To placate supernatural forces, a black bull was led through the streets of Ankobar, and the populace carried stones upon their heads as a sign of repentance.

The Reign of Téwodros
Another major epidemic occurred in the 1850s. It was particularly serious in the west of the country towards the Sudan frontier. In 1856 Flad recorded that on a two-and-a-half mile journey along the trade route from Matamma to Wahni he saw no less than one hundred skeletons, and that fifteen to twenty persons were dying daily at each of the villages he passed. People once again sought safety in flight: there was a great exodus from Matamma to the highlands, and at Wahni there were only five merchants, all the remainder having fled to the hills. An Ethiopian chronicler, Dabtara Zaneb, commented that God sent down a major epidemic and that innumerable people died all

over the country. The disease, which took the form of diarrhoea and vomiting, killed people irrespective of whether they were standing, sitting, or sleeping. Death came so suddenly that the disease was called *naftanya fangal*, because it struck down its victims as swiftly as did the *naftanya*, or riflemen. In Shawa, however, the term *agwert* also continued to be used. Another chronicler, Alaqa Walda Maryam, however, also referred to the epidemic as *naftanya*, declaring that it broke out among the emperor's troops, many of whom succumbed to this "truly terrible" disease that killed large numbers of people between dawn and dusk on a single day. The extent of the dislocation caused by this epidemic was underlined in a report by Consul Plowden who wrote on June 23, 1856, that Emperor Téwodros, then in Gojjam, had planned to march into Tegré to suppress a rebellion, but the "fatal cholera" had "disorganized the army." The epidemic, he added, "is ravaging the country, and scarce any who are attacked recover; it last appeared here twenty-two years since (i.e., in 1834), and the consternation it now causes is in proportion to the ignorance of the people, and the inefficiency of medical aid; all business, even markets, are suspended." The emperor, however, later struck camp and sought higher ground. On the way many men fell off their horses and mules, but upon the army's entering Bagémder the disease miraculously came to an end—in Walda Maryam's words, "through the goodness of Christ."

A further epidemic, which appears to have originated in the East, reached the port of Massawa in October 1865. This outbreak was "severely felt" at the port, as described by Dr. Blanc: "All those who had been suffering from insufficient or inferior food became an easy prey; few, indeed, of those who contracted the disease rallied; almost all died." The Pasha, or local ruler, "was several times on the point of death, from great debility and complete loss of tone of the digestive organs." Even the tiny European community suffered one casualty. The death toll at the port, according to Douin, a later historian, reached about 300 persons.

Faced with this outbreak at Massawa, the populace of the interior once more took immediate action to prevent the spread of infection. They cut off all communications with the coast, and refused to allow caravans to leave the highlands until the epidemic had ceased. Notwithstanding this precaution the disease soon advanced inland, first to Tegré, where according to Blanc it played "havoc," and then to other northern provinces. Shepherd reported that it "raged with great violence in Antalo and the surrounding villages," several of which were uninhabitated when he visited them a year or so later; while Munzinger, a Swiss scholar, said that the cholera also made "dreadful ravages" among the Danakil tribesmen.

Several cases of the disease were reported in May 1866 at Qorata on the south-eastern shore of Lake Tana. On hearing this news Téwodros, according to Blanc, "wisely decided" upon moving to the highlands of Begémder. Before doing so, however, he paid a brief visit to Qorata, to inquire as to the extent of the epidemic. His curiosity was, however, disastrous, for within a matter of days the disease broke out in his camp, and hundreds were dying daily. In the hope of improving the sanitary conditions of his army, the Emperor moved his camp to some high ground a mile or so north of the town; but the epidemic continued to rage with great virulence both in the camp and in the town. The church was so completely choked up with dead bodies that no more could be admitted, and the adjoining streets offered the sad sight of countless corpses, surrounded by the sorrowful relatives, awaiting for days and nights the hallowed grave in the now crowded cemetery. Smallpox and typhus fever also made their appearance, and claimed the victims cholera had spared.

Téwodros, fully conscious of the infectious character of the disease, decided on June 12 to leave for the higher and more healthy province of Bagémder. According to Waldmeier, a missionary witness, however, the march was

> very difficult. . . . We had to travel in the midst of a crowd of 100,000 soldiers, women and children. Some sick, dying and even dead, were carried in the crowd, and many others lay dead on the ground, the multitude passing over them, so that the smell became fearful, and the lamentation for the dead was heart-rendering.

By June 14 the soldiers were several thousand feet above the lake, but the cholera, smallpox, and typhus continued unabated, whereupon, according to Blanc,

> His Majesty inquired what was usually done in our country under similar circumstances. We advised him to proceed at once to the higher plateau of Begemder, to leave his sick at some distance from Dabra Tabor, to break up as far as possible his army, and distribute it over the whole province, selecting a few healthy and isolated localities where every fresh case that broke out should be sent.

The emperor acted upon this advice which accorded so closely with the custom of his own country. There was, however, no immediate respite. Waldemeier recalled that several of his own servants fell ill and died on the road, and that upon arrival at Gafat his wife was "seized with a violent attack of cholera, followed by typhus fever, which was so dangerous that she was brought to the very brink of the grave . . . the angel of death was daily claiming its victims." Conditions were so serious that Blanc was released from detention by the Emperor, and, according to the chronicler, cured many cholera victims. The policy of flight was in due course successful, however, and Téwodros "before long had the satisfaction," in Blanc's words, "of seeing the several epidemics lose their virulence, and, before many weeks, disappear entirely." This is confirmed by Waldmeier who notes that "by degrees the cholera passed away."

The magnitude of the epidemic was such that Hirsch may well have been correct in declaring it a "point of departure" for the southward advance of cholera into the country of the Gallas, who, he believes, had previously been little affected by the disease. It is interesting to note that the foreign origin of the outbreak was generally accepted. The oldest inhabitants of Tegré later told Dr. Parisis, a Greek physician in the service of Emperor Yohannes IV, that they remembered a cholera epidemic, presumably that of 1865-1866, and categorically declared that it had been brought by Indian traders to Massawa whence it had penetrated inland.

The Great Famine of 1888–1892

The last nineteenth-century cholera epidemic owed its intensity to the Great Famine of 1888–1892, which caused the population to fall easy victim to infections of all kinds. The exact history of the outbreak is unclear. An Italian physician at Massawa, Dr. Filippo Rho, believed that the disease was brought to the port in July 1890 by pilgrims returning from Mecca. A French officer, Paul de Lauribar, suggested on the other hand that cholera had already broken out in the interior some months earlier, and was actually taken in to Eritrea by destitute persons from the interior crossing the frontier in the hope of finding work. The disease, according to de Lauribar, was rampant in the colony from the end of 1889 to July 1890, and Italian *carabinieri* and native troops were continually going up and down the streets of the town burning corpses. Immigration across the border was prohibited, and many immigrants were forcibly deported. Despite the stringency of such measures, a further outbreak was reported along the Setit River in western Eritrea in 1891.

Testimony as to the extent of devastation is afforded by Bent, who, after visitng the northern province in 1893, wrote:

> Civil war, famine and an epidemic of cholera have, within the last decade, played fearful havoc . . . villages are abandoned, the land is going out of cultivation. . . . It is scarcely possible to realize, without visiting the country, the abject misery and wretchedness which has fallen upon the Ethiopian empire during late years.

The town of Dabarwa for example had been "decimated," with the result that "a few piles of stones, an almost ruined church, and a few wretched hovels" were all that was left.

The southern provinces were also seriously affected, mainly in 1892 when cholera appeared at the Gulf of Aden ports where numerous deaths were reported. A large number of the inhabitants of Bulhar, according to Drake-Brockman, were wiped out. The rate of mortality is also graphically revealed in a British consular report for 1893, which lists the number of stricken and dead at the Somali ports as shown in the following table.

Incidence of death among cholera victims at Somali ports in 1893.

Port	Number of Stricken	Number of Deaths
Zeila	369	277
Bulhar	826	686
Berbera	13	11

Many persons also died at the French port of Jibuti, among them two who attracted official attention: the colonial administrator, Joseph Deloncle, and the military physician, Dr. Aubry.

The epidemic rapidly spread inland. At Sheik Hussein no less than four-fifths of the population was reported by Donaldson Smith as having perished. Harar was also badly affected. Those infected, according to Gabra Sellasé, included persons conveying cattle from Ogaden to the famine-stricken areas of the interior. Troops sent to guard the livestock also caught the disease, and many died, their commander Azaj Walda Sadeq himself falling ill. Anxious to avoid further spread of the epidemic, he ordered that the animals be kept in Adal and that the roads be guarded to prevent the disease from advancing to Ankobar, where Emperor Menilek was then encamped. The chief then withdrew to the lowlands of Dibbi, south of Ankobar, where he had a tent erected in the forest and lived there in isolation, declaring: "If I die what matters so long as Menilek is master!" The chronicler declared that God heard these words and permitted the brave chief to recover, though few of those who caught the disease survived. One of the first of the disease's many victims at Ankobar was Walda Gabriel, a priest renowned for his chanting. Vanderheym described the population as "decimated." The epidemic came to an end only after Menilek left the city and made his way south to Entotto in September 1892. Addis Ababa, which Menilek had established as his capital a few years earlier, also suffered seriously: a British traveler, Pease, observed that the disease made "great ravages."

Cholera, according to De Coppet, at this time became known as *ya nefas basheta*, or "disease of the wind," as it was popularly thought to have been spread by the wind which blew mainly from the north-east, that is to say, from the coast where it so often first appeared.

The Twentieth Century
Greater international controls, as well as the advance of medicine within Ethiopia itself, led to a substantial disminuation of cholera in the twentieth century. The last major epidemic, which occurred in the East around 1902, seems to have reached the country in 1906 but was reported only in Wallo.

V

Typhus: Military and Civilian Outbreaks

Typhus, though less widespread and devastating than either smallpox or cholera, doubtless accounted for at least some of the major epidemics of early times. It is not, however, until the second half of the nineteenth century that its identification becomes possible.

The disease, aptly referred to in England as "camp fever," was also common among Ethiopian and foreign armies. This accorded with the pattern observed by Zinsser, the isolator of the typhus virus, who said that it was "never absent from the regions invaded by returning soldiers, who lighted fuses of infection that flickered along through villages and cities wherever chance sparked on inflammable material." The disease, which was known in Latin as *Morbus cancerorum*, or "gaol fever," was also reported in Ethiopian prisons, few of which, however, existed until modern times.

Though it is probable that typhus was responsible for the "epidemical fever" which Bruce reported among an army in Bagémder in 1771, the disease is not mentioned by name for another half-century. The earliest references are by the French traveler Arnauld d'Abbadie, who indicated that there was an outbreak of *nedad*, or typhus, at Gondar in 1842, when all the merchants in a caravan from Sennar died. He had heard of other cases of the disease in Enarya and elsewhere. Such evidence, however, is of only limited value, as it is by no means certain whether he distinguished accurately between typhus and other fevers. Emphasizing that the malady was "much feared," he stated that some Ethiopians had informed him that there was no cure for it; others told him of various supposed preventives, including hyena's excreta as well as various vegetable medicines and fumigants.

There is uncertainty, moreover, as to how typhus was referred to in Ethiopia at this time. The German missionary linguist Isenberg in his Amharic-English dictionary of 1841 listed *nedad*, the term used by d'Abbadie, but translated it generally as "burning, esp. febrile heat, fever, ague," and cited the word *setema*, equally vaguely as "a certain fever, typhus." A couple of generations later Antoine d'Abbadie equated *nedad*, also loosely, with "a feverish temperature, fever—typhus, malign fever—intermittent fever", and *setema* with "a kind of fever; typhus." To add to the confusion he quoted two other terms as being applicable to typhus: *magana*, which he described as "a kind of very serious illness—typhus?" and *badado* which he translated even more awkwardly as "typhus, smallpox." Such ambiguities render the study of the history of Ethiopian typhus hazardous, the more so as many observers may have understood the above terms as applying to typhoid or other epidemics.

Epidemics Among the Soldiers of the Nineteenth Century

The first relatively well-documented epidemic believed to have been typhus erupted in June 1866 among the soldiers of Emperor Téwodros II, then camped near Qorata by Lake Tana. The outbreak occurred, typically enough, in a situation of acutely bad sanitation: "hundreds were dying daily," according to Blanc, and heavy mortality was also reported by the missionary Flad. Following the common Ethiopian practice, Téwodros, as we have seen, ordered his men to make their way to higher land in Bagémder, with the result that the epidemic lost its virulence, and before many weeks disappeared entirely.

Another suspected typhus epidemic broke out in the early 1870s among Egyptian soldiers invading from the Sudan. The disease was described as their "most formidable enemy," and was particularly serious at the fortress of Karan where the troops lived in close proximity to one another.

A further outbreak believed to have been typhus occurred in the summer and autumn of 1876 among Egyptian forces pushing inland from Massawa into Hamasén. This epidemic was perhaps not surprising in view of the invaders' failure to take even such elementary health precautions as the speedy burial of the dead. On August 9 the Egyptian commander, Rateb Pasha, reported that typhus had spread among his soldiers, 160 of whom were hospitalized. "Four to six" were dying every day, and those entering the hospital were "more numerous than those leaving it." The greater part of the patients were Sudanese. The epidemic was so rampant among the latter that Rateb decided on August 20 to transfer one of his two Sudanese battalions from their base at Kayakhor, south-east of Asmara, to Bahr Raza further north, and replaced them by healthier contingents of Arab troops from Bahr Raza and Adi Raza. The health situation at Kayakhor was so acute that no fewer than 282 men were in the hospital on September 2 and forty-seven died within a week, after which the Egyptians decided to evacuate the sick. Many men, however, continued to fall ill. Rateb removed most of the sick from Kayakhor early in September, but conditions scarcely improved, for on reaching Bahr Raza seven or eight men were dying every day and thirty-eight were in the hospital, while at Adi Raza the sick exceeded 200. On September 16 he reported that all measures taken to arrest the plague had "proved fruitless," and the Arab battalion had begun to be affected. Even though the number of sick was "still small" the disease was "spreading more and more" among them. It also affected the "irregulars," or local Ethiopian mercenaries, three or four of whom were dying daily.

The epidemic among the Egyptian force was so serious that by September 19 no less than 384 Sudanese and 76 Arab soldiers had died. Eight to ten men were dying every day, while 416 were receiving medical treatment. Rateb was obliged to send the sick to Monkullu, just inland from Massawa, and to order their isolation. Accordingly, 260 patients were isolated on September 23, and towards the end of the month a special camp was established at Massawa. The number of cases isolated rose to 537. For a time the sitation seemed to improve, but the epidemic later took a turn for the worse, the sick roll in the Sudanese battalions rising to 594 on October 1. Respite came, however, towards the end of the month, enabling Rateb to report on November 3 that typhus had disappeared from Massawa.

Epidemics Among the Civilian Population

The typhus epidemic of 1876, though at first apparently confined to the Egyptian and Sudanese troops whose illness was the subject of official reports, later spread among the local Ethiopian population for whom no such detailed records are available. The Italian traveler Matteucci, however, later asserted that the "terrible scourge" had destroyed 25% of the population of Tegré. Adwa, the capital, was particularly seriously affected, which was not surprising since, as we have seen, it suffered from extremely poor sanitary conditions. Matteucci, finding it almost deserted, asked: "What was the cause of so much misfortune?" and replied: "A typhus epidemic, terrible in its consequences, had struck Abyssinia and especially Tegré." The blow to the town was confirmed by another Italian traveler, Pippo Vigoni, who remarked that the epidemic had resulted in "true carnage," and added: "it is calculated that more then two-thirds of the population of Adwa perished. . . . One meets almost no one, the greater part of the streets are deserted, in them one sees misfortune, death."

Such foreign observers, who wrote a generation before the discovery of the insect vectors of typhus, had no knowledge of the mode of diffusion of the disease, and therefore explained it in unscientific (albeit graphic) terms. Vigoni remarked that "a terrible famine united to the miasma produced by the thousands of Egyptian corpses left unburied, resulted in a typhus epidemic," while Matteucci, putting the blame on numerous livestock which had perished of cattle plague, observed:

> In the rainy season there rose over the city an atmosphere corrupted by the fermentation of so many animal bodies apparently dried by the rays of the summer sun, and there developed a typhus epidemic which caused carnage without regard to age or condition. In many places the corpses were not buried and became the home of new infections: the abandoned houses in great part collapsed, as if moved by pity that the human bodies lay there without honourable burial.

Later Epidemics

Another outbreak, possibly of typhus, was reported a few years later in southern Ethiopia. Massaia stated that it led to considerable mortality, notably at Ankobar.

A further typhus epidemic, together with other diseases, occurred during the Great Famine (1888-1892). This outbreak seriously affected Emperor Menilek's army which was returning in 1890 from Tegré to Shawa, and lost, as we have seen, "a good 15 per cent" of its number from typhus, dysentery, smallpox or bronchitis as Ilg reported. Typhus may also have been the cause of the high mortality reported among Menilek's armies then marching through the southern provinces.

The typhus epidemic of this period, was, however, not confined to the soldiers, but spread far and wide. In August 1889 a visiting Italian doctor, Vincenzo Ragazzi, reported that "the country of Shawa, and in general all Ethiopia" had been struck by a "murderous typhus epidemic," while a French traveler, Sylvain Vignéras, remarked that the population of Burka in the Harar area had suffered greatly from "famine, followed by smallpox, typhus and finally by cholera." Ilg's biographer Conrad Keller likewise tells of "countless persons" falling victim to typhus.

Yet another outbreak generally diagnosed as typhus occurred nearly a decade later among the soldiers of one of Menilek's principal chieftains, Ras Walda Giyorgis, who occupied Kaffa in 1897. The disease, according to the Italian physicians Carlo Annaratone and Lincoln de Castro, was subsequently introduced into Addis Ababa by the returning troops.

Cases of typhus were also reported early in the Italian occupation of Eritrea, notably at Massawa in the years immediately after its seizure in 1885, and elsewhere in April and May 1896.

The Early Twentieth Century

Though smallpox and cholera epidemics declined in the twentieth century, outbreaks of typhus continued to occur. In May 1906 the French missionary Jarosseau asserted that typhus had been raging in the Harar area for several months and that one-third of those affected had died.

The prevalence of typhus in pre–World War II Addis Ababa was later noted by Christine Sandford, as well as by an Italian traveler, Pietro Jansen, who remarked that it was a "curse" affecting the capital's little-washed inhabitants and was a danger also to European residents. Numerous cases of the disease were likewise reported in the provinces, notably by the American missionary Bergsma, and the Greek author Zervos who described it as "endemic" and the cause of "high mortality." In the late 1920s an outbreak at one of the gold mines on the Birbir river in Walaga was noted by a British engineer, Captain E.J. Bartleet, who stated that deaths were "almost a daily occurrence". Typhus was also reported in pre–World War II Eritrea. A suspected epidemic of the disease occurred in 1920, and was followed in 1927 and 1933 by two further outbreaks generally accepted as typhus. The last Ethiopian typhus epidemic prior to the Italian invasion was reported at Harar by Evelyn Waugh, who was informed in the autumn of 1935 that at the town's overcrowded prison "three or four" deaths from typhus occurred weekly.

The dreaded disease was generally known in the twentieth century as *tasbo*, an Amharic term recorded by the Ethiopian linguist Afawarq Gabra Iyasus. The word was, however, often used without much linguistic precision. The French missionary Joseph Baeteman, though a lexicographer of repute, translated typhus as *Hedar basheta* (i.e., "illness of the month of Hedar"), thus confusing it with influenza which, as we shall see, struck the country in the month of Hedar, (November–December) 1918, though he also equated the latter term with "influenza" and "influenza-typhus". This medically impossible correlation was repeated by the Italian scholar Cerulli in a dictionary published as late as 1940.

Numerous cures for *tasbo* were known to traditional Ethiopian practitioners. Medicines in common use, as recorded in the notebook of *dabtara* (or lay cleric) of Bagémder, included the roots of *waginos* (*Brucea antidysenterica*), *gumaro* (*Capparis tomentosa*), *giséwa* (*Withania somnifera*), *zamato* (?) and *tult* (*Rumex steudelii*), and the shoots of the sycamore.

Dysentery

Dysentery, which was due mainly to pollution of drinking water, was fairly widespread in warm weather and, as Courbon, Blanc, and Mérab noted, was common in many regions, among them the Red Sea and Takazzé areas and various parts of the plateau, including Adwa, and Ogaden.

Epidemics of dysentery were reported on several occasions, notably at Harrar at the time of the Egyptian occupation in the 1870s, and at Addigrat in May 1905 when Martini, the Italian governor of Eritrea, stated that the outbreak, which he thought was due to bad water, resulted in the death of two or three persons daily.

VI

Influenza: The *Hedar basheta*

Influenza, which may have been responsible for several unidentified epidemics of early times, can be documented in Ethiopia for over a quarter of a millennium.

Perhaps the earliest reference to the disease is in Ludolf's Amharic-Latin dictionary of 1698 which lists *gunfan* or "catarrhus" and *gunfanam* or "catarrhis obnoxius." The former probably referred then, as now, to both the common cold and influenza; the latter probably more specifically to influenza.

Eighteenth-century chronicles tell of two *gunfan* epidemics, which, in view of their severity, must have been influenza rather than the common cold. The first, in 1706, is mentioned in the annals of Emperor Iyasu I, which record that because of the outbreak the emperor's son and heir, Takla Haymanot, was obliged to leave his residence, while "many people fell ill" and died. The second attack, in 1747, was also deadly. The chronicle of Iyasu II states that "many illnesses" then raged in Gondar "and in all the country," where the dead were so numerous that people to bury them could not be found. "Many people died suddenly," and there was "no one who did not fall ill of *gunfan*."

Foreign travelers, who constitute the principal source of information on the epidemics of the early nineteenth century, were conspicuous by their absence in 1803, 1833, 1837, and 1847, the years which witnessed the principal influenza outbreaks of this period in other parts of the world. The Ethiopian chronicles of this time are also particularly defective. There is therefore no means of assessing how far these international epidemics impinged on the country.

Despite this dearth of documentation, there are several references to the outbreak of fevers and "pernicious miasmas" which may have been influenza.

Towards the end of 1835 or beginning of 1836 there was an epidemic of "cerebral fever" which carried off a "large number" of the inhabitants of Mahdara Maryam in Bagémder, thereby obliging Empress Manan to flee the town, and in April of the following year a "terrible" epidemic "decimated" the inhabitants of Massawa.

Dr. Petit's Reports

The first strictly medical account of an Ethiopian influenza epidemic was written in 1839 by Dr. A. Petit, a member of the French scientific mission, who witnessed it at Adwa. He noted that this outbreak was far less serious than others remembered by the inhabitants, who, perhaps referring to local manifestations of the international outbreaks of 1833 and 1837, said that earlier attacks had been "more grave, and could even become fatal."

The epidemic of 1839, which came in two waves, began, according to Petit, "at the beginning and end of the rains," that is to say in July and September, when Adwa was "the theatre of an epidemic illness." By the middle of July "the greater part" of the city's inhabitants had fallen victim to the disease. It began with a feeling of discomfort, lassitude in the limbs, weakness, and an inability to move. Soon afterwards there developed an acute inflammation of the pituitary membrane of the nose with considerable secretion in the eyes and nasal chambers. The latter was also the seat of strong tingling, while the front sinus was characterized by discomfort and constriction. The inflammation often extended to the laryngo-pharyngeal mucous membrane, thereby producing angina. It many cases the irritation subsequently descended into the bronchus and gave way to catarrh with coughing and expectoration. At the same time, or more often several days later, an intense cephalalgia (headache) developed, while the general weakness became more acute and the patient felt "inexpressible discomfort." The pain seemed to be situated on the exterior of the head, almost in the skin of the hair, as evident from the fact that strong pressure reduced or even removed it. Discomfort usually extended as far as the ears and teeth, which became extremely sensitive. The pulse was usually slow, full, and vibrant, though sometimes almost normal. The skin was hot and dry in the first case, and moist in the second. The tongue became large and yellowish and the belly sluggish. In certain cases there was a desire to vomit, though the movement of the bowels was almost always normal. Finally, there was a feeling of discomfort in the limbs, particularly in the legs and shoulders.

The second outbreak occurred two months later, in September, when the disease seemd to have been modified: neuralgic pains showed themselves only in exceptional cases, and the cephalalgia was normally limited to one side of the head or face. The disease was observed by Petit to have responded to emetics with ipecacuanha and saline purgatives, though it was sometimes necessary to have recourse to bleeding.

The Late Nineteenth and Early Twentieth Centuries

Ethiopian influenza, being little different from that in other countries and normally mild, received scant attention from foreign travelers of the second half of the century. There is, however, evidence of a serious outbreak in 1889–1890 during the Great Famine when the starving population also fell easy prey, as we have seen, to other epidemic diseases. This influenza outbreak probably formed part of a world epidemic. Dr. Wurtz recorded that at the end of 1889 there was a "murderous" influenza epidemic which "decimated the population," and quoted Ilg as stating that there were more than 20,000 sick men in the army, many of whom died of severe influenza.

Influenza and the common cold were alike referred to in nineteenth-century Amharic as *gunfan, gumfan,* or *genfan,* as recorded in the dictionaries of Isenberg and d'Abbadie, though linguists of the early twentieth century indicate that the form *gunfan* was by then normal. A common saying of this time was: "He who with *gunfan* catches a dog, a child or a goat, cannot remain hidden."

Early Twentieth-Century Outbreaks and Cures

The frequency of influenza epidemics in early twentieth-century Addis Ababa was recorded by Dr. Mérab, who stated that in 1908 and 1914 the town suffered from several outbreaks. Most cases he had seen were gastro-intestinal, and to a lesser extent pulmonary, for the nervous variety was exceptional. There were also minor forms of the disease, referred to as *mech*.

Influenza, Mérab stated, was popularly "attributed to the influence of the sun," as in Europe to that of the cold. Some people on the other hand thought it was caused by the "evil eye," while others said it might result from a dead cat being thrown by an evil-disposed person on one's bed or into one's room or courtyard.

Traditional cures included the roots of the rue plant, *téna Adam* (*Ruta montana*), mixed with *barbaré*, or red pepper, marshmallow leaves, and other plants, boiled together with *taj*, or honey wine. Use was also made of a concoction from the root of a plant called *baglat* (?) or sheep's tail, a kind of convulaceae with cathartic properties, which was both drunk and rubbed on the body. Another remedy was the juice of a secret plant which was placed in the ears and nose, and supposed to produce an almost instant cure. Also popular was a steam bath made by boiling the bryony. Patients taking this treatment were supposed not to leave their houses until they had changed their *shamma*, or toga, failing which it was believed that the illness would return. One last cure was an unidentified emetic, which, according to Mérab, was used in cases of gastritic influenza.

The *Hedar basheta* of 1918

Though most outbreaks of influenza are but poorly documented, records of the epidemic of 1918 are by contrast remarkably rich, and can, moreover, be supplemented by the testimony of survivors. This epidemic, the last prior to the introduction of modern medicine, provides a dramatic case study of the advent and impact of a killer disease in a still largely traditional society.

The influenza epidemic of 1918 made its appearance in Ethiopia, as in most parts of the world, in two distinct waves: the first in the spring and summer, and the second in autumn. The first wave, which was mild and never properly diagnosed, manifested itself as early as April. A Swedish Protestant missionary, Karl Cederqvist, reported from Addis Ababa on April 22:

> Many persons are ill here in the town and some of them that have come from the western Galla provinces have been taken ill on the road. Still all of them have succeeded to reach us. I also suffer from fever, but have up till today been able to keep on foot and at work.

However, he succumbed soon afterwards and on May 6 wrote to Stockholm that on account of illness he could not send a report to his mission director.

Continued fever, which for lack of accurate diagnosis was widely assumed to be typhus or smallpox, became increasingly prevalent in the ensuing months. On July 21 the Italian governor of Eritrea, De Martino, telegraphed to Rome that the Italian minister in Addis Ababa, Count Colli, had telephoned to say that a "fierce variolic epidemic" was raging in the Ethiopian capital, and that the Ethiopian government had requested assistance. He accordingly dispatched a physician, Dr. Pasquale Vetuschi, who traveled via Jibuti with 100,000 doses of smallpox vaccine—which were of course quite useless for an attack of influenza. The disease meanwhile failed to abate. One of the earliest known victims in the capital was a Greek youth, Stamatios Ghanotakis, who passed away on August 7. This phase of the outbreak was later recalled by Gerald Campbell of the British legation who stated that "many" people died, and, because of the dearth of grave-diggers, were interred only "about 6 inches under the surface." The foreign legations protested against such burials at St. George's Church, which lay just above the market, and an order was accordingly given "that only churchyards outside the town should be used."

By the latter part of August the epidemic was widespread. On August 27 it struck down the regent, Ras Tafari Makonnen (later Emperor Hayla Sellasé). Four days later, on August 31, he wrote to the French missionary Monsigneur André Jarosseau in Harar to inform him that he was "suffering from a kind of fever" which was "becoming worse," and begged him to pray for him. Tafari was treated by an Armenian physician, Dr. Ohanes Devletian, but, following long-established Ethiopian practice, also made numerous gifts to the churches, and presented them with money "according to the size of their *sabaka*," or parishes. News of the regent's illness duly reached the foreign diplomatic community. On September 2, Major J.H. Dodds of the British legation telegraphed to the Foreign Office that Tafari was "suffering from a form of typhoid which is prevalent in Addis Ababa," but added, "At present his condition does not give cause for anxiety." On the following day he nevertheless sent a further telegram to state that because of the ruler's sickness it was "impossible" to do business with the Ethiopian government. Two days later the governor of Eritrea telegraphed Rome that the Italian minister in Addis Ababa had informed him that the Ras was "seriously ill," and was suffering from "a form of typhus most widespread at this moment in Addis Ababa."

The epidemic had by now gained increased ferocity. In the first week of September it carried off numerous victims in Addis Ababa. One of the first was Ababa Yebsa, a young educated nobleman employed in the palace treasury, who died on September 6. His death was but one of many. Alaqa Kenfa, an Ethiopian cleric who kept a diary, observed that the number of persons going to funerals was at this time "greater than those who did not go," and that the living "shivered with fright like a wounded beast," for "a person seen today might not be seen tomorrow."

The regent's health meanwhile was fast deteriorating, and was so critical on Sunday, September 8, that he felt it necessary to receive Holy Communion. Alaqa Kenfa commented, "people pitied him because he was so young." He was in fact twenty-six years of age. Dodds telegraphed that day that Tafari had "suddenly" become "worse," but that the doctors still had "hope." Discussing this development he later reported that "the condition of the Ras on the 7th and 8th . . . gave cause for great anxiety, and, although it was only known to a very few, he hovered between life and death on those days." The problem, Campbell subsequently claimed, was that the ruler had been "touched in one lung." Tafari's illness created such concern in government circles that orders were given for the minister of war, Fitawrari Habta Giyorgis, then on an expedition to Walamo, to return to Addis Ababa immediately. The patient's health reached its lowest ebb on September 8, after which, however, it began to improve. Dodds noted that "it was with a feeling of great relief" that he received a "reassuring report" from the regent's French physician, Dr. Le Pape, on the morning of the ninth. Tafari's condition nevertheless remained critical for many more days. Fitawrari Hapta Giyorgis duly arrived in the capital on September 17, but, although his return was designed to ensure the government's security, he himself "soon fell a victim" to the epidemic, and was for a time "in great danger" and "at death's door."

One of the first prominent foreigners to die of the disease, on September 17, was the regent's physician, Dr. Assad Chaiban, a Lebanese, whose demise greatly shocked the foreign community. His death, Dodds commented, introduced "a touch of the dramatic," for he had been "untiring in his attendance on the Ras." Chaiban's death was also recalled fifty-six years later by Alfred Abel, an old-time Austrian resident of Addis Ababa, who informed the present writer that it was "rather a mystery" at the time as the doctor was only thirty-five years old (an age confirmed by the gravestone later erected by his grateful royal patient) and "in perfect health. He died within two or three days." The cause of death, Abel claimed, was not widely realized until the middle of October, "when the real epidemic broke out. Then naturally we knew that he had died of what we called Spanish influenza." His imposing gravestone tersely states that he was a "victime de son devoir."

The epidemic was by now affecting increasingly large numbers of the city's inhabitants. Alaqa Kenfa reported that "many people were dying in Addis Ababa," and sadly commented:

> Just as a brother would walk over the corpse of his brother on a battlefield so nobody troubled to bury the dead by the roadside. They simply walked by. There were no more graves in the churchyards so it was decided that people would be buried by churches that would be built later.

The earlier ban on burials at St. George's was then abandoned, for, as Campbell cynically observed, it "did not suit the priest in charge . . . so he had a dream in which St. George patron of this Church told him that he claimed the dead for himself." Alaqa Kenfa claimed that so many people were dying that they exceeded those who attended funerals, and that because of the shortage of grave-diggers people began burying their relatives in other people's graves. Many corpses, according to Campbell, were interred "on top of those who died in the August epidemic." Writing of St. George's church, he added, "The priest got his backsheesh and even the dogs got a feed, as parts of various bodies were hardly even covered. In the midst of the influenza we were thus faced with a very probable outbreak of cholera or other disease."

Many people, in accordance with long-established custom, now began fleeing from the city, or shut themselves up in their houses and refused to receive visitors. "One of the first to flee," according to Campbell, was Abuna Matéwos, the Egyptian head of the Ethiopian Orthodox church, who established himself in seclusion on the mountain of Managasha. His abandonment of the capital, and of Empress Zawditu and Regent Tafari, according to Alaqa Kenfa, made a bad impression on the inhabitants of Addis Ababa, who murmured that the prelate had left them to die without spiritual support. "Many minor chiefs," Campbell records, nevertheless followed the *abun*'s example, among them the Kantiba (or Lord Mayor) Wasané Za Emanuel, who was, however, "eventually brought back" to govern the town.

Most survivors of the first wave of the epidemic, among them Ras Tafari, were by now on the road to recovery. The latter achieved a fairly rapid cure. His doctors, Dodds reported on September 17, stated that he was "out of danger" and that in the absence of unforeseen circumstances he would be "well enough to resume his duties in about six weeks' time." Despite this the ruler's indisposition led to the wildest rumors. Dodds that day reported:

> That the Ras himself died in the Palace about three weeks ago is firmly believed by a large number of people, and it is with a view to give the lie to this report and reassure the population that it is proposed to exhibit Ras Tafari on the balcony of the Palace at Mascal (i.e., September 27).

> Had Ras Tafari died there is little doubt that there would have been serious
> trouble throughout the country, but with the Ras on a fair way to recovery . . . there
> is every hope that Mascal will pass off quietly.

Public order, Dodds explains, was in the hands of Kantiba Wasané, who, since his return, had been "controlling the town in the name of the Ras."

In a move to calm the city the regent made a public appearance a week or so later, and, according to Alaqa Kenfa, joined the company of his fellow nobles on September 30. On that day De Martino telegraphed from Eritrea that Tafari had "easily" overcome his infection, while the diarist, recalling the regent's previous gifts to the churches, piously reflected, "God pardoned him, and he was cured." The patient himself subsequently observed in his autobiography that he had been "seriously ill," but "by God's goodness survived."

The public appearance of the regent was, however, short-lived, for, fearing reinfection, he attempted as far as possible to isolate himself from outside contact. According to Campbell, "no sooner did he realise the gravity of the situation than he shut himself up in the Ghebi (i.e., palace) with his wife and family and a small garrison and no one except the doctor was allowed in or out."

The second, and more virulent, wave of the epidemic began in many parts of the country in October. Much of the infection is thought to have reached Addis Ababa by way of the Gulf of Aden coast. In British Somaliland the senior medical officer, F.E. Whitehead, reported that there were "a few sporadic cases" in October, but the disease was not "noticed to be epidemic" until "early in November." Giving it as his opinion that "the first cases in Berbera where the disease was first noticed", were "in all probability" brought by steamer from Aden, he states that "the first few cases that came to Hospital for treatment were amongst Somalis, and were not a first recognised as influenza." From Berbera "the disease spread very rapidly," and reached "outlying stations" in the Protectorate within "about a fortnight." Elaborating on the progress of the epidemic, he remarked:

> From Berbera the disease spread in all directions along the caravan routes, and
> presumably by dhows and vessels also, to practically every part of the occupied
> country. The wave still advancing probably met and mixed with waves which were
> advancing from other centres, in French Somaliland and Abyssinia.

Explaining that it was "impossible to say with any exactitude how many people actually suffered," Whitehead observed that "many native inhabitants were suffering and dying from the disease," though there had been no deaths among Europeans. In some places there had been "partial disorganisation" among his staff on account of their falling sick themselves. In some areas "50% of the Somali population suffered, and of those suffering 5% died," and taking an average of all stations, the mortality seemed to have been "about 7% of those contracting the disease." The "large majority of deaths" were due to "pneumonia complicating the disease," though "a few died from sheer exhaustion and some apparently from fright." Among 800 Indian troops 499 (over 60%) caught the disease and 53 (over 10%) died, while among 550 Somali troops 336 (approximately 61%) were affected and 15 (almost 5%) died. The Somali police, 131 strong, suffered three deaths (around 2%), while the subordinate administration staff, which consisted of 67 persons, reported 27 cases of infection (over 40%) and three deaths (approximately 2%). The prison population of Berbera was "the last to get influenza, probably because they were more or less isolated," but out of 125 persons 70 (55%) were affected, and two died (1.5%). Mortality in the camp for the destitute was, predictably, higher, for out of 232 persons, 120 (50%) caught the disease and 20 (8%) perished.

In French Somaliland the epidemic made its appearance at about the same time. An Indian informant, Savak J. Mistry, who lived there as a youth, told the present author that the disease, which was probably brought in by French vessels visiting Jibuti, broke out "a week after Amistice Day," November 11. A week after the celebrations he, his sister, and his mother all fell ill, and his mother died "within a week" (actually on November 26 according to official records). Jibuti mortuary figures, which are available only for foreigners and military personnel and do not mention the cause of death, indicate that the death rate was running at this time at about eight a month, but the number of Somalis dying of the disease, to judge from the situation in nearby British Somaliland, must have been infinitely higher. Mistry estimated that "more than five hundred died." There were, he recalled, only two doctors in the town, and many people lacking medicine ate onions, in the belief that they had preventive or curative properties.

From the coast the epidemic made its way to the Ethiopian capital with great rapidity. Mistry, who worked on the railway and believed that this was the route by which the disease reached Addis Ababa, observed that the journey took three days and that the disease was felt in the city "within a week." Nagadras Jemaneh Yameru, then an official in the law courts, likewise claimed in 1874 that news of the epidemic at Harar reached Addis Ababa by telephone, and that the infection itself arrived only a few days later. Abel, an informant with precise memory, suggested on the other hand that the epidemic may actually have begun in Addis Ababa slightly earlier, for he recalled that "between the tenth and fifteenth of October several rather mysterious deaths took place," while Alaqa Kenfa tersely notes that the disease "killed a number of Arabs, Indians and *faranje*," or Europeans.

The rising death rate heralding the second phase of the epidemic commenced in Addis Ababa around the middle of October when, according to Abel, it "started to become very bad," and there were "many cases of death." The situation grew far worse, however, in the month of Hedar (which began on November 10). Alaqa Kenfa stated that "from Hedar 1 the disease struck many people," while Emperor Hayla Sellasé also later dated the beginning of the epidemic from that day. This chronology is substantiated by the meager church records available. At the Catholic church at Dire Dawa, burials had on average been taking place only every other month in the summer of 1918, but subsequently increased in frequency, with one in September, two in October, one in the first fortnight of November, and seven within the next two weeks. At the Catholic church in Addis Ababa there had been only three burials in August and none in September or October, but in November they increased to twenty-six. All but three were registered as due to influenza. At the Greek church in the capital, burials, which had occurred at the rate of about one a fortnight since August, rose to ten between November 12 and 27. Mortality among the much larger Ethiopian Orthodox and Muslim population must have been far greater, but passed statistically unrecorded.

Victims dying around the beginning of Hedar included Wallata Berhan Joséf, the daughter of the Ethiopian consul at Jibuti, who succumbed on November 10; her sister Yashimabet was to die five days later. The regent's Armenian physician, Ohanes Devletian, the second medical man to perish of the epidemic, passed away on November 11. Less than a week later, on November 17, the epidemic carried off its third victim from among the capital's small medical profession: Dr. W.A.M. Wakeman, an Anglo-Indian physician formerly attached to the British legation who was about to start a private medical practice. His death was a great blow to the local Indian community, "several" of whose members were then dying.

The virulence of the epidemic now amazed all observers. Nagadras Jamanah reported that some of the modern educated Ethiopians, such as Kantiba Gabru and Nagadras Zewgé, speculated as to whether the infection had been caused by the use of poison gas during the European war, while Dr. Jacob Zervos, a Greek physician in the city, described the disease to Abel as "like a sort of bubonic plague." The Austrian, recalling this description half a century later, comments, "naturally if you hear the word plague you get frightened. I was terribly frightened."

The foreign diplomats were also appaled by the situation. Count Colli telegraphed to the governor of Eritrea, on November 16, that the outbreak was "very extensive" in the capital where there had been "most numerous" deaths, many of them Europeans, and that no less than sixty of the Italian legation's Ethiopian staff had perished. Campbell, who believed that this phase of the epidemic opened on November 14, observed three days later:

> With the suddenness approaching that of a volcano the epidemic was upon us. On November 13th we were all proceeding with our work as usual; from November 14th onwards the Gebbi was closed and the Government ceased to exist. Chiefs were either fleeing or hiding in their houses, postal and telegraphic services were suspended, the town was deserted save for funeral parties by day and . . . thieves by

> night . . . the Legations had to give up work and set to tending the sick and dying among their communities.

Though emphasizing that the epidemic was "serious," Campbell was still fairly confident, for he observed on November 17 that though "several Indians" were dying, Europeans were "not seriously affected" if they took "proper precautions." He was nevertheless careful to advise his minister, Wilfred Thesiger, then on leave, not to return to Addis Ababa until the illness had abated, for there was "every danger" at Aden and Jibuti. On the following day he telegraphed a further warning against Thesiger's coming, and declared:

> Influenza epidemic widespread especially along railway. Incubation only 24 hours and immediate precautions are essential, otherwise results fatal. On railway precautions are impossible. All work here suspended.

The seriousness of the situation led to the rumor, reported by Colli, that Empress Zawditu was about to abandon the capital and move to Ankobar. In the same message he stated that the minister of war, Fitawrari Habta Giyorgis, was severely ill and on November 27 warned that "his death would have political consequences of some gravity."

The disease meanwhile continued to advance, in Alaqa Kenfa's words, "like a forest fire" which "never seemed to stop. Many houses were completely closed because the owners and families were dead," and "people took communion and were reconciled with their enemies without the need of intermediaries" for there was no knowing how long anyone would remain alive. The epidemic, he claimed, killed almost without distinction, for its victims included "newly married couples and those betrothed, foreigners, doctors, Arabs, camel drivers and slaves." The Swedish missionary Cederqvist drew a similar picture. Declaring that the epidemic "swept across the whole country like a ruinous brush," he observed that it took with it "both old and young, educated and uneducated in thousands." Charles Rey, a subsequent British visitor, recalls that Ethiopia at this time "suffered perhaps more than its share" of the "virulent illness," and that "victims in Addis Ababa died like flies."

The political situation in the disease-ridden capital was, in the British legation's opinion, still critical, for the regent, Campbell reported on November 17, was still "in danger," though the presence of his cousin, Ras Kassa Haylu, provided the assurance that in the event of Tafari's death "revolution may be prevented." Ras Kassa, however, himself soon contracted the disease, whereupon he immediately asked the Italian envoy for a carriage to take him back to his country of Salalé. He wished, as Aleqa Kenfa puts it, "to die in his own home." The Ras was thereupon given a cart constructed by an Italian telegraphist called Bertolani which transported him over the flat land, but on rough terrain was obliged to travel on muleback.

The climax of the epidemic, according to contemporary opinion, came a week or so later, after the feast of Hedar Mika'él, on November 22, when, as Alaqa Kenfa stated, "many more" people died, and

> The epidemic was accepted as a relative. . . . It afflicted whole families. As a group of drunkards laugh when they fall together, trying to pull each other in different directions, so were neighbours afflicted when they visited each other.

A particularly serious aspect of the epidemic noticed by Cederqvist was that it swept away many priests and educated people, as a result of which the people's natural leaders were decimated, and it was "not easy to get any help."

The death toll in this final phase included a number of notables. Kantiba Wasané, the chief earlier appointed to control the metropolis, died on November 27, as recorded on his impressive grave at Sellasé church. Ato Gezaw, a Catholic intellectual whom the regent had entrusted with translating the French civil code, passed away on November 30, before completing this work. Other prominent Ethiopians who succumbed included Dajazmach Abreha Araya, a nephew of Emperor Yohannes and sometime governor of Tegré, who had been imprisoned in Salalé until 15 days before his death, and Alaqa Walda Giyorgis, the former father confessor of King Takla Haymanot of Gojjam and high priest at St. George's Church in Addis Ababa, whose church's desire not to be excluded from the burial of victims may have been his undoing. Among others dying of the disease were two of the small band of modern educated Ethiopian women: Ayahelush, wife of the intellectual Mika'él Beru of Walqayt, and her daughter, Asagadach Mika'él.

Several prominent foreigners also perished. They included Dr. Le Pape, one of the physicans treating the regent only a few months earlier, who passed away on November 26, the fourth member of the profession to die in the Addis Ababa holocaust; a Frenchman, Gabriel Vorrières of the prospecting firm of Achille Bayart, who died on November 20 or 22; and an Austrian merchant, Oskar Reich, who died on November 25. The extent of the epidemic was recognized four days later by Campbell who reported that the outbreak was "widespread and virulent," and that "mortality among all classes" was "disquieting." Though the British legation staff and families were "not seriously affected as yet" he noted that no less than 50 of their "native servants" were ill. Later, on December 2, he reported that Dodds had seen the regent on the previous days, and that the latter had agreed that Abyssinia was "finished."

One of the few clinical accounts of the epidemic is afforded by Campbell, who remarked that the symptoms were

> . . . very similar to those obtaining in other parts of the world; viz. fever, headache, sore throat, cough, pains in the back. . . . patients who took the immediate precaution of going to bed and staying there . . . generally reached a stage of convalescence characterised by considerable weakness and depression within a

week to ten days. Those who did not take precautions quickly developed pneumonia and in nearly every case terminated fatally.

Alaqa Kenfa states that the majority of victims "used to cough, and if they had no phlegm spat out whatever they could find in their mouth. They had no appetite. . . . Those who could spit out their phlegm were cured." Abel, who himself had a mild attack, recalled over fifty years later:

> The symptoms I remember very well. You had difficulty to breathe, and terrible headache, and stomach trouble, and you were quite stiff, and had a temperature. I had a very hot head. . . . I had no appetite. I did not feel very ill. I just felt *abattu*— just tired, and I wanted to lie down, but the trouble was if you were lying down your heart was beating very fast.

The epidemic from the outset placed an impossible burden on the capital's meager medical resources. Abel recalled there were "very few doctors in Addis Ababa in those days"—no more than eight by the present writer's computation, far too few to treat ordinary cases of illness, let alone an outbreak of epidemic proportions. The handful of medical men proved unable to cope with the calamity. Most, Rey subsequently claimed, "worked day and night most valiantly fighting the disease," but, as already noted, no less than four, Chaiban, Devletian, Wakeman and Le Pape, succumbed to the fatal virus. The good Swedish missionary Cederqvist, shocked by this mortality, sadly exclaimed, "what surprised thinking persons was that God first took the doctors. . . . and after that swept away the people." Avedis Terzian, an old-time Armenian resident, commenting on this half a century later, exclaimed, "the doctors, who didn't know the cure for the disease, couldn't even save themselves!" Two of the four surviving doctors were also incapacitated. The Greek Zervos was at Jibuti when the epidemic broke out, and, on returning to Addis Ababa, caught the disease on "the second day," as Campbell notes, and was "in his house ever since." His services, moreover, were limited, for he "considered it his duty to attend Europeans first and Indians and Abyssinians afterwards." A sixth physician, Dr. Landau, a Pole, was, according to Abel, completely demoralized by the epidemic and "disappeared" at an early stage. "Dr. Landau," he recalled, "was my neighbour and had an Austrian, Oskar Reich, staying at his house. . . . When he died," on November 25, "Dr. Landau closed his door, and didn't want to see anyone." By the latter stages of the epidemic most of the medical profession were thus either dead or had ceased to function.

Only two doctors in fact served the people of Addis Ababa throughout the epidemic. They were Dr. d'Antoine de Bosas, a Frenchman, who contracted the disease, and Dr. Hamid Nia, an Indian. Both did signal service. D'Antoine, Campbell later reported, was "so overwhelmed with work that his breakdown was expected daily," but "he stuck nobly to his task throughout the epidemic, although suffering part of the time from cough and headache and thus risking his life as he well knew." His devotion late won the commendation of the British minister, Thesiger, who wrote that

> even when suffering himself . . . he refused to give in and continued his work, although, as a doctor, he was fully conscious of the risk he ran. Even when most overworked, Dr d'Antoine never failed to respond to applications for advice or assistance . . . his work throughout was beyond praise.

Aid to the sick was also afforded by several other dedicated persons. One of the best remembered was the Swedish missionary Cederqvist, who, Mérab says, "combined the functions of doctor of the body with those of a doctor of the mind." He "went about from hut to hut," Friede Hylander records, and "did well and helped everybody." Another man to gain reputation for humanitarian service was Major Dodds of the British legation who devoted himself to the sick, particularly among the British Indian and Arab communities for whom he was responsible. He "did very notable work," Campbell notes, and was "indefatigable" in his "endeavours to alleviate suffering." Also highly spoken of was Mr. J.G. Mody, an Indian Parsee photographer, who, according to Mistry, looked after the sick among his fellow Indians, as well as Greeks and others. Mody's dedication was confirmed by Thesiger who states that "on his own initiative and moved entirely by a conscientious sense of duty" he "took upon himself the work of caring for such of his fellow countrymen who were ill and devoted himself wholeheartedly to his self-imposed task." His service was later recognized by the British Indian government which awarded him the title of Khan Saheb.

Though this handful of dedicated persons did valiant service, mainly for the foreign community, Colli telegraphed significantly, on November 27, that it was possible to do "almost nothing for the native population."

Treatment was also gravely handicapped by dearth of medical supplies. Addis Ababa then possessed only one hospital, the Menilek II, and no more than two or three pharmacies. The latter, like other shops, closed down early in the epidemic. Abel, who remembered the near impossibility of obtaining medicines, declared:

> The pharmacies were closed. I remember very well I sent a messenger to 'Doctor' Zahn (proprietor of the principal pharmacy) who was a friend of mine, and asked him if he could not get me a few aspirins, at least for myself and my household. (In those days people had enormous households—perhaps even fifteen people.) He did not even reply. His was the best pharmacy: you could get everything at his place, but he closed down when the epidemic broke out, and one could not get hold of him.

The result of the closure of pharmacies, Abel concludes, was that there was "no medicine, no aspirin, absolutely nothing."

Even the foreign legations suffered from a lack of medical supplies. The British legation, according to Campbell, was "very short" though it succeeded in obtaining a small amount of "asprin," pyramidon and eucalyptus oil in the town. Writing as one of those attempting to provide relief at the legation, he declared: "Once anyone got seriously ill we were done, and so was he poor beggar." The shortage of supplies is corroborated by Thesiger who later observed that "the necessary medicines gave out" and that "for some time only ill-adapted substitutes were available." It should be pointed out, however, that, in this era—before the advent to antibiotics—drugs even if available would not have been very efficacious, for, as the Royal College of Physicians in London observed, no medicine then invented had "proved to have any specific curative effect" against the dreaded disease.

For lack of medicines many who could afford to do so had recourse to spirits, a dubious form of treatment in that the Royal College of Physicians warned that "alcoholic excess invites disaster." Wayzero Zanabach, an elderly woman of Tegulat, recalled that *araqi* was drunk, supposedly as a medicine, and Campbell stated that at the British legation "the doctor ordered spirits as a tonic for the servants who were ill and as a preventative for those who were working," while for the British he ordered wine which then cost no less than seven Maria Theresa thalers a bottle. The widespread drinking of alcohol was confirmed by Abel, who recalled:

> I was drinking a lot of whiskey because Dr. Zervos was a friend of mine and I sent a message to him, and he actually came to my place on a mule, and he said, "Well, I have no medicine. I can't help you; the only thing is to drink whiskey or cognac."

Musing on his own illness, he added:

> We did not know what to do. The doctor said you should drink whiskey or cognac, and eat what you liked as long as you had an appetite, but that probably you would have no appetite.

The use of alcohol as medicine is corroborated by Terzian, but Abel stated that supplies of it were soon exhausted.

Another popular medicine mentioned by several informants, among them the Armenian, was the leaves of the eucalyptus trees which Menilek had introduced to the Ethiopian capital a generation or so earlier. These leaves were boiled in water and used as a disinfectant. Mention is also made of the eating of garlic which was reputed to have prophylactic powers.

Many people, as we have seen, reacted to the epidemic by shutting themselves in their houses or by fleeing from the areas thought to be worse infected. At the palace, Empress Zawditu tried to cut herself off from her subjects as far as possible. Campbell reports that "from November 14 onwards the Ghebi was closed," while Alaqa Kenfa agrees that "nobody could go in or out," and that Zawditu herself never left her residence. This isolation continued well into December, for the British envoy reported on the eleventh that though the epidemic "had by then abated" the palace gates had "not yet been reopened." The regent, as already mentioned, also isolated himself.

According to Alaqa Kenfa he did not venture out of his palace. Campbell confirms that he had "shut himself and his men up in the Ghebi and was not even told who was ill or dead as it might worry him" and "no one except the doctor was allowed in or out." Ras Kassa followed a similar policy and "shut himself up" in his house in the capital before leaving for his fief.

While the empress, the regent, and others remained in the capital in isolation, Campbell noted, others, including "many chiefs," followed the *abun*'s example by fleeing the town. Some of these refugees, the British envoy noted on November 17, traveled along the railway, thus, he believed, "spreading the infection" all along the line into Ogaden. The futility of such flights was noticed by Cederqvist who reported that many people sought refuge at Dire Dawa and Jibuti only to fall victim to the disease there. Those fleeing by railway included many Indians, who, Campbell said, left "in panic," as well as a considerable number of Armenians, who, Terzian recorded, made their way to Aqaqi, though "this did not help them" as the epidemic caught up with them there.

The uselessness of flight from the seemingly omnipresent epidemic led to the composition of a *qené*, or poem, in Ge'ez based on Pslam 129:7–8:

> Whither shall I go from thy spirit? Or whither shall I flee from thy presence?
> If I ascend up into heaven thou art there: if I make my bed in hell, behold, thou art there.

The *qené* declared:

> Where can we go from your spirit, full of fear.
> And where can we flee from your face, O Creator, death?
> We cannot go up to the heights,
> We cannot go down to the lowlands,
> For there is the plague.

One of the consequences of the epidemic was that Addis Ababa in the last months of 1918 was deserted by a large proportion of its inhabitants. Campbell observed: "Of all the numerous officials and chiefs, so conspicuous in normal times, only one remained at his post, namely Ato Heroui of the Municipality. He had very little authority and could not do much unaided." Administration, consequently, was virtually suspended. Colli telegraphed on November 27 that the gravity of the situation had been enhanced by the "ignoble carelessless of the Government and chiefs, who, seized by panic, had shut themselves up in their houses or abandoned the city." Three days later, on November 30, the British legation starkly wired, "Abyssinian Govt. utterly disorganised as a result of influenza epidemic."

Administrative chaos was by then so great that the Italian minister communicated to his government, as Campbell reported on December 6, that it was "no longer possible to regard Abyssinian Government as a serious organisation with which the Powers can satisfactorily treat." Recalling the

Tripartite Treaty of 1906 which had partitioned the country into three spheres of influence, Colli went so far as to propose that the three Powers should "discuss effective and prompt method of imposing their will." He had suggested that the regent should be used as a "figure-head who can be led but cannot direct." Failing this the Italian minister requested to be recalled. Campbell for his part commented, "I fully share his disgust at complete collapse of this Government."

Addis Ababa meanwhile was also abandoned by many of its poorer inhabitants, as was recorded by Thesiger, who remarked, "after the first few days the labouring classes fled from the town." The peasantry in the surrounding countryside moreover ceased to come to the capital to bring cattle, grain or other provisions. Campbell observed that consequently the price of grain "became prohibitive" while Terzian later remarked:

> The whole town was dead. Shops were closed, some of them even without a lock. . . . The market was dead. Nobody came to town; there were no Gallas or farmers bringing in supplies. It looked like a dead city. Everyone was isolated.

Abel likewise recalled:

> There was no shopping, everything was closed. There was no bread after a few days, and I remember I was eating *enjara*—the servants always had enough *tef* at home—but you couldn't get any vegetables or butter. The shops were all closed—so of course was the bank. . . . The peasants did not bring in supplies from the countryside because they were afraid, so we couldn't get any vegetables or milk.

Social life was similarly disrupted. Alaqa Kenfa observed that "people became strangers to one another," while Abel, recalling that he "must have stayed at home at least two or three weeks without leaving the house," declared:

> We were in a state of desperation. You couldn't visit friends. You couldn't get a mule or horse because your servants also were ill, or were afraid of being ill. There was a real panic. . . . Social life came to an end completely, absolutely.

Emphasizing the apathy which characterized his own household, he continued:

> The servants were all demoralized, they refused to do anything, they were all lying down. Some perhaps ill, but others were afraid, demoralized, thinking, "We must all die, all of us we shall die, what's the use of doing anything. I'll just lie down until death comes."

A kind of paralysis thus gripped the capital. The telegraph, Campbell reported on November 28, had been "suspended," and the operation of the railway was "likely to cease owing to illness of employees." The courts of law and police likewise no longer functioned. Alaqa Kenfa remarked that "there was no justice in those days," while Terzian observed that the police, hitherto stationed around the market, "ceased to be operative." The disintegration of the police, according to Campbell, led to a breakdown of public security.

Looting took place every night "as there were no policemen" and "the thieves, emboldened by the knowledge that all the police were ill, committed in all some 25 robberies, and the owners, ill in bed, were helpless as experience had shown that they ran the risk of pneumonia and death if they went out into the night to defend their property."

Mortality in Addis Ababa at the height of the epidemic reached considerable proportions. Alaqa Kenfa stated that one hundred or "at least seventy or sixty" persons were buried at each church every day (as well as smaller numbers at the remoter churches), while Campbell declared that "at one Church alone from 100 to 150 were buried daily and there are ten or more other Churches." Colli reported on November 27 that the town was "decimated," with the death rate running at four hundred a day. Further evidence on the extent of the epidemic was afforded by Campbell, who reported that "the greater part of the European, Indian and Arab communities were laid low," and that the death toll by December 2 included "about 30 Indians and Arabs," besides "I suppose 15 to 20 Europeans." Turning to the much more serious impact on the Ethiopian population he declared that at the British legation "practically all the servants fell ill and were totally incapacitated from work." Many "dropped like flies." No less than ten out of seventy servants died, but he and his compatriots were "proud of this" as the Italian legation had suffered thirty deaths. (Colli himself, it will be recalled, actually reported 60.) Mortality may have been greatest among young persons, perhaps because they had built up less immunity, for Alaqa Kenfa remarked that the disease "did not kill many old men or women."

Burial was a major problem throughout the epidemic and became increasingly acute as mortality rose. A major difficulty, noted by Thesiger, was that as a result of the flight of the "labouring classes no one was available to dig the graves." Alaqa Kenfa, confirming that "there was no one to bury the dead," remarked that the number of people to be interred was so great that the Muslims would transport two or three corpses at a time by camel for burial, while the Christians for lack of carriers would take their dead by mule or donkey. Several corpses would often be packed into a single hearse, with the result that sometimes while the grave-diggers were at work the hearse would split open, thus attracting the vultures which filled the sky. The story was told of a man who dug a grave by himself only to find, on returning with the body he had intended to bury, that someone else had been hastily interred in the hole. "There was no weeping and mourning," Alaqa Kenfa commented, "for even to find a grave was an achievement." Corpses in many cases were left unburied for as much as four days while others were allowed to rot in their houses. Because "people could not bury their dead, the dogs and vultures ate the corpses by day, and the hyenas did so by night." Such statements are corroborated by Colli, who telegraphed on November 27 that the dead were abandoned in their houses and along the roads, and by Thesiger, who recalled that "even the pretence of burial ceased and in many cases the dead were frequently left in the deserted tukuls or thrown out in the ditches to the mercy of the dogs and hyenas, thus polluting both air and water."

Acts of individual kindness, however, were also reported. Alaqa Kenfa recorded that when a mother carrying her dead child on her back reached the churchyard and cried for help, some people who had gone there to inter one of their own relatives dug a grave for her and helped her bury her dear one.

Burial problems were likewise recalled by Abel, who was then living just south of the market, and observed:

> There were deaths every day and in the morning one heard people call "Guragé, Guragé"—now they would say, "Coolie, coolie"—to bury their dead. This means that every morning there were people to be buried. It was difficult to find coolies; funerals were quite a problem. There were no coolies to dig properly, and people were buried near the surface; naturally everyone was afraid there would be cholera. It was a great problem to bury people.

The demand for coffins was so immense that the local carpenters, mainly Greeks, who were no doubt themselves short of labor, took advantage of the situation, according to British reports, to charge as much as 500 Maria Theresa thalers for the "simplest coffins"—an immense sum for those days.

Burials were carried out with scarcely any ceremony, as Cederqvist recorded. Abel, also recalling this fact, reported that burials were no longer conducted with reverence for the deceased, for people "just wanted to get rid of their dead. . . . they wanted to get them away because they were thought to be a source of infection." Remembering the death of his colleague and neighbor Oskar Reich, he continued:

> . . . we were so apathetic that although he was a great friend of mine and my compatriot I did not go to his funeral. There were no funerals. People were just thrown on a sort of *alga*, and brought to Giyorgis, not to Gulalé—that was out of the question. Giyorgis was the nearest cemetery, and people were buried there. . . . Sometimes people had to lie twenty-four hours or more at the place where they died.

The difficulty of carrying out burials was confirmed by Terzian, who observed that in the case of the Armenian community there were only two able-bodied men not affected by the disease—Kourken Pogharian and Hrant Krikorian—and they assumed the responsibility of burying their compatriots.

Inadequate burials, which created a considerable health hazard, continued to cause much concern among foreign diplomats. Campbell, reporting on "the insanitary method of burial" whereby bodies of victims dying in October and November were "placed a few inches under the surface and on the top of the corpses of those who had died during the August epidemic," commented:

> This happened in the churchyards in the most populous parts of the town and especially in that at the head of the market-place where dogs were seen rooting up and devouring portions of bodies. Furthermore these churchyards being close to

the streams and sources from which come the main water supplies of the town, a great risk was being incurred of the water becoming contaminated and causing a further and far more serious epidemic.

Campbell stated that he enlisted the sympathy of his diplomatic colleagues in this "urgent matter." Colli, who was doyen of the diplomatic corps, accordingly visited the regent, "from whom all tidings had been kept," and "rated him soundly." The Italian "asked for a chief to be placed in charge of the town with whom the legations could deal, and for responsible officers to be appointed to each cemetery to see that graves were properly dug and that lime was transported and used as occasion demanded." The regent "expressed his inability" to deal with the situation "as he had no chiefs to carry out his orders," but "offered to see what could be done." Subsequently "an ex-Russian Officer employed in the Public Works Department came forward and had lime transported to two out of the twelve cemeteries." Dr. d'Antoine de Bosas, according to his compatriot Stévenin, also supervised burial procedures, while the graves, Campbell stated, were "dug deeper." (The present writer, on inspecting Addis Ababa graveyards of that period, was informed at Sellasé church that the area in which the dead were buried extended far beyond the precincts of the present churchyards and that much use was made of lime.)

Campbell, however, was still not satisfied, for he complained, on December 11, that the lime was "even now . . . only sprinkled on the outside of the graves," and added, "we are just trusting the climate and altitude to preserve us from plague, cholera and other evils." Emphasizing the seriousness of the matter he remarked with trepidation: "it remains to be seen whether we are in time. If not, it means everyone leaving Addis Ababa and finding a new capital."

In the absence of statistics, the total number of persons who died of the epidemic in Addis Ababa must be a matter of speculation. Campbell, writing on December 11, put the number at "from 4,000 to 5,000," while Thesiger on December 31 quoted an estimated "ten thousand" out of "a total population of fifty thousand." The figure of ten thousand was subsequently accepted as a modest estimate. Alaqa Kenfa stated that mortality in fact exceeded that amount, while the regent later wrote that "more than ten thousand people died."

The deadly epidemic soon spread to most parts of the country. As in the capital there were many places, Stévenin stated, where the survivors were unable to bury all the dead, many corpses being left to the hyenas and jackals. The northern provinces were badly affected. Colli reported on November 27 that the disease was "spreading northwards." Tegré was soon seriously affected. The manner in which the disease may have reached Adwa was suggested to the present writer over half a century later by Dr. Harold Nystrom, an old Swedish physician who was there in his youth, and is convinced that this *gunfan*, or influenza, "definitely came from the south" around the middle of December. He believes that a certain Lej Tassaw, sent from Addis Ababa to supervise the local telegraph, arrived with the infection. "I remember," stated Nystrom, "he came to our house, and said he was not feeling well." He died of influenza a few days later, after which the epidemic "spread like anything in Adwa, Maqalé and Aksum, especially Aksum where it was very bad because it was not a clean town." Many people, he explained, considered the disease a punishment from God. Reiterating his own belief that the infection had come from the south he stated, "News came from Addis warning people that there was a *basheta*" or illness "coming all over the country." The people, he adds, knew the disease had originated abroad, for they said, "*kawuch agar matta*" (i.e., "it came from outside"). The incidence of infection in Adwa was also high, as Nystrom knew from personal recollection. Talking of the days before Christmas 1918, he observed:

> We were a family of seven: five children and my parents, and they fell ill, all of them except me; my sister and I were up nursing the others, but then my sister fell sick also, so I was alone. I never got it.

Recalling that he "seldom got colds," and probably enjoyed some kind of immunity, Nystrom declared, "many people in the town died. . . . Christmas 1918 at Adwa was not merry at all." The general feeling in the town, however, was that the epidemic was not as acute as in Addis Ababa. "What we heard about Addis," he recalled, "was something terrible. They said they were dying like anything in Addis. When they talked about Addis, they said, '*hullu hullu saw alqwal*,' 'everyone, everyone is finished' ". Nevertheless, mortality in Adwa was by no means negligible; Nystrom guessed that it amounted to perhaps 100 or 200 in a population of 5,00 or 6,000.

The principal medicament employed in Adwa, according to the Swede, was, as elsewhere, the leaves of the eucalyptus tree which was learned of from Addis Ababa. It was, he explained, popularly held to be the "only *madhanit*," or medicine, "that was effective." The leaves were taken from trees which had been planted some years earlier in the former garden of Emperor Yohannes, the sole place in the city where they were to be found. The most common practice was to put the leaves on the fire to disinfect the house with the fumes; some, however, boiled the leaves to make an infusion which they could drink. Nystrom's father, a missionary doctor, had no medicines with which to treat the epidemic but gave his approval to this use of eucalyptus.

The epidemic apparently reached the Italian colony of Eritrea towards the end of the year. The governor, De Martino, reported on December 7 that the epidemic, though "widespread," was "mild" and not of the Spanish variety, but this soon proved an over-optimistic opinion. The records of the Swedish Evangelical Church at Belesa, the only mortuary figures available, show that the number of deaths among this small community from all sources rose from one in November to six in December, four in January 1919, and six in February. A Swedish Protestant missionary, J. Iwarson, reported from Asmara on December 31 that conditions at Christmas had been "unusually serious." Three members of his community had died and urgently needed burial, while fifty more were ill and just as urgently needed care. He added that he had only one boy and a servant not affected by the disease. Iwarson hilmself fell sick on the following day. In a letter of January 30 he observed:

> . . . just about the New Year an epidemic of influenza started at our highland stations. Those who were not themselves affected by it had to devote their time to take care of others. I myself had to go to bed on New Year's Day, but I recovered so much after ten days that I was able to get up. Pastor Svensson was ill, but he is better. In Asmara there were some 50 sick within the community, so the Iwarsons were very busy.

In a subsequent report Iwarson declared that distress was very great, and that many people had dropped dead in the market to which they had gone in quest of bread. Mortality had been so extensive that there were numerous unsupported widows and orphans. The Italian government and the missionaries had both attempted to dispense charity, but the relief they could offer was insufficient to meet the need—the more so as destitute persons in a constant stream were flocking to Asmara in search of aid. Many were the cries of *meskin* (literally, "destitute", a term used in begging) and *Maryam Maryam tehabkum* (i.e., "May Mary give it to you!").

The epidemic continued in the Asmara area throughout January 1919. Another Swedish missionary, Nils Nilson, who had also been in bed with influenza on New Year's Day, reported on January 13 that "many of the local people have died." Among the small Protestant community one family had lost father and mother within a month. The latest victims had come from the family of a certain Haylamika'él Kidan, all of whose members had caught the disease. The six-year-old son Menasé had died on New Year's Eve, Haylamika'él himself on New Year's Day, and his sixteen-year-old daughter Astér four days later. The epidemic continued throughout the month, and Iwarson stated on January 30 that the illness was "still active" among the population of Asmara and appeared to be "coming back" among the Protestant community.

Neighboring parts of Ethiopia were similarly affected in the Spring of 1919. On February 8 De Martino reported that the infection had "spread widely in Wallo and other regions of the north, including Tegré," though the disease there was "generally" of a "mild character."

The epidemic spread to western Eritrea, which in the autumn of 1918 had been suffering from a harvest failure. A Swedish missionary, K. Rodén, reported on December 2 that influenza had broken out, as a result of which the Italian authorities had prohibited groups of people from assembling. This prevented the missionaries' school at Galab from opening and on January 10, 1919, it was still closed.

The epidemic also led to high mortality in the southern and western provinces. Cederqvist, writing of the south, stated that many landlords ordered the peasants to bury their dead but the people "were very much afraid of the sickness and did not dare to enter the huts in which there were dead bodies. They therefore pulled the huts down from the outside, and covered both the dead and the wood of the houses with soil and stones." The slave trade was likewise affected. Charles Hobley, a British provincial commissioner in Kenya, claimed that the epidemic "swept off many thousands of slaves," and led to a decline in slave-raiding in the frontier zone between Ethiopia, the Sudan, Uganda, and Kenya.

The disease also created ravages in the far west where towards the end of 1918 Dajazmatch Beru, one of the chiefs near the Sudan frontier, appealed for help from a British official at Gambela. The official, knowing of the presence of an American Protestant missionary, Dr. Tom Lambie, at Nasser, several days' journey down the Sobat river in the Sudan, telegraphed requesting his assistance. Lambie duly opened a hospital at Sayo, or Dambidolo, in Walaga province, but later transferred his activities to Addis Ababa where, as we shall see, he established a mission hospital.

In the east of the country mortality was also high. From Dire Dawa, according to Campbell, the infection swept up to Harar which, by December 11, was "suffering," and then spread "throughout the provinces" of the east, though it was not as "malignant" there as in the capital. De Martino nevertheless reported on February 8 that the disease had extended into the Dankali lowlands where the death rate was "somewhat higher" than in the north. Léon Erzingatzian, an Armenian merchant living in Addis Ababa, told the present writer that at Dire Dawa people of all nationalities brewed or burned leaves of eucalyptus trees obtained from Harar and around Aramaya.

In the Somali area the disease continued to rage with intensity. The British commissioner and commander in chief, G.F. Archer, reported on December 6, 1918, that the 5th Light Infantry, no less than 370 men, had suffered 41 deaths at Berbera and Las Kherai, while the Somali Camel Corps had lost nine more men. Mortality among the handful of British officers was "nil," but it was estimated that there had been "1,000 deaths" among the Somalis "during the last 14 days," though "everything possible had been done by the inadequate medical staff."

The British in Somaliland at this time believed that the epidemic would make its way throughout the Somali region. Whitehead, the senior medical officer, observed that there was "little doubt" that the disease would "reach the Mullah's dervish followers (if it has not already done so) when we may hear rumours of 'plague' or 'cholera' amongst them." The ensuing medical history is obscure, but it should be noted that the mullah, Muhammad Abdullah Hassan, died of some kind of fever, generally assumed to have been influenza, a couple of years later, the date of his death being variously reported as November 23 or December 2, 1920, or January 5, 1921.

The terrible plague which had wrought such destruction throughout the land burned itself out with almost miraculous rapidity. Alaqa Kenfa, who attributed this to supernatural intervention, claimed that the acute mortality ended on the feast of St. Mary, Hedar 21 (November 29). Four days later, Colli telegraphed that the disease showed a tendency towards being attenuated; a week afterwards, on December 10, Campbell wired "epidemic of influenza abating," adding officiously that the "Abyssinian Government" was still "completely disorganised and incapable of attendance to official business at present."

The rapidity with which the epidemic came to an end is attested by the meagre statistics available. Jibuti records show that the number of foreigners and military personnel dying from all causes dropped from nine in December 1918 to three in January and two in February 1919. Roman Catholic burials in Dire Dawa likewise fell from eight in November and four in December 1918 to only one in January 1919. In Addis Ababa the Catholic and Greek churches, which in November had registered twenty-six and ten deaths respectively. reported none in the next two months. One of the last identified persons to die of the infection was an Armenian, Mennous Savadjian, who passed away on December 1. Two days later Mrs. Thesiger, wife of the British minister, telegraphed from the Ethiopian capital to Sir Reginald Wingate, governor of the Anglo-Egyptian Sudan, requesting him to "implore" her husband not to continue his journey to Ethiopia where the influenza was "widespread and very severe," but on the very next day she wired that the epidemic was "abating." The epidemic was in fact almost certainly over a little before the end of Hedar, probably on or about December 9, the date given for its ending in Hayla Sellasé's autobiography.

The relatively sudden ending of the epidemic left a deep impression. Alaqa Kenfa claimed that "Our Lady intervened, and all the patients recovered. The power of the disease decreased, and the death of one man after that date was equal to the death of eleven before then." The dramatic ending of the plague was later recalled by Abel, who stated that late in November "there were fewer cases" of the disease, and "people became more lively." He remembered particularly that:

> . . . one evening thee was terrific shooting all over Addis Ababa from about eight o'clock until midnight, and the people said they were shooting to disturb the evil spirits. . . . You wouldn't believe it, but the next morning the situation was much better. . . . The people thought they were shooting at the Devil.

Subsequently when people met each other they would express thanks to God that "I am still alive" and that "you have escaped."

The disease also passed away rapidly in the rest of the country. A British Somaliland report of January 4, 1919, stated that by then the epidemic had "almost abated at all stations," and on January 6 the British commissioner and commander in chief noted that it had "entirely abated." In Eritrea mortality among the Swedish evangelical community at Belesa likewise fell from six in

February 1919 to one in March, and no further deaths from any cause were reported in the next two months.

The great influenza epidemic, for all its virulence, was thus of short duration. By the end of the year in Addis Ababa, those patients who had not died were well on the way to recovery. Life in the capital—and in the country at large—began returning to normal fairly quickly. One of the most notable patients then recuperating was Abuna Matéwos, to whom the regent wrote on December 18, expressing his happiness that the ecclesiastic's health and that of his assistants was improving.

The process of postepidemic normalization of trade was described by Abel, who recalled how the shops gradually began to reopen:

> I remember my servants came and said you could get bread—that was perhaps three of four days after the shooting—and then vegetables came. It took about a week, perhaps a fortnight, until life become more or less normal, for the shops to open, until you could get aspirin, etc.

Fears for the future were still present, however, for, as Abel also recalled, "We were afraid of cholera because people had not been buried in a proper way." Soon afterwards, however, "the Municipality began reorganizing the graves," and that concern too receded into the past.

The miseries through which the country had passed seemed to have had a chastening effect on Ethiopian society. The regent wrote on December 14 to Haji Ahmad Abon, a land functionary in Harar, stating that even before the pestilence he had intended to exempt the Muslim population around the city from paying the grain tax of previous years, but that now, because of the people's "illness and stricken condition," he would not ask them to pay even for the current year. He requested the persons exempted to pray for him.

Memory of the evil days also had the incidental effect of fostering the growing public sentiment that marriage reform was needed. On December 22, Ras Tafari wrote to Abuna Matéwos, recalling that "differnt kinds of sins" had been practiced in Ethiopia, and that marriage regulations had been "completely disobeyed," even by the clergy, as a result of which "God after much toleration, started to bring all kinds of misery upon us, time and again. More than that God these days brought severe misery and consequently many people, children and the rest, are terrified and most probably it is the will of God to establish this question of marriage."

Though the great epidemic gradually came to an end, it bequeathed to the Amharic language the term *ya Hedar basheta* or "disease of Hedar." The formula seems to have become current within a year of the outbreak, for Nystrom claimed to have heard it used in Adwa before his departure from the town in October 1919. Though the epidemic was part of the world influenza outbreak, the word *Hedar basheta*, as we have seen, was later sometimes incorrectly associated with typhus. Thus the French lexicographer Baeteman translated the term as "influenza, typhus?" while Cerulli claimed that "illness

of November" was used in Shawa for "abdominal typhus." In more sophisti-
cated Ethiopian circles, on the other hand, it was fashionable to refer to the
epidemic by the French loan-word, "*grippe*," commonly rendered as *grip*
(e.g., in the writings of Blattengéta Heruy Walda Sellasé and later in Hayla
Sellasé's autobiography).

VII

Syphilis

Veneral diseases were probably the most important nonepidemic diseases in Ethiopia, not only because of their prevalence but also because of their effect on fertility.

Origins and Linguistic Data

The origins and early medical history of syphilis in Ethiopia cannot be established. Nineteenth-century popular belief, however, held that the disease was introduced into the northern provinces by the Portuguese after the wars of Ahmad Gragn in the sixteenth century and was later diffused by Arab merchants who traveled widely throughout the land. Some support for such theories can be found in the evidence of subsequent foreign observers. Arnauld d'Abbadie noted in the middle of the nineteenth century that old people in the north declared that syphilis had been "feared in their youth" and had made its appearance only "very recently, 50 or 80 years ago at most." Kirk likewise reported from Shawa in the 1840s that the disease had "only been known in southern Abyssinia during the last 40 years."

Linguistic data on syphilis is available for the last quarter of a millenium, and, though collected by persons with little medical understanding, is not without interest. It suggests firstly that, as elsewhere, the disease was believed to be related to smallpox, and secondly that it was considered to be of foreign origin.

Similarity between the two diseases, which in England led to the use of two related terms (*pox* and *smallpox*), had interesting though very different linguistic consequences in the Ethiopian languages. Within a century or so of its assumed importation, syphilis was referred to in northern Ethiopia by the word which served in the south of the country to denote smallpox, a disease known to have existed in the country since time immemorial. Though it is tempting to conclude that syphilis, the imported disease, was given the name earlier used for smallpox, the indigenous disease, this cannot actually be established on the data available.

Our first reference to syphilis in Ethiopia, from a period when popular belief regarded it as little more than a century or so old, appears in Ludolf's Ge'ez-Latin dictionary of 1699 which indicates that the disease was then referred to as *fantata*. The German scholar describes the complaint as "morbi maligni vel acuti genus" (i.e., "a serious or acute type of disease"). A variant of the term, as noted in the early nineteenth century by Pearce and Isenberg, was also used in Tigrinya, the language of northern Ethiopia, and the one closest to Ge'ez. In the Amharic-speaking areas to the south, on the other hand, the term *fantata* served to denote smallpox, as recorded by Isenberg and later by Dillmann, and early in the twentieth century by the Italian lexicographer Guidi.

Smallpox in Amharic, however, was also referred to as *kufagn*, a word listed in Ludolf's Amharic-Latin dictionary of 1698. The word was subsequently employed in an Amharic medical text belonging to King Walda Giyorgis Wassan Sagad of Shawa (died 1812), now in the British Library (Orient 828), which equated it with *fantata* in the latter's Amharic meaning of smallpox, for the text expressly declares, "*kufagn fantata naw*" (i.e., "*kufagn* is *fantata*"). The ambiguity resulting from the use of the same word in different parts of the country for two completely distinct diseases seems to have led to the adoption —perhaps in the late eighteenth or early nineteenth century, the period of the assumed expansion of syphilis into central Ethiopia—of new terms for venereal disease. Thus in Amharic, the term "*ya Adal fantata*" (i.e., "*fantata* of Adal," referring to the low-lying region east of Shawa) emerged. The word is found in a Ge'ez-Amharic grammar and vocabulary of this time and was subsequently also mentioned by Antoine d'Abbadie. The designation *Adal*, according to the latter, was taken to mean syphilis. Use of the name Adal suggests that the disease was thought to have reached Shawa from the east, presumably along the trade route from the coast. The term "Adal smallpox", however, was soon abandoned in favor of the more usual Amharic word *qitegn* which was already given in an eighteenth-century medical text in the British Library (Orient 11,390), as well as in the medical book of King Walda Giyorgis. The word was also cited subsequently by Pearce, Isenberg, d'Abbadie, and other lexicographers.

Notwithstanding the assumed late arrival of syphilis in the south of the country it is curious, and perhaps significant, that the word *fando*—the standard Oromo name for the disease—was already known to the informants of the German scholar Karl Tutschek who listed it in his dictionary of 1844.

Despite the abandonment of the name "Adal smallpox" the supposed alien origin of syphilis was still occasionally referred to in later times. Thus, according to Massaia, in the middle of the nineteenth century it was the practice in the south-west to speak of syphilis as the "Muslim disease," presumably because it was believed to have been introduced by Muslims, who were the principal merchants trading with foreign lands. Borelli likewise reported that he had been told by both Amharas and Oromos that the infection had been spread by the Arabs. A somewhat similar view was later expressed by Parisis, a Greek physician in the north of the country, who stated that syphilis was spoken of in Tigrinya as *habe farange*, or "European disease".

Though such appellations have long since disappeared, the two principal Semitic languages of Ethiopia still have different designations for syphilis. The relations between them, and the popularly assumed history of the disease, is well summed up by Kidana Wald Keflé, a traditional Ethiopian scholar, who remarked in a postwar Ge'ez dictionary, "The Tegreans when they wish to say *qitegn* say *fantata*; and the Amharas also call the *qitegn* by euphemism *fantata* . . . the *qitegn* comes from sexual relations, it is a disease of the sexual parts . . . The *qitegn* appeared at the time of Gragn. It is said that it was the Portuguese who brought it."

Prevalence of the Disease

Nineteenth-century travelers suggested that syphilis attained its highest incidence in the north of the country and was far less widespread in the south, where, we have seen, some felt it had only recently been introduced. In the 1840s, for example, Kirk declared, "The Gallas are still generally exempt from the scourage, but it is at length beginning to attack the tribes bordering on the Amhara districts." Two generations later, Soleillet claimed that the disease was common among the Amharas but rare among the Gallas, while Massaia stated that isolated Galla areas were free from infection, though large towns such as Jimma, which were frequented by traders, were badly affected. The worst areas in Shawa were similarly in the vicinity of the capital, trade centers, and army camps. At the end of the century Donaldson Smith likewise declared that though the disease was "rampant" in the north he had seen scarcely any evidence of it in the far south, except at Gumba where the population was much affected. A generation later Mérab agreed that syphilis was uncommon among the Gallas though gonorrhea was prevalent. Little syphilis was reported in other areas: Munzinger stated that it was "quite unknown" among the Dankalis, while Rabbi Nahoum later reported that the Falashas were "entirely free" from it.

Syphilis, which was widespread throughout the northern plateau, was often encountered in its most serious forms. Pearce remarked that the disease was "very common" in the north, where it resulted in the ruin of innumerable people, and Parkyns that it was more or less incurable by traditional means. The result, according to Rüppell, was that, for lack of adequate treatment, the disease was often met with in an advanced stage. Dr. Kirk stated that syphilis was also "exceedingly common" in Shawa where it committed "great ravages." It attacked "all ranks and all ages," from "the lowest beggar to the immediate relatives of the King" and "infancy and decrepited old age" both offered "frequent evidences of the disease." Both Courbon and the French scientific mission of the 1840s related that it was common, and visible in all known forms. A detailed breakdown of the varieties of sites of infection in a typical syphilitic population is given in the table below. In addition, 11 children were brought in suffering from syphilitic sores about the pudenda and nates.

Sites of infection in 305 syphilitic patients examined by Dr. Kirk at Ankobar between December 1, 1841, and March 20, 1842.

Form of Syphilis	Males	Females	Total
Primary	38	13	51
Affections of nose	40	31	71
Affections of throat and palate	30	21	51
Affections of throat and nose	21	28	49
Nodes	4	4	8
Syphilitic ulcers (secondary)	16	23	39
Cutaneous syphilitic affections	17	9	26
Syphilitic rheumatism	5	5	10
Total	171	134	305

The prevalence of syphilis is further evident from the observations of later writers. Blanc in the 1860s stated that 90% of the persons he treated in Bagémder suffered from the disease, and Cecchi that it was common in Shawa, where he had seen it even among girls not more than nine years old. Italian doctors in Eritrea told Bent in the 1890s that the incidence of syphilis among the Christian population was "appalling," while early in the twentieth century Hayes reported that it was "extremely common" around Lake Tana. Dr. Mérab later estimated that venereal disease was three times more widespread in Ethiopia than in Europe and accounted for 27% of his poorer patients, with an even higher incidence among the aristocracy. Subsequent observers, such as the Phelps-Stokes mission, Fan C. Dunckley, and Rey, agree that syphilis was common in Addis Ababa, while a Swedish doctor informed Harmsworth that it was responsible for 75% of his cases. Franz Pedar, a Hungarian physician in Harar, estimated that together with eye disease syphilis accounted for 90% of his casework, and Dr. Lanzoni, an Italian in Goré, recorded that it was "widespread in a startling manner among the better class, the poor, the townsfolk, and the country folk."

Attitudes to the Disease

Available evidence suggests that syphilis in Ethiopia bore no greater stigma than any other disease. Early in the nineteenth century Pearce asserted that it was "never kept secret," for, "as soon as it was discovered, those afflicted make it known to all their friends and neighbours, and thus it becomes public throughout the district in which they live; and every friend will pay a visit, and, if the disorder has fallen upon some man or woman of consequence, they will often meet upon a day appointed, and keep a cry at the house, as when a person dies." The British surgeon Charles Johnston likewise noted in the 1840s that syphilis was "admitted and spoken of without reluctance or shame." Superstitious persons claimed that it originated from such causes as eating diseased fowls or living in the neighbourhood of someone more than usually afflicted. Great care was taken, accordingly, when purchasing fowls in the market, to learn whence they came. The possibility of contagion was, however, also accepted, for it was held that the disease was "communicable by the simplest contact," so that "those who are suffering from it are . . . carefully avoided, except by their own relatives, and for years after they are quite cured, a reluctance to eat or drink with them, except with certain precautions, may be observed."

The above-mentioned attitudes to syphilis were deeply ingrained. Cecchi remarked that people would open declare, "I have syphilis," while early in the twentieth century Mérab recorded that a patient would "have no shame in calling himself syphilitic; it is for him, as it should be for us, a disease like any other." Emphasizing this point, he noted that he had known Ethiopians who would say, "It was the year of my syphilis," or "When I had my syphilis. . . . " Far from being embarrassed, an infected person would often show his sores to his friends, as it was felt that one had to confess one's illness before it could be cured, otherwise it would "remain in the body like a secret on the heart." Persons believing themselves infected would seek the advice of everyone, and would count opinions, but would not begin treatment until there were unmistakble signs of infection. Despite this lack of shame, persons affected with the disease were afraid of being shunned, though it was believed that this could be avoided if the infected person urinated in the hollow of his hand.

Traditional Treatment

A wide range of cures was used in the treatment of syphilis. One found in the Ge'ez and Amharic medical textbooks of the late eighteenth and early nineteenth centuries was based on inoculation, a practice well known, as we have seen, in relation to smallpox. This cure made use of the patient's pus and the juice of a plant called *toppya* (*Calotropis procera*), the bark of which was still employed in syphilis treatment in the twentieth century. An early prophylactic prescription read as follows:

> Having mixed the juice of *toppya* with barley flour you dry it on a cooking plate and grind it into powder. Then you knead it with the pus, and swallow three pieces as big as a thumb, and remain in the sun. This causes vomiting and strong diarrhoea. When you are exhausted the antidote is chicken. This treatment will bring about a cure before 40 days.

Inoculation for syphilis was also reported in the early twentieth century by Mérab, who spoke of a medicine consisting of "a mixture of the juice of plants and syphilitic pus."

Most of the oral medicines for syphilis, like the traditional European pharmacopeia in general, were drawn from the vegetable kingdom. Some of the most widely used were purges, in many cases in fact taenicides. "To cure this disease," related Pearce, "they take strong purgatives, bulbs, roots, herbs, flowers, and barks." The use of such medicines constitutes an interesting parallel with pre-Renaissance Europe, where, as the modern medical historian Castiglioni recalled, treatment of syphilis "at first consisted of purgatives."

Ethiopian medical textbooks, which are replete with prescriptions for the cure of syphilis, reveal the importance placed on such purgatives. Those preparations in most common use included the latex of the *qwolqual* or *quencheb* (*Euphorbia candelabrum*), the roots or leaves of the *makan endod* (*Phytalacca dodecandra*), the bark or seeds of the *besanna* (*Croton macrostachys*), the flowers of the *kosso* (*Hagenia abyssinica*), the roots of the *qachamo* (*Myrsine africana*), the *michamicho* (*Oxalis anthelmintica*), and the *endukduk* (*Euphorbia schimperi*).

The latex of the *qwolqwal* or *quencheb*, described by the Italian Cacciapuoti as a "drastic purgative," was mentioned in prescriptions of the late eighteenth and early nineteenth centuries. One of them declares: "Having extracted the latex of the *qwolqwal*, having clarified honey, and having mixed them together, when you take them with a spoon it is good."

The roots or leaves of the *makan endod*, which also served as a taenicide, were recommended "so that one does not contract syphilis through touching or sweat." An early twentieth-century prescription, which, like many others, contained an element of magic, stated that "seven young shoots should be put in a mortar laid on three stones, and pounded in a place far from the house where neither man nor animal can reach it," The same text further recommended:

> Make (the patient) drink it with the milk of a cow that has the same colour as her calf. Measure the milk by the digit of your small finger. Make him vomit, drinking *agwat* (butter milk). The liver of hen is its antidote. If he cannot bear it let him wash with cold water.

The bark, wood, and seeds of *besanna* were likewise widely used in the treatment of syphilis. Pearce referred to this plant as "a very strong purgative" and taenicide. Another early twentieth-century prescription, which claimed to be good for both syphilis and leprosy, stated:

> Gather the seeds of *besanna* in large quantities, and dry the kernels: mix them and bury them in the fire-place in a small pot. Bury it in a hole where no one can reach it. On the seventh day eat it measuring by spoon; not much. . . . Vomit, drinking butter

milk, or *tabla* (linseed oil) if you cannot find butter milk. The antidote is the liver of a chicken.

The flowers of the *kosso* tree, the most popular Ethiopian taenicide, likewise served, according to Pearce, for the treatment of syphilis. Almost a century later Mérab observed that it was still common practice to take this drug every other day for four or five months while Masucci, an Italian author, noted its use during the fascist occupation. Subsequently, after World War II, D. Lemordant of the Institut Pasteur in Addis Ababa confirmed that *kosso* and *besanna* were "associated . . . in the treatment of syphilis." A typical prescription recorded by Taye Haile, a student of the University College of Addis Ababa, reads as follows:

> Crush the bark of *besanna* together with *kosso*. Take one tablespoon of *besanna* powder and mix it with two tablespoons of *kosso*. Dissolve the powder in a glass of *talla*, or beer, prepared solely from barley. Then drink the solution. The germ comes out either by diarrhoea or vomiting.

Patients following such treatment often would be made to eat handfuls of *barbaré*, or red pepper.

Purgatives for syphilis were also frequently used by the Somalis. Burton in the early nineteenth century observed that such medicines included *senna*, the dried leaves of the *cassia*, and colocynth, or the dried pulp of a kind of cucumber.

Several other medicines for syphilis were taken orally. Perhaps the most popular was the root, bark, and wood of the *gatam* (*Heptapleuram abessinicum*), which was recommended in an early text that observed, "Chew the roots of *gatam*. If one lies with a woman infected with syphilis it does not touch one." A subsequent early twentieth-century prescription given by a *dabtara* (or lay cleric) at Entotto gave the following instructions as to how the root should be obtained and administered:

> Dig out the root of *gatam* to the depth of a *senzer* (or palm). Leaving the upper part, remove the bark of the lower part. Dry it, reduce it to powder, mix it with water. Let the patient drink it, and not spit it out.

The importance attached to *gatam* can further be seen from a text that gave the following directions: "Remove the bark using a knife with a handle made of olive wood. Pound the inside with a pestle and mortar. Dry and pound. Mix with *talla* (or beer), and let the person drink." The prescription added, somewhat optimistically: "Both males and females will be safe even if they touch the blood or have intercourse with a person with syphilis. If a baby is given this powder mixed with butter he will be immune from syphilis until old age." This prescription or a similar one was known to the twentieth-century Ethiopian intellectual Agegnew Engeda of Bagémder, who stated that the *gatam* bark constituted "an efficacious remedy." Introducing an element of magic into his account, Engeda stated that the bark had to be cut by a young boy who had to hold a knife with a horn handle in his left hand, and declare, "In this way remove the syphilis from so and so." He had to do this from a tree which could not be reached by cattle, for otherwise the remedy would be worthless. The bark had then to be dried and crushed with honey to form seven or nine balls, to be taken once daily.

Another widely used plant was the *qabarecho* (*Echinops*) which was also reputed to have magical value against thieving. An early prescription offered these instructions: "Having extracted its roots you weigh a *waqét* (or ounce) and boil it in seven cups until it becomes only two. Then you drink it, one cup at dawn, and one in the evening. Do this for forty days."

Other herbal cures include the roots of the *cheferg* (*Sida*), *gabar embay* (*Solanum*) and *yameder embay* (*Citrullus colacynthis*), the flowers of the *yameder kosso* (*Parochaetus communis*), and *wodel asfes* (*Vigna luteola*), the leaves of *azamer* (*Schmidelia africana*), the leaves and seeds of the *degetsa* (*Calpurnia subdecandra*), and various parts of the *amadmado* (*Chenopodium album*) and *waginos* or *ashkella* (*Brucea antidysenterica*).

Although most of the medicines taken internally for syphilis were herbal, two mineral substances, copper sulphate and sulphur, sometimes also were used. Copper sulphate, which was known as *kebra samay* and was probably imported, was referred to in a late eighteenth- or early nineteenth-century text that reads, "Drink *kebra samay* for three days. Having weighted 4 *waqéts* of *qabarecho* boil it in seven cups of water until it becomes only two. Drink one at dawn, and one in the evening." Sulphur was mentioned in an early twentieth-century text advising the patient to "buy large quantities of sulphur" which were to be boiled with water and butter and drunk for three days. Another nonherbal cure in common use among the Somalis was the fat of a sheep's tail melted down as a beverage.

Syphilis was also treated externally, often with medicines made from the same plants as used for oral medicine. These included the latex of the *qwolqwal* or *qencheb*, the leaves of the *gatam*, the root of the *cheferg*, the leaves of the *degetsa*, and the fruit of the *waginos*. A typical remedy using euphorbia recommended: "Having gathered the latex of *qencheb* in a pot, apply it each morning for three days while the sun dries the affected parts. On the third day, if there are still sores, dress them with cow's butter. It cures the syphilis." The use of *gatam* is also referred to in a later text which observes, "If he has sores dry the leaves, steem them in *nug* (or niger oil), boil it, and anoint the sores." Another passage, advising the use of *abalo* (or *waginos*), remarks, "Crush a fruit . . . shave the genital region, the eyebrows and the beard, and anoint one's whole body with this fruit and fresh butter."

Another much favored treatment was a maceration of the bark of the *enkoy* (*Ximenia americana*), the identity of which, according to Mérab was kept a "great secret." The medicine made from it was so highly rated that it was applied to the nose, ears, mouth, and genital organs before coitus, as if of prophylactic value. Syphilitic sores were also treated by sprinkling them with cold water freshly drawn from the wells, or, better still, from the river "before the bird had wetted its beak." Ulcers were often cut away with a razor or other sharp object and then cauterized with a hot iron. Among the Somalis, on the other hand, it was common practice, according to Burton, to "leave the patient all night in the dew."

Though most medicaments for external application, like those for internal use, came from the vegetable kingdom, several prescriptions recommended preparations containing iron slag or rust; one medicine was even made from a moth called *kolo*, the exact identity of which is obscure. Syphilitic ulcers were likewise washed with a solution of copper sulphate, while among the Somalis it was not uncommon to anoint the body with sulphur boiled in ghee, and expose it to the sun.

Another widespread practice, which went unmentioned in the Ethiopian medical texts, was the use of thermal baths. Early in the nineteenth century Kirk remarked that they were "held in high repute," and this was also confirmed, as we shall see, by other nineteenth-century observers. Such baths continued to be widely used in the twentieth century, as illustrated by an Amharic poem in which a prospective patient declares: "If I catch syphilis I will go down to Felwaha," (i.e., to the "boiling water" of the thermal springs). This cure would often be combined with other treatments. A patient thus might take *kosso* for four or five months before going to Felwaha, and invoke the great saint Abbo who lived in the monastery on the nearby mountain of Zeqwala. Alternatively, visits to the baths might be combined with a little magic: many patients would complete their cure with the sacrifice of a young goat, which would then be consumed to the accompaniment of certain exorcisms.

In the Matamma area near the Sudan frontier use was also made of "a sort of whitish-coloured earth" called *toureyba*, which, according to the Sudanese medical historian Dr. Ahmad Bayoumi, contained iodide of mercury and was "either taken orally in water or applied dry to the ulcers." Mercury, it should be recalled, was also recognized in other parts of the world as efficacious against syphilis.

The meat and blood of the wild pig, according to Plowden, was also used for therapeutic purposes. This was confirmed by Parkyns, who related that when he shot a wild sow an Ethiopian soldier "ran up to her, and, piercing her neck with his lance, greedily drank the blood which poured out." Parkyns hypothesized that "the idea of the flesh and blood of a swine being medicinal," which was "common in Abyssinia," originated when Ethiopians witnessed Europeans using lard in the making of mercurial ointment. It would seem more probable, however, that the pig had been chosen long before for psycho-logical reasons, because it was abhorred and regarded with superstitious awe. Porcine-based treatments continued until recent times. In the early twentieth century Dr. De Castro reported that syphilitic sores were treated with the application of pork fat, while a medical text written by an Ethiopian church scholar, Abba Gared of Kambata, claimed that to cure syphilitic rheumatism one should "eat the meat of the wild boar." Another variation of this cure, as well as a hint to its rationale, was given by the French linguist Marcel Cohen, who stated that the raw meat of the pig and the raw liver of the hyena—"two kinds of food specially repugnant to the Abyssinians"—would be mixed together and given to the syphilitic patient; immediately afterward, the patient would be informed what he had consumed and the resulting "astonishment and disgust" was supposed to effect the cure.

In addition to such aggressive treatments, amulets against syphilis were often worn. Instructions for their preparation and use are commonly found in Ethiopian medical textbooks. The following is a typical example:

> *Lawz* (or almond nuts), *maqmaqo* (*Rumex abyssinicus*), iron slag (or rust?) and *barbaré* (*Capsicum frutescens*) (or pepper), put them in an amulet. It is good. Do not eat *delleh* (or spicy pepper sauce) for seven days. For half that time do not eat at all, it is not good.

Another prescription recommended the practitioner to prepare the amulet with his left hand while reciting the Lord's Prayer seven times. Some amulets contained such diverse substances as the flesh of lizards, birds, and local plants, among them the roots of *sansal* (*Adathoda schimperi*), *zarch embay, embaya ade* (?), and *embobamasqal* (?).

Magic was also employed. When a person discovered that he was infected with syphilis, he might seek a cure by sacrificing a few-weeks old goat and eating it with cooked red peppers together with the entire contents of its stomach and entrails. A similar custom was followed using goat flesh, which was considered to have remarkable medicinal properties: a person with syphilis might go to market, obtain a black he-goat, kill it, and drink its blood. He would then expel the contents of the intestines, mix them with blood, and consume them. He would also eat the "twelve parts" of the animal, on the premise that the disease would thus be driven from each corresponding organ of his own body. The goat was selected in order to avail oneself of the curative powers of all the plants which existed, which could be done by consuming the flesh of an animal—such as the goat—that grazed everywhere. Popular belief dictated that the patient should not eat anything he had not tasted before falling ill, for if he did so the complaint would return.

VIII

Leprosy and Leper Mendicants

Ethiopia suffered since time immemorial from a high incidence of leprosy, and indeed has been said to be one of the countries most seriously affected by the disease. The Portuguese priest Francisco Alvares testified in the sixteenth century that the country was inhabited by "many lepers." The more numerous observers of the nineteenth and early twentieth centuries indicate that little had changed in the intervening years. Pearce, a British resident in Tegré, declared in 1831 that infection was "very common among the lower class" and that there were "thousands who had lost their fingers and toes" and whose bodies were "covered all over with large white spots." A decade or so later the French scientific mission of 1839-1843 reported that the disease was "very common" in the north, while the German explorer Rüppell, writing of the same area, described persons with open sores on their feet, the bones of which gradually degenerated so that their toes fell off. Travelers to the southern provinces told similar tales. Rochet d'Héricourt, a French visitor to Shawa, referred to leprosy in the 1840s as one of the most common complaints (though he admitted that he had not himself seen many lepers). In Ankobar, the British diplomatic mission of 1841-1842, which treated 717 patients, found that twenty-six were suffering from the disease. Numerous cases were also reported later in the century by other observers, who noted significant regional variations: the French traveler Borelli, the Italian missionary Massaia, and the Italian physician De Castro all stated that leprosy was most widespread in Gojjam in the north-west, while another Frenchman, Soleillet, believed it was much more common among the Amharas than the Oromos, or Gallas,—a view shared in the early twentieth century by Dr. Mérab, the perceptive Georgian proprietor of Addis Ababa's first pharmacy.

The extent of leprosy in Ethiopia struct most foreign visitors. The disease was described as "very prevalent" around Lake Tana and in the west, and common in most towns, including Dasé to the north, Goré to the west, and Harar to the south-east (where Dr. Mérab saw about a hundred lepers), but seems to have been relatively rare at the old capital, Gondar.

The first tentative estimate of the country's leper population was made early in the twentieth century by Capuchin missionaries at Harar, who put it at 8,000. A decade later, Mérab suggested a substantially higher figure. Arguing that there must have been between one and three lepers per thousand people of the general population, he estimated that there were at least twenty thousand among the country's ten million inhabitants. Some of his Ethiopian friends believed that many lepers concealed their disease, and that therefore there were perhaps between five and ten lepers per thousand population or a total of at least 50,000. Menilek's interpreter, Hayla Maryam, had indeed spoken of no less than 100,000, but Mérab considered this an exaggeration. His own "conservative figure" of 30,000 was nevertheless considerable, for it compared with an estimated 130,000 in the Indian subcontinent, 40,000 in Japan, 15,000 in Indochina, and 8,000 in Madagascar.

Terminology

Leprosy, from early times, was known in Ethiopia as *lamts*. This term is found in the Ge'ez Bible, which was translated between the fourth and sixth centuries A.D., and also appears in several medieval texts. The word is likewise current in Amharic, as well as in Tegrenya as *lamtsi*. Leprosy was, however, often designated by more general terms, which were also applicable to elephantiasis or other serious skin diseases. Thus in literature as well as in common parlance, such words as *qwesala sega* or *sega dawé* (i.e., ulcerated or diseased *sega* [body]) and the even more ambiguous term *talaq dawé* (i.e., major disease) were used with reference to leprosy. On the other hand, leprosy was also frequently referred to more explicitly as *qumtena*, an Amharic word derived from the verb to amputate. This served to describe persons who had lost limbs, either on account of the disease or (in former days) as a punishment. A similar concept probably lies behind the Galla, or Oromo, word for leprosy, *kurchi*, which may well have its origin in a verb meaning to cut or break.

Biblical Ideas and Values

Ethiopian Christians paid considerable attention to statements on leprosy (*lamts*) in Holy Writ, and were well aware of the Old Testament belief that lepers were "unclean," as stated in God's injunction to Moses and Aaron in Leviticus 13:44–46: "He is a leprous man, he is unclean: the priest shall surely pronounce him unclean. . . . All the days wherein the plague shall be in him he shall be defiled; he is unclean: he shall dwell alone; without the camp shall his dwelling be." And the similar ideas in the Lord's command to Moses, in

Numbers 5:2-3, that the children of Israel should "put out of camp every leper. . . . Both male and female shall ye put out, without the camp shall ye put them, that they defile not their camp." This stern approach was mitigated in Ethiopian eyes, however, by Christ's miracle described in Matthew 8:2-3, Mark 1:40-42, and Luke 5:12-13, in which "there came a leper, and worshipped him, saying, Lord, if thou wilt, thou canst make me clean. And Jesus put forth his hand, and touched him, saying, I will; be thou clean, and immediately his leprosy was cleansed."

Texts such as the latter made a deep impact in Ethiopia, and found their way into numerous legends. One such legend, found in both the *Synaxarium* and the *Miracles of the Holy Virgin* and illustrated in numerous manuscripts, tells how Mercurius, a bishop afflicted with leprosy, was reminded by St. Zacharias that, because the Bible had called his condition "unclean," the priesthood was "not fitting" for him as long as the disease was upon him. Mercurius however, subsequently went to a church dedicated to St. Mary, where he prayed before her picture, after which, in a dream, he saw her hand rubbing his body and, on awakening, found himself "cleansed."

Miraculous cures of leprosy are a recurring theme in Ethiopic literature. They are attributed to Christ, the Virgin Mary, and various saints. St. Zacharias is thus reported to have healed a deacon of leprosy by ordering him to fast and pray, Abba Macarias to have cured a female leper by letting her touch his face, and Abba Bifamon to have healed a blind leper by smearing the latter's eyes and body with his saintly blood. St. George of Lydda is said to have cleansed a leper by anointing him with oil from a sanctuary lamp, while Abba Matthew is held to have healed, and later baptized, a "pagan" leper woman by smiting the earth with his staff and making the sign of a cross on the ground. Cures, it was believed, could be achieved only if sinners repented. One leper woman, guilty of both incest and murder, learned this at the cost of her life, for, though she washed in holy water by a church and appealed to St. Basil, she did so in vain; the *Synaxarium* claims that the earth was rent and swallowed her up, because, without any change of heart, she had "dared to sacrifice in uncleanliness to the Church of our holy Lady the Virgin Mary."

Leprosy, though susceptible to miraculous cures, was also thought to be called down from heaven on wrongdoers. For instance, the prophet Elisha's curse of his servant Gehazi (reported in 2 Kings 5:27) was repeated and embellished in the *Synaxarium*, which tells how Gehazi, his sons, "and all his seed" became lepers. Another legend held that Emperor Diocletian while destroying a sanctuary was splashed by a drop of its holy oil, whereupon leprosy broke out on that spot and caused him to die.

Manuscript illuminations, mainly in *Miracles of the Holy Virgin*, dating from the seventeenth and early eighteenth centuries, reveal that Ethiopian artists depicted leprosy in three different ways. Sometimes the victim was painted with dark patches (as in British Library Oriental [BL Orient.] MSS. 508, 510, 590, 639, 647, 649 and 653), and sometimes with white ones (as in

BL Orient. MSS. 639, 641, 645), while in other cases almost the entire body was white (as in BL Orient. MSS. 520, 635 and Additional MS. 24,188). An even more graphic representation is found in an early nineteenth-century biography (BL Orient. MS. 718) of the medieval saint-emperor Lalibala, who is depicted as a child with a group of lepers. The latter have dark areas on their skin, and the victim in the foreground has lost all his fingers and toes.

Ethiopian Attitude Towards Leprosy

Legends and beliefs such as the above reflected and helped to mold the Ethiopian attitude towards leprosy. Perhaps because of belief in the possibility of miraculous cures, Ethiopian society seems to have been considerably more tolerant of lepers than were societies in the West, where "total ostracism" of lepers in the early medieval period had been followed by their rigid detention in "houses of Lazarus." Toleration in Ethiopia may also have resulted, as Parisis argued, from the fact that people did not consider leprosy contagious.

The Ethiopian attitude to the disease can be seen in the country's traditional code, the *Fetha Nagast*, or Law of the Kings, which took as empirical and humanitarian a view of the disease as possible. A characteristic passage declared that a leper could not serve as a priest, but hastened to explain that this was not due to his being "unclean"—the concept found in both Leviticus and the *Synaxarium*—for such was "not the case" once he was baptized; rather, it was feared that, if he officiated, this could cause priests to be despised, presumably on account of the opprobrium with which the disorder was popularly regarded. A leper was likewise excluded from being a patriarch, not by reason of uncleanliness, but because his condition would prevent him from "associating with people under his jurisdiction." It was similarly stated that a judge had to be free of leprosy, but, again, only because the disease would "keep away many people who have (to come) to see him." As for marriage, the code rejected the idea that leprosy was a disability, and affirmed that whether or not to marry a leper was a decision entirely for the would-be spouse. In cases where the condition developed after marriage, two different rulings were handed down. The first established that the infection did not entitle the healthy party to separate from the diseased one. The second ruling, which is described as the better, stated that a man who wished to separate from a wife with the disease could do so if he gave her a complete outfit and dowry, but if he did not wish to separate he could live with her on condition that he provided her food, "since what befell her was not by his or her will."

The nonsegregation of lepers implied in the *Fetha Nagast* impressed Alvares, who claimed in the sixteenth century that persons afflicted with the disease did not "live away from the people," but with them. He added that there were, moreover, "many people" who "out of their devotion" washed lepers and tended their sores with their hands. A sterner approach to leprosy may have developed later, possibly as an indirect result of Muslim teaching which advocated the isolation of lepers. Nevertheless, the French Saint Simonian travelers, Edmond Combes and Maurice Tamisier, were favorably surprised by the humanity shown in Ethiopia. They declared that in that country lepers, "whom the Jews put outside the camp" and who in Europe were "excluded from society," were "allowed to communicate with everyone. Those who have families remain with them, and, when a leper is rich, he never lacks servants." Lepers were indeed seen at all festivities, and people displayed no reluctance at drinking from cups used by them. The Frenchmen even claimed to have encountered a group of leper priests, with whom the village chief was on good terms, on occasion sharing the horns from which they had drunk.

However, later nineteenth-century evidence suggests that by that time lepers were often isolated from the rest of society. The reason for this, according to Massaia, was that the disease was considered "dishonourable," not only for the victim but also for his or her relatives to the seventh degree of consanguinity. The result was that lepers were supposed to avoid contact with healthy persons, even members of their own families, and had to remain in their own separate quarter, far removed from either towns or villages.

Massaia's report is confirmed by other observers. Borelli noted that lepers "lived in groups separated from the rest of the inhabitants" and "married among themselves," while the German traveler Rohlfs agreed that lepers could only approach within a certain distance of an ordinary settlement and were then expected to make themselves known (for example, by shouting in a loud voice). If they failed to keep the required distance they rendered themselves liable to attack by healthy members of society, and could even be killed. The latter statement, however, is not supported by other testimony and may have been the case only in Tegré province, where the segregation of lepers probably was stricter than elsewhere. That they were treated with some humanity is clear from Rohlfs' statement that people, though avoiding unnecessary contact with lepers, put out food or other alms for them to collect. At Mandera, a major commercial center in the Muslim west of the country, there was in the late 1880s "a special isolated quarter to which lepers were relegated."

Lepers, though largely isolated from the rest of the population, were never regarded as objects of horror, Mérab insisted, but rather of pity, even of sympathy, particularly among Christians who remembered Christ's kindness to them. They were therefore treated with toleration, and, to the surprise of many Western observers, were allowed to appear at royal courts, and to beg with impunity.

Lepers at Court

Ethiopian rulers, whose style of government was essentially paternalistic, raised no objection to the arrival of numerous lepers at their courts. Dejazmach Webé, the early nineteenth-century ruler of Tegré, used a leper monk as a messenger to the French traveler Arnauld d'Abbadie. The latter recalled that the man, a native of Gojjam, had lost some of his fingers and toes, which caused him wryly to declare that God was "taking his body bit by bit." King Sahla Selassé of Shawa also treated lepers with "especial charity," and received them at his palace. The Frenchman Rochet d'Héricourt noted that they were in receipt of state charity, while the British envoy Harris saw there the "miserable spectacle" of many "leprous" and "scrofulous" persons, besides others whose limbs had been amputated as a punishment. This "horrible and revolting" mass of humanity, as the Englishman chose to term it, was composed of "the old, the halt and the lame, the deaf, the noseless, and the dumb, the living dead in every shape and form." A similar picture was presented by Johnston, a British surgeon, who observed that on entering the palace compound he "passed, for about twenty yards, between two rows of noisy beggars, male and female, old, middle-aged, and young; who, leprous, scrofulous, and maimed, exhibited the most disgusting sores, and implored charity for the sake of Christ and the Holy Virgin."

Such sights were frequently seen at other royal capitals. The German missionary Stern, who did not share the Ethiopian compassion for lepers, declared that Emperor Téwodros, "from motives of mistaken piety," encouraged the "social bane" of leper mendicancy, with the result that in the vicinity of the palace at Dabra Tabor there were "hordes of mendicants, clad and unclad, sound and diseased, some smitten with the curse of leprosy, others with virulent scrofula." They were lying in "promiscuous confusion," but, on seeing him, "all stretched out their withered hands, or ghoulishly came hobbling near, and in the name of *Kedus Michael, Tecla Haimanot*, or some other noted saint, almost forcibly demanded our charity." This "mode of soliciting food or alms," he commented, was "in perfect harmony with the beggar's trade," and "a man's Christianity" would indeed be "suspected" if he rejected such appeals for alms.

Such scenes were far from rare. The Greek physician Parisis, on visiting Dabra Tabor in 1885, found that its 25,000 inhabitants included over a hundred lepers who had come from the provinces to beg for alms. The majority were males between the ages of twenty and forty; he had in fact seen none below that age. Many men and women had lost several of their fingers, and had flattened noses which caused them to utter hoarse sounds that evoked in him a feeling of intense pity.

Large groups of begging lepers were still common in the first decades of the twentieth century, when Mérab reported that no less than a thousand would sometimes assemble and receive alms from Emperor Menilek and his chiefs.

Lepers with the Army

The toleration afforded to lepers was such that large numbers of them accompanied rulers on campaign. Emperor Téwodros, Stern complains, was "invariably" followed by "bands of professional *fakirs* on mules and horses" who "clog[ged] his steps and his ear with their perpetual whine." This phenomenon continued, as noted by Soleillet and others, throughout the century. Borelli, describing the return of Menilek's army from Harar in 1887, notes that it had among it many lepers who came to importune him during the night by chanting and displaying their "terrible malady," with the loss of fingers, feet, and hands. Menilek's forces advancing on Adwa in 1896 are likewise said to have been accompanied by many lepers.

Leper Mendicants

Lepers, as well as persons suffering from other serious diseases, Pearce noted early in the nineteenth century, were "great beggars." This was confirmed by Antoine d'Abbadie, who stated that they were known as *hamina* (i.e., *cantastorie*, or minstrels), and recalls that in Gondar in the 1830s he heard the "plaintive voice" of lepers, as well as of itinerant monks and students, begging from door to door in the name of Christ, the Holy Virgin, Takla Haymanot, or whatever saint was celebrating that day. Blanc, a British physician who traveled in the north-west in the 1860s, similarly reported that he was "at all hours of the day surrounded by an importuning crowd" of lepers, and persons suffering from syphilis, elephantiasis, and other complaints, while the Napier expedition of 1867–1868 reported seeing some 1,500 beggars, including blind, lame, and diseased at Adwa.

Later in the century Soleillet estimated that the lepers of Shawa numbered two or three hundred men, women, and children, who "lived in bands" and traveled throughout the province. They were, he said, nocturnal visitors, who, spending the day in various isolated places, entered the villages at midnight, singing beautifully in chorus. He adds that on one occasion Menilek's uncle, Ras Dargé, had been accompanied by a crowd of no less than 300 lepers, and that they often followed the great lords about in bands in a very bold manner, sometimes even threatening to lie in the beds of those who refused them alms.

Bands of lepers were also known in Tegré, where Rohlfs recorded that, forced to live in isolation, they formed "companies of beggars" and purchased old horses on which they rode far and wide. To awaken pity they sent the most repulsive among them to beg. One group consisted of "truly pitiful creatures, hollow-eyed and hollow-cheeked, some covered all over with spots, others with open wounds," and rode on nags almost equally miserable. On Rohlfs' approach, the party halted at a distance, their hands raised towards him, gesticulating for alms. Never had he seen so appalling, so frightful a sight. The situation in Eritrea was not dissimilar, as Francesco da Offejo reported from that colony in 1904 that lepers were importunate and would take charity almost by force, cursing the family of anyone who hesitated to give them alms.

Leper beggars similarly abounded in early twentieth-century Addis Ababa. Boyes, a British traveler, said that they "were to be seen by the hundred . . . many of them wrecks of humanity, some with arms or legs missing, and others suffering from all kinds of diseases." The subsequent "rapid growth" of the city's population after World War I may well have resulted, as Christine Sandford believed, in a substantial increase in the number of lepers. Rey, at about this time, observed that such "remnants of humanity" were "allowed to wander about at will." They were "great beggars," and when the disease became too bad for them to walk they procured old ponies and rode from house to house soliciting alms. He told of a "well-known Greek, *not* a connoisseur of horse-flesh," who "bought a pony, and was surprised to find it continually stopping at houses *en route*. Inquiry elicited the fact that it had originally belonged to a leper and had so acquired its habit of house-to-house visits!"

Begging lepers were still generally regarded with great consideration. Boyes, who felt that Ethiopian society treated them "rather generously," reported that the citizens of Addis Ababa on going to market rarely passed them "without dropping something at their feet," perhaps "a few sticks of firewood, something to eat, or whatever they were taking to market." Mérab took a similar view, observing that lepers were seldom turned away, for the Ethiopians were a "charitable and generous" people who always gave at least something, a piaster, a bullet (then much used in lieu of money), a piece of cabbage, a handful of barley, or a little cotton cloth.

Lepers in former days begged with almost total impunity. Pearce, in the early nineteenth century, claimed that they were sometimes thieves, and often "very insolent," and would even abuse passing governors, who, in accordance with the custom of the country, would never take any repressive action against them. Such statements were confirmed by later observers. Stern wrote of the "bluster and arrogance" of what he termed "indolent and often vice-tainted vagrants," while Soleillet described lepers begging every morning from house to house. They were scarcely ever refused, for they would return on the following night to curse any houses where they had been rejected. One of their most frequent threats was, "I will lie on your bed!"

A vivid impression of the lepers' exactions is provided by Massaia, who recalled being accosted by a leper who insisted on being given, as his right, one of the neck-cords traditionally worn by Ethiopian Christians. "If you do not let me have it," he menacingly declared, "prepare yourself to sleep with me tonight!" The Italian, knowing the immunity enjoyed by lepers, felt compelled to comply with this request, whereupon the beggar, with the same threat, demanded a dollar, which the missionary firmly refused. The leper then petulantly advanced on him, and attempted to caress him with his hands covered with sores, and was only prevented from doing so by some local peasants, after which Massaia felt it expedient to make peace with his persecutor by presenting him with a bar of salt, equivalent to one-tenth of a dollar. Emphasizing that such incidents were not uncommon, the missionary observed that lepers had total liberty to do what they liked, and that no one was able to restrain them. They accordingly entered any home, demanding whatever they pleased, abusing whoever failed to yield to their caprices, and committing sundry acts of violence against persons and property, for no authority dared admonish or punish them. On one occasion a group of lepers appeared at a country market, and menacingly asked for some honey and butter exposed for sale. When the vendors refused, the lepers thrust their hands into the pots, thus rendering the wares unsaleable. The lepers' unbridled liberty had reached such a point that many persons not actually affected by the disease joined them to enjoy their unrestricted privileges.

Abuses of this kind seem to have been brought under control subsequently, for we have had no reports of them in the twentieth century. Lepers, in many cases on horseback, continued, however, to beg for their sustenance. Rey tells of lepers in the Addis Ababa of the 1920s wandering around, exhibiting "revolting sores and stumps of legs and arms." He himself saw "one of these unfortunates, lacking hands and feet and part of his face, mounted on a donkey as miserable-looking as himself, chanting outside the huts . . . until he literally blackmailed the wretched people into giving him a piastre or two to get rid of him."

Lepers, and other sufferers, traditionally flocked to the more important churches in quest of alms or miraculous cures. One of the largest concentrations of lepers was in the sacred city of Aksum, where Alvares in the sixteenth century reported the presence of "more than 3,000 cripples, blind men and lepers." Four centuries later, the Italian physician Annaratone wrote in similar vein of "about a thousand lepers arriving at Aksum for a great festival from 'all parts of Ethiopia,' " while a British traveler, Bent, described "a ghastly mass of beggars," including "lepers innumerable, with decaying limbs," who came "to get alms from the rich monks."

Lepers were also a familiar sight at other places of worship, including those of Addis Ababa and Dasé, and many built their houses in the vicinity to churches and convents.

Popular Ideas on the Causes of Leprosy

Traditional Ethiopian society had little knowledge of the cause or mode of transmission of the disease. Mérab, who enquired diligently into popular beliefs, asserted that the Ethiopians attributed leprosy to a "thousand and one causes, each as fantastic as the other," among them a blow from the Devil, entry into a church sanctuary reserved exclusively for priests, and "violation of the marriage contract by moonlight." The latter belief was slow to die, for a study of 1975 reported that some people asserted that the disease developed "after sexual intercourse in the open, when there is a moon, or when the woman has her period." Infection was also sometimes said to result from spirit possession.

Notwithstanding the limited isolation of lepers, and their threats to sleep in the beds of persons who failed to provide alms, there appears to have been little real awareness that the disease could be transmitted from person to person. Perhaps not surprisingly in view of its long incubation period, many Ethiopians, according to both Parisis and Mérab, believed that it was not contagious. This view, which helps to explain the toleration afforded to lepers, was evident from the fact that though people avoided drinking from a horn touched by the lips of persons suffering from syphilis, they took no such precaution in the case of those with leprosy. The Ethiopian belief in the noncontagious character of the disease was reinforced by the popular view that it was inherited. This was asserted in such popular sayings as "A leper is the son . . . or the grandson and great-grandson of a leper." By the early twentieth century, however, Addis Ababa opinion was beginning to recognize occasional cases of contagion, among them of one or two Europeans, including an Italian in Harar. Old beliefs, however, were not easily abandoned, as is evident from the fact that the Agaw people of Bagémder were reported in the 1960s as still maintaining the opinion that leprosy was an "inherited disease." An Ethiopian health officer commented that this was "no wonder," for the complaint "certainly 'runs in families'."

Prayers, Vows, and Amulets

Many Ethiopians, as we have seen, believed in miraculous cures. Sick persons accordingly spent much of their time in prayer, and would vow to make generous gifts to the church if they recovered. British consul Plowden claimed in the 1850s that miracles were not infrequent, for whenever offerings slackened, the priests saw to it that "a leper is cleansed, or the blind are restored to sight."

One of the saints to whom prayers were frequently offered was Gabra Krestos, also known as 'Abd al-Masih. This son of Emperor Theodosius of Constantia, according to the *Synaxarium*, was afflicted by a skin disease and his sores were licked by the dogs in his father's courtyard. Though his illness was not specified in the text, popular belief has often identified it with leprosy. An observer of the 1970s was thus informed by a leper that the saint, wishing to "live a blessed life," gave "all his wealth to the poor people and asked God to give him leprosy to suffer like Jesus Christ." The Lord accordingly "gave him leprosy," and as a result lepers revere him as their patron saint.

The use of amulets against leprosy, which were worn around the neck, was also customary.

Medical Treatment

A variety of traditional medical cures for leprosy were in widespread use. Ethiopian medical texts, the earliest dating from the late eighteenth century, indicate that the disease was treated both internally and externally.

Medicines for internal use came, like the greater part of the local pharmacopeia, mainly from the vegetable kingdom, and consisted of roots, bark, leaves, fruit, and seeds of a multitude of plants, many of which also served in the treatment of syphilis and other complaints. The most popular specifics against leprosy included the leaves, fruit, and root of the *mesanna* (*Croton macrostachys*), the fruit and roots of the *gizéwa* (*Withania somnifera*), and the roots of the *gamaro* or *gumaro* (*Capparis tomentosa*). Medicinal use was also made of the *midaqwa*, or wild antelope, which was believed to possess great curative properties.

Medicines for external application were even more numerous. Most were based on plants of one kind or another, among them the roots of the *améra* (*Lonchocarpus laxiflorus*), *messerech* (*Crotalaria platycalyx*), *dadaho* (*Euclea schimperi*), and *maqmaqo* (*Rumex abyssinicus*), the leaves and fruit of the *degetsa* (*Calpurnia subdecandra*), and the leaves, seeds and small branches of the *waginos* (*Brucea antidyssenterica*). Other remedies included the crowfoot, or ranunculo, from which a blistering paste was made, and such common condiments as red pepper and mustard. Many medications also contained butter, while others were made with honey, white-of-egg, fig-juice, or the latex of the *qwolqwal* (*Euphorbia candelabrum*). Though most medicines for external applications were largely herbal, some included such varied items as spiders' webs, cow-dung, birds' droppings, burnt dog's excrement (preferably, according to some prescriptions, that of a black animal), the stools of a black cat, a monkey, and a cock, the burnt horn of a black goat, and the fat of the *chelat* bird, as well as salt, sulphur, and soot. Other popular curses are said the have included an ointment made from the powder of a burnt toad, during the application of which the patient was supposed to refrain from all sexual intercourse, and, according to one otherwise unsubstantiated account, the blood of a newly born child (a specific also said to have beem employed by Constantine the Great). Some of these medicaments were far from cheap. One traditional practitioner at Gondar in the 1920s, Ato Balay, is said to have charged a fee of 30 to 40 Maria Theresa thalers for a cure.

Use was also made of vapor baths, a long-established mode of treatment in Ethiopia, where patients would be closeted in a small hut, and various medicinal plants, among them the aforementioned *degetsa* and *gizéwa*, would be inhaled.

Thermal Baths
Lepers also took good advantage of the country's thermal waters, which, as we shall see, bubbled out of the ground in many areas and were widely used in the treatment of many complaints.

IX

Rabies

Hydrophobia was not uncommon in Ethiopia and on one occasion in the early twentieth century, it took on the proportions of an epidemic. Notwithstanding some supersititions and misconceptions, the disease, its method of contagion, and its incubation period were relatively well known, and traditional practitioners employed a wide variety of supposed cures, some of which— being identifiable for well over a century—illustrate the well established character of the traditional pharmacopeia.

Early nineteenth-century travelers, the first to discuss the incidence of rabies, were by no means unanimous in their assessment. In the 1830s the German explorer Eduard Rüppell, who reported seeing a mad dog at Adwa, declared that rabies was "by no means uncommon." The Frenchman Rochet d'Héricourt, a decade or so later, told of an apparently rabid dog that bit a soldier and three other dogs at Dabra Tabor. His compatriot Antoine d'Abbadie agreed that hydrophobia was "not rare" and mentioned that a rabid dog had attacked two of his brother's servants, one of whom died, and cited the case of another dog who bit four persons. He believed that the disease was more widespread in Ethiopia than in other Middle Eastern countries because the country's cool climate prevented people from sweating, and sweat tended to act as a disinfectant in case of bites by rabid animals.

Other commentators took a somewhat different view. The French medical observer, Alfred Courbon, believed that rabies was "very rare," while the British envoy, Walter Plowden, observed that it was "not very common," though "more prevalent in Gojjam than elsewhere." A generation or so later, in the 1880s, the Italian geographer Antonio Cecchi stated that hydrophobia was "not serious," at least in Shawa, while Nicholas Parisis, a Greek doctor in Tegré, agreed it was "rare among the Abyssinians." The French trader, Léon

Chefneux, who had spent thirty years in the country, was similarly quoted early in the twentieth century as declaring that he had never seen anyone dying from the disease.

The first and only recorded rabies epidemic occurred in Addis Ababa in August 1903, and, according to Dr. De Castro of the Italian legation, lasted for "a few months." He adds that this was the only such occurrence during his ten-year residence from 1901 to 1911, that in fact hydrophobia was not seen every year, and that frequently the disease was "completely absent for long periods." Dr. Mérab likewise expressed his doubts as to the frequency of the disease. He believed that this was not surprising as the local dogs were of the same race as those of Constantinople, which he knew from personal experience were but rarely affected by hydrophobia.

Nevertheless, rabies was considered so important that Menilek's palace had a traditional practitioner who provided treatment, entirely free of charge, to anyone in need. At least one patient came every week. Cures at the palace were supposed to be a hundred percent successful, which Mérab thought was not surprising, for most patients had never really been exposed to any risk of rabies. Usually, they had in fact been only touched by a rabitic dog, or bitten by a healthy one.

Incidents with dogs were also reported in other parts of the country. The situation in Gondar was summed up early in the twentieth century by an Italian physician, Amleto Bevilacqua, who stated that though dog bites were "most common" and reached a "truly extraordinary number," rabies "did not seem to be known." A couple of decades later it was reported that there was in Gondar a traditional practitioner called Warqu who specialized in curing persons bitten by mad dogs, but took no recompense, for, he said, "It is for my soul."

Serious cases were occasionally reported, however. Fan C. Dunckley, an Englishwoman residing in Addis Ababa and writing of the late 1920s, told of three separate incidents which occurred in a single year, immediately after the rains. In the first, a dog kept as a pet by some farmers outside the capital developed the disease and bit three people; in the second, she and her husband were attacked in Addis Ababa by a pi-dog, or stray-animal, but managed to hold the animal at bay; in the third, a Greek woman in the interior was bitten by her pet and, being twenty-four days' journey from the capital, was unable to obtain treament in time and so "died a terrible death." Discussing these incidents, Mrs. Dunckley noted: "rabies in Addis Ababa was far more frequent after the rains than at any other time of the year. Various theories have been put forward for this— one being that the dogs drank from the puddles of the road, paths, etc., and that a germ got into the water and the dog drew in the germ while drinking."

Rabies was likewise reported in Eritrea where the Italian resident in Adi Quala later declared that the area suffered "a great deal" from it as rabies was "prevalent amongst the wild animals."

The significance of the disease is further evident from the continued existence of traditional specialists in post–World War II Ethiopia. One of these, Zawgé Takla Maryam of Kasima near Dabra Berhan in Shawa, who was interviewed by the present writer in 1969, claimed to receive as much as thirty to forty Ethiopian dollars for a course of treatment or five dollars from poorer patients, and said that he was treating a minimum of six cases a month in Addis Ababa.

Ethiopians were traditionally well aware that the bite of a rabid dog was often fatal. Ethiopian medical texts, in both Ge'ez and Amharic, dating from the eighteenth and nineteenth centuries, recognize that the bite of a mad dog was a very different matter from any ordinary bite. Nineteenth-century travelers, such as d'Abbadie and Cecchi, confirmed that Ethiopians knew that the bite of a "mad dog" was dangerous and required speedy treatment, while De Castro in the twentieth century stated that "the natives say that even the saliva (of a rabid dog), without biting, is fatal." Despite such awareness, Dr. Mérab believed that diagnosis by traditional practitioners was often faulty and that Ethiopians often confused relatively minor ailments with rabies, particularly in cases where the patient had previously been bitten or had had some contact with a dog. Such confusions, he argued, also accounted for the apparent efficacy of all sorts of traditional cures.

Ethiopian ideas on the length of the incubation period coincided with—and may well have been influenced by—those in other countries. Two nineteenth-century medical texts stated that treatment should continue for forty days, while d'Abbadie delcared that "the Abyssinians say, like us, that there is no more danger after 40 days," and Cecchi that it was the practice in Shawa to treat patients within forty days of their being bitten. Zawgé Takla Maryam likewise told the present writer that after receiving an advance payment at the beginning of his treatment, he collected the bulk of his fee after the fortieth day.

Some popular ideas on rabies were entirely fantastic. In Shawa, for example, according to Cecchi, it was widely believed that "when an unfortunate was bitten by a rabid dog this produced in his belly puppies which grew day by day." Patients were often treated with medicines that caused them to vomit, after which there would be a discussion as to which part of the animal had been ejected. One person would claim to recognize a leg, another a shoulder, a third a part of the breast, and the discussion would be halted only when the practitioner gave his own equally naive verdict.

Rochet d'Héricourt, on the other hand, was informed that a rabies victim when properly treated released "microscopic worms" in the urine, while Dr. Mérab reported that it was thought that successful medicine expelled small white worms which were held to be the offspring of the mad dog who had bitten the patient. Zawgé Takla Maryam, who endorsed this view, stated that seven days after being bitten the victim began to vomit dark worms, which also came out in his or her stool, and that about twenty days after the biting they more and more resembled the shape and color of the dog from which the infection emanated.

Traditional Treatment

Ethiopians traditionally employed a wide variety of treatment in cases of bites by dogs believed to be rabid. Though attention was primarily centered on human patients, dogs and other domestic animals were also treated. Many cures were based on purging. Some medical texts stated that in the case of a bite by a dog, donkey, or mule—but above all by a mad dog—the patients had to drink a medicine which would cause the poison "to go out in the diarrhoea", and added: "If one makes it go out quickly the poison does not reach the heart." A not too dissimilar view was put forward by Saw Aganyahu, a traditional practitioner in Gondar, who stated that the objective was to prevent the poison from "working in the belly," while Alaqa Gabra Wald, an old-style physician from Farasbét Madhané Alam in Gojjam, wrote of the need to apply special medicines "so that the poison does not go to other parts of the body."

The importance of purges in old-style treatment was underlined by d'Abbadie, who bluntly declared that Ethiopians cured hydrophobia by purgatives, while Rochet d'Héricourt described a treatment that resulted in evacuation of the bowels, release of urine, and vomiting. Other cures reported by Cecchi were based on the use of emetics.

Treatment sometimes was conceived in terms of innoculation, which, as we have seen, was also employed with a fair measure of success as a preventative for smallpox. Careful attention was also paid to the cleaning and disinfection of wounds made by rabid dogs.

Most traditional medicines for rabies came from the vegetable kingdom. Early nineteenth-century texts listed the following medicines for persons bitten by a mad dog:

1. The roots of the *zarch embay* and *meder embay* (types of *Solanum campylacanthum*), *gamaro* (*Capparis tomentosa* or *C. persicifolia*), *changar zabaquel* (?), *talanj* (*Achyranthes aspera* or *A. argentea*), *asarat* (*Mandragora officinarum* ?), *makan endod* (*Phytolacca dodecandra*), *chaqma* (*Ricinus communis*), *samag* (?), *améra* (*Lonchocarpus laxiflorus* ?), *sera baji* (?), *harag resa* (?) and *yasét qast* (Asparagus aethopicus), the bark of the *mesanna, esa zarwé* (*Croton macrostachys*), and the leaves of the *degetsa* (*Calpurnia subdecandra*), *lemmech* (?) and *qatatena* (*Verbascum sinaiticum*). The text added somewhat cryptically that the *dennech zakalb*, or wild potato (*Coleus edulis*), was "better" than all roots, but "had to be taken with water."
2. The wild cucumber *dembushesh*, of which one prescription stated, "when you make him drink it he is cured."
3. The roots of the *amerá, esa menahé* (?), *esa zarwé* (?), *enzarazay* (?), *asarat* (*Mandragora officinarum* ?), and *sara baji*. These roots had to be dried,

crushed, and mixed with citron water when intended for a human patient, milk for a dog, or plain water for any other domestic animal.

4. The leaves of the *zarch embay* (*Solanum campylacanthum*) and *makan endod* (*Phytocacca dodecandra*). The leaves of the former had to be dried, ground into a fine powder, mixed with honey, and tasted on the thumb; the leaves of the latter had to be crushed and drunk in a small cup of milk.

5. The leaves of the *makan endod* was also taken by itself. One text stated that the juice of these leaves had to be drunk in small quantity for 40 days, while the patient recited the religious words of the *Habeka Qeddasé*.

6. The roots of the *endahabella* (*Kalanchoe quartiniana*), collected in three different places, *asarat* (Mandragora officinarum?), *chefreg* (*Sida ovata*), and *jebarra* (*Tupa rhynopetalum, Tupa schimperi,* or *Rhynocopetalum montanum*). These roots had to be boiled for a short time in steer's urine placed in a new clay pot on three stones.

7. The root of the *tacha* (?) mixed with that of the *grar*, or acacia (*Acacia abyssinica*), and boiled, the decoction thus made being drunk.

8. The roots of the *ablalit* (?) and the *qabarecho* (*Echinops*), which were to be finely ground and eaten with *enjera* bread.

Other cures were mentioned by several foreign observers. Rochet d'Héricourt learned of one based on a *cucurbitacae*, or kind of gourd, the roots of which were dried and ground into powder, after which 12 to 13 grains were administered in a small spoon of honey or milk. During the next hour and a half, this induced many evacuations of the bowels, vomitings, and the release into the urine of "microscopic worms." The patient, weakened by this treatment, was then given whey, and later the flesh or gizzard of a chicken, well-peppered and roasted in butter. D'Héricourt, who had first heard of this treatment from Ras Ali, the ruler of Bagémder, reported that when a dog at Dabra Tabor bit a soldier and three other dogs the chief said to him, "Now you will see the efficacy of the remedy of which I spoke." The ras had the dogs separated and, when the attacker was calm, had it swallow the medicine in a spoonful of honey, after which it allegedly recovered. Eight days later one of the dogs which had been bitten developed signs of madness, but was allegedly cured in the same manner. On the twelfth day similar symptoms appeared in a second dog which was likewise supposedly cured, but the third animal, which for purposes of control was not treated, died after 42 days. The soldier, for his part, became ill nine days after being bitten. His head was heavy and very hot, and he seemed dull, spoke little, slobbered at the mouth, and became angry when offered a glass of hydromel. On the following day he was given the medicine in a spoonful of milk and was, it was claimed, quickly cured. The validity of this treatment was later questioned by Courbon, who considered the assertion of its infallibility "entirely false."

The traditional practitioners of Derita, Gojjam and the lands south of the Blue Nile, according to d'Abbadie, all had their own cures. In Derita, the cure consisted of some unidentified leaves, which were placed in fresh milk to produce a strong purgative, while in Gojjam people pulverized a root "not generally known." In another cure, seven fruits of an unspecified plant were placed in milk or beer to produce a purgative.

Two other cures were reported by Plowden. In the first the leaves of the *qarat* (*Osyris abyssinica*) were rubbed on the patient for three days and "divers ceremonies performed." In the other, the patient was to eat large quantities of garlic, which was supposed to be remarkably efficacious; a man already raving from the disease was reported to have been cured in this manner.

Several other specifics were later reported by Mérab. One consisted of a handful of crushed roots of the *améra* (*Lonchocarpus laxiflorus*, already cited in a nineteenth-century medical text) and of the *wahi* (?), which were to be drunk in beer. In a second, the patient ate a root of the *meder embay* (*Solanum campaylacanthum*), mentioned in several medical texts, and a root of the *ayt-joro* (?), each about the size of a thumb, and kept a diet of leavened bread. In a third cure, the powder of the *assereb* (?) and that of the *manahé* (?) were boiled in *taj*, or mead, with the powdered foot of a crab or lobster, and a soupspoonful of the potion was given internally for seven days. A fourth cure, the one used at Menilek's palace, was made from the roots of the *ahaya* (*Salix subserrata* or *S. alba*), which was drunk in combination with water or other liquid.

An early twentieth-century medical text drawn up by Alaqa Gabra Wald contained the following specifics for persons bitten by a mad dog:

1. The roots of the *waynageft* (?) and *asarkush tabatabmush* (*Cissus adenatha* ?), which had to be ground into powder and eaten with unleavened bread.
2. A variation of this prescription stated that the patient should drink a decoction made from the root and leaf of the *wagnageft* (?) with a little water.
3. The *meder embay* (*Solanum campylacanthum*) which had to be eaten with *enjara* bread made from black *téf.* (It is probable that the prescription referred to the root of the plant as recommended in the nineteenth-century texts, though this is not stated.)
4. The roots of the *gotech* (?), which had to be dug up by a small boy wearing a silver ring and using a horn-handled knife and an olive stick, and be taken from seven different places on a Friday and Wednesday (i.e., a fast day). The root was to be measured with the digits of the boy's small finger, pounded on three stones, and given to the patient who had to drink it from a new vessel with the milk of a cow who was the same color as her calf.
5. The powdered roots of the *meder embay* and *zarch embay* (types of *Solanum campylacanthum*), to be drunk by humans and dogs as a prophylactic. (The roots of both plants, as we have seen, had earlier been mentioned in nineteenth-century texts.)
6. In the case of a child with rabies, it was recommended that he or she be beaten on the back of the neck with a branch of the *daga abalo* (*Terminalia*

glaucescens or *Crotalaria lachnocarpoides*?), the length of a cubit and a span. This had to be carried out three times, but not by a pregnant woman.

A different prescription also using the above-mentioned *abalo* was later collected in Gojjam by Alemayehu Mogus, a scholar of the postwar generation. This prescription stated that the *abalo* fruit should be dried, ground, and mixed with the roots of the *meder embay* (*Solanum campylacanthum*), a medicament long cited in connection with rabies. The mixture was to be taken with honey in the treatment of people, or raw meat in that of dogs. Another informant from Gojjam reported to the present writer that a potion consisting of parts of the *qarat* (*Osyris abyssinica*), *abesh* (*Trigonella foenum-graecum*), and *ted* (*Juniperus procera*) mixed with hyena droppings was sometimes used as a prophylactic. The use of *qarat*, it should be noticed, had earlier been reported by Plowden.

The treatment given by Zawgé Takla Maryam was based on a mixture of no less than nineteen plants, several of which were mentioned in earlier manuscripts. Zawgé's prescription consisted of the roots of the *alblabit* (?), *dog* (*Ferula communis*), *faras zang* (*Veronia adoensis*), *shenat* (*Trichelia volkensii*), *aheya joro* (?), *embay* (*Solanum*), *agam* (*Carissa edulis*), *asarkush* (*Cissus adenatha*), *gabarecho* (*Echinops*), *achefa* (?), *shehare* (?), *zarazay* (?), *qatatena* (*Verbascum sinaiticum*), *esa zawi* (?), and *zarch embay* (*Solanum campylacanthum*), the bark of the *besanna* (*Croton macrostachys*) and *taferado* (?), the leaves of the *ahaya* (*Salix subserrata*?), and *zerat chefar* (?), and the sap of the *qwolqwal* (*Euphorbia abyssinica*). Patients, who were supposed to remain alone in a "clean house" (i.e., without sexual intercourse), had to take this medicine with yogurt, or, on fast days, with beer made from barley or black *téf*. The dose was three spoonfuls, to be taken every fifteen days for six months. Dogs, on the other hand, had to be administered four spoonfuls with bread, also made from black *téf*, every twenty days for forty days. Mad dogs had to eat lemon rind with unleavened bread made from black *téf*.

Another treatment, reported by Grazmach Asregdaw Borja, consisted of the leaves of the *etsa faris* (*Datura stramonium*), which were crushed, and the resultant juice given to the patient to drink with the milk of a cow of the same color as its calf. The antidote for this poison was said to be the liver of a chicken.

Other vegetable cures were mentioned by foreign scholars of recent times. The Italian botanist Fabrizio Cortesi tells of the use of the root of the *eniderobaia* (*Cucumis ficifolius*), which was also subsequently mentioned by his compatriot Raffaele Cacciapuoti. The latter says that the juice of the crushed leaves of *etsa faris* or *mestenager* (*Datura stramonium*) and the *tirufra* (*Datura metel*) also served as a prophylactic. D. Lemordant, a Frenchman and sometime director of the Ethiopian Pasteur Institute, mentioned the use of the *améra* and *ahaya*, both earlier mentioned by Mérab, as well as three other plants. These were *asarkush tabatabkus* (*Cissus adenantha* ?; earlier cited by Alaqa Gabra Wald), the dried roots of which were mixed with flour, *messerech* (*Clerodendron myricoides*), and *damakasé* (*Ocimum menthaefolium* or *Ocimum lamifolium*).

Another specific, the use of which can be documented for almost a century, was made from a species of black beetle which was said to have purging qualities. D'Abbadie in the early nineteenth century stated that in Enarya "they cure the man bitten by a mad dog by making him take a kind of black scarab (*bombi*) which is found in September in the fields of *mashilla* (i.e., sorghum). The dose consists of 12 scarabs well pulverised and swallowed in water. The patient is strongly purged and almost always cured." This purge was "very violent," and he had been assured that it had "killed a man in Gudru". Use was also made of another black insect, about the size of a bee, seen on the leaves of beans. On the third day after being bit by a rabid dog the patient would swallow two-thirds of this insect, the tail of which was first pulled off. Two of these insects produced three doses. The insects were pulverized, and eaten "in pure honey, fresh cheese, or, according to some, citron water. If the powder touches the tongue it blisters. This remedy provokes plentiful evacuations of urine—sometimes for 2 whole days. Afterwards the patient complains of hunger and is cured."

The black-beetle cure, interestingly enough, was recorded a century later in an Amharic medical treatise in the possession of a *dabtara* (i.e., lay cleric) at Entotto. This treatise stated that a person bitten by a mad dog should swallow a finely-ground *wajbit*, which was described by Marcel Griaule as a black coleopteran or beetle found in potatoes attacked by dampness. The cure being apparently a powerful purge, the text further declared that the effects of the treatment could be halted by taking *baso*, a gruel made of grilled barley. Further confirmation of this treatment comes from Alemayehu Mogus who recorded that it was common practice in Gojjam to administer the *wajimbit* beetle, the head and legs of which would be removed. Persons bitten by a dog suspected of being rabid were supposed to eat this insect with honey, and suspect dogs were to eat the same with milk.

Several superstitious practices were sometimes connected with rabies treatment. Dr. Mérab reported that it was said that some hairs of the rabid dog should be placed on the wound of its victims. It was also widely believed that the rabies patient should avoid crossing any river which contained water throughout the year, for such waters were thought to be inhabited by demons who would destroy the efficacy of any cure. Zewgé Takla Maryam also stated, quite independently, that a patient should not enter a river and, if obliged to cross, should be carried over and not allowed to stand at the water's edge.

Inoculations based on the eating of rabid material were reported in the early twentieth century by De Castro, who learned from Emperor Menilek that Ethiopians would make a rabid dog bite a cow, which would then be slaughtered and its meat eaten by the persons who had been bitten. De Castro, who was not impressed, commented that this did not prevent the victims from succumbing to the terrible disease. A somewhat different treatment was later reported by Lemordant, who said that persons bitten by a rabid dog would sometimes be required to eat the animal's liver with *barbaré*, or red pepper, while Alice Morton, and American anthropologist, reported that when a cow became rabid at Bishoftu in 1970 its owner refused to have it destroyed and sold its flesh as a preventative for rabies.

The cleaning and care of wounds inflicted by dogs, as well as horses, donkeys, mules, monkeys, and hyenas, received considerable attention in traditional medical texts. Some texts specified that the wound should be "burnt with the boiling oil of *nug*," or Niger oil (*Guizotia abyssinica*), after which a hot poultice made of cloth soaked in the yolk and white of an egg beaten up with fresh butter and *nug* oil was to be applied for three days. One prescription claimed that a wound would heal if covered with salt, honey, or onion and honey, and that a mixture of peas and honey was also good. Another passage stated that two heads of garlic should be mixed with *nug* oil and put on the fire to produce a liquid which was then placed on the wound, while a third text declared that in case of either dogbite or snakebite the wound should be burned.

The prescriptions of Alaqa Gabra Wald also recommended how the wounds of rabid dogs should be treated. One passage stated that seeds of the *wanza* (*Cordia africana*) should be powdered with fig leaves and applied to the wound which would "then be cured." Another passage stated that a decoction made from the root and leaves of the *waynageft* (?) mixed with salt, water, and garlic should be tied to the wound "so that the poison does not go to other parts of the body."

Traditional "cures" were thus very varied—but many can be seen to have been used consistently for at least several centuries.

X

Tapeworm and Taenicides

Taenia, or tapeworm, has been known in Ethiopia since early times. The infestation originated in the custom of eating raw meat, which had been considered a delicacy in the highlands since at least medieval times. The consumption of raw meat was first mentioned in the early fifteenth century by the Arab historian Maqrizi and was described in the following century by Alvares. The widely held belief that the practice began during the wars of Ahmad Gragn, when people supposedly were afraid of lighting fires, is therefore clearly apocryphal.

Prevalence of Tapeworm

The prevalence of taenia, which was reported in the seventeenth century by three Jesuits, Manoel de Almeida, Manoel Barradas, and Pero Paes, was later discussed by the Czech monk Brother Remedio Prutky, who noted in the mid-eighteenth century that the Ethiopians "once a month" were "much troubled by the presence of worms in their stool." This statement was echoed a generation later by Bruce, who stated that "the Abyssinians of both sexes and all ages" were "troubled" by what he called this "terrible disease"; but he also noted that "custom" had enabled them to bear it with "a kind of indifference."

The high incidence of tapeworm also struck most subsequent foreign observers. In the early nineteenth century, the French physician Dr. Petit observed that only a small percentage of the people of Tegré were free of taenia, while Johnston, a British surgeon, noted that the entire population of Shawa was "dreadfully" infected. Parkyns, a British resident in the north, declared that out of forty servants, male and female, whom he had ever employed, only two were exempt, while the French envoy Rochet d'Héricourt noted that the parasite was found in children as early as the age of four. Such statements were confirmed by later travelers, among them the Italian missionary Massaia, who stated that it was "difficult to find a person not affected"; the Protestant missionary Sterm, who wrote that the tapeworm was a "national" disease from which "scarcely one in a hundred is exempt"; and Dr. Mérab, who declared that every honest Ethiopian had it, had had it, or would have it. Ascarides and other types of internal worm were also fairly common, particularly among children, as testified in the mid-eighteenth century by Plowden and almost a hundred years later by Mérab.

Traditional Taenicides

Ethiopian society responded to the challenge of tapeworm by developing a wide variety of taenicides, thus bearing out the Latin adage, *ubi malum, ibi remedium*.

Kosso

The commonest traditional taenicide was the blood-red flower of the *kosso* tree, a powerful and very bitter purge, so generally employed that its name, as Almeida noticed in the seventeenth century, was used to refer to the parasite. *Kosso* played so extensive a role in Ethiopian life that Mérab in the early twentieth century remarked that to mention it was to cover a quarter of the country's pharmacopeia.

The *kosso* tree, which was seen throughout the Ethiopian highlands, grew best in areas of considerable elevation. It was found, according to Almeida, in "nearly all the high and cold parts" of the country. This was confirmed over a century later by Bruce, who stated that the tree was "an inhabitant of the high country" and often planted with cedars in the vicinity of churches. Later observers stated that *kosso* was found most frequently above eight thousand feet; according to Johnston, it often marked the site of abandoned as well as occupied villages.

The medical use of *kosso* can be traced back at least to the sixteenth century. The Ethiopian monk Bahrey wrote in his *History of the Galla* that Bifole, the fourth Oromo *luba* (or chief) adopted the habit of taking the medicine during his term of office (which ran from 1546 to 1554). *Kosso* drinking, Bahrey explained, was then already customary in the northern provinces where the inhabitants took the drug "to kill and rid their stomachs" of certain worms. The use of *kosso* was also mentioned early in the sixteenth century by Almeida, who stated that it was "an excellent medicine" with which to kill the worms that "constantly breed in these people."

Despite such commendation, *kosso* was by no means fully effective. Though a strong and indeed violent purge, it frequently failed to eject the tapeworm completely: the head of the parasite would remain in its host's intestines, and from it the worm would grow again, attaining its former size within a couple of months. This factor, together with the extensive consumption of raw meat and consequent reinfection, obliged large sections of the population to take *kosso* repeatedly, usually at intervals of only one or two months. Though the relationship between the eating of raw meat and the prevalence of tapeworm was obvious, the only prominent Ethiopian known to have abstained from the traditional diet was Empress Mentewwab in the eighteenth century, who, according to the Armenian traveler Tovmachean, "did not eat raw meat." Most other people, according to Mérab, took the view that the parasite was sent by God and that its prevention was beyond human control.

Kosso drinking was so widespread that Ethiopians were said by Bruce to have alleged that "the want of this drug" in other lands was the reason why they did not travel, or, if they did so, left their country only for short periods. The medicine was, however, available at that time in Cairo, where it was sold "for the use of Abyssinian and Nubian slaves and others."

Kosso was consumed in such immense quantities that it constituted a major article of trade. In early nineteenth-century Shawa, the drug was "taken in considerable quantities" to market where it was exchanged, Johnston said, for grain or cotton, "a handful of the latter, or a drinking-hornful of the former, purchasing sufficient for two doses, two large handfuls." The French physician Courbon, who confirmed the medicine's commercial importance, stated that packets containing about thirty-five grams, or enough for one dose, were available in several markets of Tegré. The mother of Emperor Téwodros was described as having been a *kosso* dealer, an occupation which, despite the medical importance of the drug, was considered dishonorable. *Kosso* it should be emphasized, was at all times very cheap. Mérab reported in 1912 that a piaster or one-sixteenth of a Maria Theresa thaler would purchase enough for three or four doses.

Nineteenth- and early twentieth-century evidence indicates the extent to which *kosso* drinking was an integral part of traditional social life. Courbon, for example, noted that "men and women, all and sundry, in this country . . . take *Kouzzo* regularly every two months," while De Cosson declared that "all the Abyssinians are in the habit of taking monthly doses of kousso." *Kosso* is said to have been drunk by persons above six or seven years of age, regardless of their social class. Royalty were not excepted. De Cosson noted in his diary that Emperor Yohannes "received no one this morning as he had been taking kosso," while the Italian explorer Cecchi states that when Menilek took the drug his palace was closed, with admission granted only to important dignitaries. A generation or so later the bimonthly event of *kosso* drinking was described by Mérab as a virtual holiday for the patient, who withdrew from all normal activity. The statement, "the master has taken his *kosso*," was synonymous with saying "he cannot receive you today." *Kosso* drinking indeed was an accepted excuse or justification for not keeping appointments. It was used by the debtor who did not wish to meet his creditor, by the accused who wished to avoid going to court, and by the official who sought to delay answering a summons from the emperor. A popular song contained the words: "The soldier, who was afraid, said to his wife, 'give me *kosso!*' to release him from going to war". The taking of *kosso* continued well into the twentieth century. One the eve of the Italian invasion of 1935, Rey reported that it was "a regular and understood procedure for one's servants to take a day off once a month" in order to drink *kosso*, and "quite common" to be told that an important official could not receive one "because he has taken *kosso.*" It is therefore not surprising to learn from Mérab that the first modern pharmacy was popularly referred to as the *kosso-bét*, or "*kosso* house."

Methods of preparing this most extensively used of all Ethiopian drugs varied slightly from family to family, but were basically uniform. The usual procedure, as described in the eighteenth century by Prutky, was to infuse eight drams of powdered *kosso* flowers in eight drams of *taj*, or mead. Patients, who had to abstain from food or drink, would drink this potion in the evening, after which "all night until the fifth or sixth hour of the morning" they would be "purged with staining and loss of blood," after which they would "lie like the dead, utterly exhausted, having voided a great quantity of worm." At length, having rested a while, they would rise and eat a dish of gruel made from chick-peas, after which they would be restored to health—and start eating raw meat again. "The Abyssinians," he said, "practise this cure monthly, and if they travel through the provinces for commerce and other purposes they always go supplied with *kosso* powder."

Variants of this procedure for preparing *kosso* are suggested by later travelers. Bruce, for example, reported that it was normal to place a handful of *kosso* flowers in about two quarts ot *talla*, or beer, and to steep it overnight, after which the brew was ready for use. Petit, in the early nineteenth century, stated that a large handful of *kosso* flowers would be placed on a stone, pounded, and mixed with water to form a paste which would then be dissolved in unfermented beer, or in some cases *taj*, the resultant liquid being filtered before being drunk.

A more detailed account was afforded by Johnston, who suggested that the less scientifically minded often had to resort to certain mystic rites. He declared:

> The fruit of the *cosso* is gathered before the seeds are quite ripe and whilst still a number of the flowerets remain unchanged. The bunches are suspended in the sun to dry, and if not required for immediate use are deposited in a jar. . . . When taken it is reduced upon the mill to a very fine powder, having previously been well dried upon a small mat, upon which for some superstitious reason or other, several bits of charcoal are placed. The largest drinking-horn being produced, the powdered *cosso* is mixed with nearly a pint of water, and, if it can be obtained, a large spoonful of honey is also added. When everything is quite ready a naked sword is placed flat upon the ground upon which the patient stands. The nurse then takes between two bits of sticks as a substitute for tongs a small bit of lighted charcoal, and carries it around the edge of the vessel three times, mumbling a prayer, at the end of which

the charcoal is extinguished in the medicine which is immediately drunk off by the patient, who all this time has been pulling most extraordinary faces, expressive of his disgust for the draught. The operation is speedy and effectual, and to judge by the prostration of strength it occasioned in my servants, when they employed this medicine, it must be dreadfully severe.

Almost a century later Mérab reported that the *kosso* flowers would usually be beaten and crushed in the vertical hand-mill used for grinding grain or pepper (*barbaré*) and would then be thrown in a cup of warm water or (perferably) mead, beer, or whey, and left there for 15 minutes, after which the liquid would be swallowed.

The normal custom, as explained by Plowden in the nineteenth century and by Mérab in the twentieth, was for the patient taking *kosso* to abstain from all food until the worm was ejected. This practice is confirmed by Yohannes Walda Gerima, a post–World War II student of the plant, who observed that the medicine was "taken before any food, and nothing . . . eaten until a mass of segments of the worm has been discharged with the stool." Abstention from sexual intercourse on the previous night was also required, Mérab and Yohannes Walda Gerima both explained, and it was believed that failure to comply with this rule would endanger the cure.

The actual dosage was not precisely determined, and seems to have varied with circumstances. In the nineteenth century, Rüppell wrote of about 28 grams (i.e, the weight of a Maria Theresa thaler), Kirk of 21 to 28 grams, and Courbon and Fournier of 20 and 35 grams, respectively. It was generally agreed, however, that the drug led to the almost total evacuation of the stomach in only a few hours.

Though *kosso* was most frequently administered alone, sometimes it was also mixed with other taenicides. A typical prescription, according to the nineteenth-century botanist Schimper, might thus include linseed or mallow seed, a half-handful of the root of the *botto* (*Gnidia involucrata*), three or four leaves of the *wayra* (*Olea africana*), a small handful of *tambelel* or *habi tsalemm* (*Jasminum abyssinicum*), several fruits, especially of the *endod* (*Phytolacca dodecandra*), a half-handful of the root of the *tirraha* (*Verbascum ternacha*), leaves of the *haffa falo* (*Pirconia abyssinica*), tips of the *matari* or *amfar* (*Haffa falo polystacha*), the powdered leaves, flowers, and fruit of the *Euphorbia handukduk*, and a small piece of the root of the *Euphorbia andandash* or *Euphorbia depauperata*, or, occasionally, of the *Eudor-dorken* (*Euphorbia petitiana* or *schimperiana*).

Opinions as to the *kosso*'s medicinal value differed. Rüppell thought that it might be found a purge of great value in Europe, and a number of French and other doctors encouraged by Rochet d'Héricourt adopted it in the treatment of tapeworm, which was then common in both France and England. *Kosso* flowers to a value of 200 Maria Theresa thalers were exported through Massawa in 1840. Most observers of the drug, however, were more critical of it. Kirk, who believed that its frequent use resulted in prolapsus ani (protrusion of the rectum), exhaustion, and sometimes death, believed that it "must shorten the natural period of existence." Johnston, who considered it a "vile drastic cathartic," observed that it occasioned "frequent miscarriages, often fatal to the mother," and that men had "been known, after a large dose, to have died the same time from its consequences." Plowden thought that repeated dosing was "exhausting on some constitutions." De Cosson told of a soldier who "had taken his dose of *kousso* in the morning, and before twelve hours had elapsed . . . was dead from weakness." Mérab, no superficial observer, agreed that the effects of drinking *kosso* were sometimes "absolutely disastrous," for it often produced gastritis and had fatal consequences. Actual cases are on record. The early twentieth-century noble Ras Nadew and the latter's wife both died, according to Bartleet, from overdoses of the drug, while Tereffe Walda Tsadiq, a modern Ethiopian scholar, recorded that Mardasa Joté, a ruler of Walaga, passed away "one day after taking *kosso*."

Emperor Menilek, conscious of such problems, was said to have advised the preparation of a milder and more pleasant type of *kosso*. According to Keller, the emperor, noticing that honey produced by bees who visited flowering *kosso* trees had a peculiar character, surmised that this type of honey would be useful as a taenicide. Nothing came of the idea, however, and the population at large continued, like their forebears, to rely on frequent doses of this extremely bitter and far from satisfactory drug.

Other Taenicides

Though *kosso* was widely available over much of the country, many patients employed other types of taenicide, largely, as Johnston noted, "to escape" the "punishment" inflicted by *kosso*. A score of such medicines can be identified.

One of the most popular was made from the bulb *Oxalis anthelmintica*, known in Amharic as *michamicho* or *ya yefat qetal* and in Tigrinya as *abba chego*. This drug, which Courbon considered much superior to *kosso*, was in Plowden's opinion "agreeable to the palate," but "not strong enough to be certain in its effects". The bulb, like most other taenicides, was used in a number of different ways. It might be chewed in the mouth, crushed on a stone and drunk with beer or mead, eaten with lentil purée, or grilled on a hot iron or in the cinders of a fire. The normal dose consisted of almost sixty grams, and patients were required to abstain from all food while taking the cure. An unusual feature of this medicine was that it was slow to take effect; according to Petit, no less than twelve to fifteen hours were required before an evacuation occurred.

Another much favored taenicide was made from the powdered bark of the *mesanna* (*Albizzia anthelmintica*) or *besanna* (*Croton mascrostachys*) trees, which, though botanically different, had similar properties and were therefore often confused. The medicine was made from their bark, which, according to Yohannes Walda Gerima, would be dried in the sun and then "either pounded or ground until it became a powder," after which it was eaten in gruel or with bread or drunk with water." The drug had the reputation, according to Plowden, of being milder than *kosso*, though its results were still "somewhat violent" and were felt for several days, "frequently attended by rheumatic pains and, for twenty-four hours, with weakness and constant thirst." Schimper, writing specifically of the *Croton mascrostachys* (known in Tigrinya as *ambukh* or *tambuk*), stated that it was, however, little more than a laxative, and effective as a taenicide only if mixed with *kosso*. Mérab, though stating that it sometimes produced violent pains, nevertheless claimed that this drug was often successful, and usually ejected the tapeworm in three or four hours without any inconvenience, while the later Italian scholar Baldrati considered it much safer than *kosso*. Another advantage of the *mesanna/besanna* was that it was almost tasteless, though difficult to swallow. It could moreover be taken without the necessity of abstaining from food; on the contrary, "free living" and the drinking of "ripe or well fermented mead" was said to Plowden to have been recommended.

This medicine was taken with honey, butter, linseed oil, mead, beer, or even water, or might be added to flour in the making of bread. Two teaspoonfuls, according to Plowden, constituted a sufficient dose for a person unaccustomed to this drug, but Courbon wrote of two handfuls, or about 60 grams, as an average dose.

The *Maesa picta* or *lanceolata* (variously known in Ethiopia as *soaria, kella, kelhoa* and *kalaba*) was also used as a taenicide. It, too, was administered in various ways. Johnston stated that the berries were usually eaten by themselves, but Schimper said they were often powdered and mixed with cream cheese or bean or pea puree, 32 or 44 grams comprising an average dose. This medicine, Baldrati recorded, could be purchased in many local markets of Eritrea.

The *Myrsine africana* (in Amharic *qachamo* or *fealfej* and in Tigrinya *zadsé* or *zosso*) was also a highly regarded taenicide. The medicinal properties were found in the fruit, which, according to Mérab, would be crushed between two stones and the resultant paste drunk in water; a normal dose, according to Fournier, was 15 to 20 grams.

Persons with a tendency to diarrhoea, according to Schimper, often preferred to take a medicine made from the seeds of the *Embelia schimperi* or *Combretum acuelatum* (known in Amharic and Tigrinya as *enqoqqo*). This was a climbing plant with red berries, which Johnston saw in a forest at the foot of Qundi hill near Ankobar, and which in the early twentieth century was reported by Azais and Chambard to have been on sale at most Ethiopian markets. This taenicide, which was first mentioned by Prutky in the eighteenth century, had the advantage of being almost tasteless. It was therefore often mixed with honey or pieces of bread and given to children who would have refused *kosso*. The *enqoqqo* had moreover a particularly good reputation. The nineteenth-century missionary Stern described it as an "infallible antidote" for taenia, while Mérab stated that it was often taken by persons who had failed to get rid of a tapeworm by means of *kosso* and that it had no side effects. Yohannes Walda Gerima dissented, however, claiming that the drug was "very strong and at times dangerous." Several modes of preparation were employed. Johnston stated that the berries were "swallowed whole, like pills," and a "very great number" were required "to produce the desired results." Mérab, on the other hand, said that the seeds—two doses of which could be obtained for a piaster—would be boiled for two or three hours, after which they would be crushed and mixed with water. Yohannes Walda Gerima noted that a handful of dry seeds would be removed from their husks and broken, the semi-ground seeds then soaked in beer or mead for a night or so, after which the solution was filtered and drunk before breakfast. Whole seeds were sometimes employed, which stopped the liquid from reaching the kernel, thereby preventing the potion from becoming very strong.

The *Jasminum abyssinicum* (in Amharic *tambalal* and in Tigrinya *habi tsalem*) was also much favored. Its leaves, according to Courbon, would be ground between two stones and mixed with water to produce a medicine which was then drunk.

The *Celosia anthelmintica* (known in Amharic as *belbilla* or *belbelto*) appears to have been particularly potent, for its leaves, flowers, and fruit, according to Schimper, were all used. The early nineteenth-century French travelers Ferret and Galiner, however, described this medicine as "dangerous" and liable to produce acute pain.

The *Punica granatum* or pomegranate (known in Amharic and Tigrinya as *roman*) was held by many to be the best of all taenicides. Where possible it was made from the roots, 30 to 40 grams of which, according to Fournier, would be boiled in a liter of water. Because of the difficulty of obtaining the roots—which necessitated the destruction of the tree—they were used only by important persons, among whom they were very highly rated, for, according to Mérab, it was believed that they ejected the parasite whole. Most people, however, were obliged to make do with a medicine brewed from the bark and branches of the tree and from the pith of the fruit.

The roots of the *Silene macrosolens* (in Amharic *waggart* and in Tigrinya *ogkert* or *sara sara*) were also highly regarded. They were said by Mérab to have been considered also as one of the most effective taenicides. The normal dose consisted of five or six pieces crushed with oil-seeds and then mixed with water.

Other popular taenicides were made from the fruit of the *Albizia gummifera* (known in Tigrinya as *kachiona*), the *Buddleja polystrachya*, called in Amharic *amfar* and in Tigrinya *matari*), the leaves and bark of which were also used, the fruit of the *Mollugo glinus* (known in Tigrinya as *kossala*), and the seeds of the pumpkin *Cucurbita maxima* (locally called *dubba*) and, much more rarely, of the soap tree *Phytolacca dodecandra* (in Amharic *endod* and in Tigrinya *shebti*). The dosage of this last plant, according to Fournier, was about seven fruit. The root of the *Verbascum ternacha* (known in Amharic as *tirraha* and in Tigrinya as *zengé adghi*) was also used, often, according to Fournier, mixed with *kosso*. Other taenicides which are recorded, but with little data, include the flower of the *sangla*, reported by the Armenian traveler Dimothéos as growing largely in Lasta, the *semezza* or *semala* (*Adhatoda schimperiana*?), the *katsam* reported by Parisis, and the *ya faras zang* (*Leonotis rugosa*) listed by Lemordant.

The above drugs, it will be perceived, all come from the vegetable kingdom. There is evidence of only two other types of taenicide. One was *tasma kosso*, the wax of a type of bee which lived in the ground, which was traditionally mixed with chick-pea flour and shaped into small pills, seven of which constituted a single dose. This medicine was so strong, according to Mérab, that overdoses could be fatal. The other nonvegetable cure was thermal water which Massaia testified was drunk in Kaffa as a cure for tapeworm.

Despite this considerable variety of taenicides, *kosso* remained secure as the country's principal drug for the treatment of tapeworm. None of these medicines, however,—not even *kosso*—were able to substantially decrease the incidence which accordingly has been described as the classical disease of Ethiopia.

XI

Traditional Medicine and Surgery

Our knowledge of traditional medicine and surgery in Ethiopia owes much to the existence of a small but important corpus of medicoreligious and medicomagical literature, written in both Ge'ez and Amharic, dating back at least to the second half of the eighteenth century and containing thousands of prescriptions for a wide range of diseases.

This literature often makes no clear distinction between its medical and extramedical aspects. Diseases are thus treated as scarcely different from any of the other problems of human existence. An early twentieth-century medical text written by a *dabtara* (or lay cleric) of Entotto thus contains not only prescriptions for the treatment of epilepsy, fever, syphilis, rabies, skin disease, kidney trouble, hemorrhoids, constipation, diarrhoea, dysuria, itching, coughing, snoring, and sterility, but also magic formulas to assist in dealing with such varied concerns as averting the evil eye, overcoming demons and other evil spirits, defeating the machinations of human enemies, escaping arrest or prison, preventing the escape of slaves, acquiring money and royal honors, learning to play the harp, and obtaining a long life, clear sight, good memory, a large family, and a faithful wife.

A methodological difficulty with Ethiopian medicoreligious/medicomagical literature is that it is impossible to tell how far the treatments recommended in it were in fact followed by the population at large. To obtain even a rough picture of the actual medical practice of the past, one therefore has to draw also on the writings of foreign travelers, which, though in a sense less authentic than the local texts, have the advantage of describing cures actually employed rather than those merely recommended. It is significant in this connection that several traditional practices, including bleeding and cupping, variolation, cautery and bone-setting, as well as the use of steam and thermal baths, are described in the travel literature but do not figure in the local texts.

Methods of Prevention

Traditional medicine in Ethiopia in many cases was concerned with both the prevention and the cure of disease. Well aware of the infectious character of many diseases the Ethiopians, as we have seen, took steps to control the spread of epidemics, above all of smallpox, cholera, typhus and influenza. At such times, as explained in earlier chapters, people were prevented from traveling from areas of infection to other parts of the country.

Precautions against the spread of cattle disease were likewise recorded. A British traveler, the Earl of Mayo, reported that when advancing inland from Massawa in the 1870s he was prevented from entering Asmara so as "to stop our baggage-bullocks from coming any further than the top of the hills." On enquiring as to the reasons for this action he learned that "there was cattle disease among the herds of the Shoho . . . , and an order had been issued all through Abyssinia that no cattle were to travel, or be allowed to go to or from infected districts." Impressed by this regulation, he commented: "This is worthy of the notice of our sanitary commissioners at home."

Flight from disease, as noted on a number of occasions on previous pages, was also a traditional practice, substantiating Ludolf's assertion that on the outbreak of a pestilence people often retired to the mountains, "putting all their security in flying from the contagion."

In the case of smallpox reference has also been made to the "draconian policy," whereby certain groups of the population were reported to have attempted to prevent the spread of infection either by burning the sick alive in their own houses or by leaving them to be consumed by hyenas.

Inoculation

The principle of inoculation, as seen in Chapter III, was important in the traditional treatment of smallpox, but was also attempted, as we have seen, in the cure of rabies.

The Traditional Pharmacopeia

The traditional Ethiopian pharmacopeia, which was extensive, came, as already suggested, mainly from the vegetable kingdom, and comprised the leaves, flowers, seeds, bark, sap, and roots of a wide variety of plants. The animal kingdom provided four main articles of medicine: honey, butter, sheep's fat, and certain insects with medicinal properties. Honey was used in the treatment of colds and sore throats, as Pearce and Johnston both reported. Melted butter served as a specific against smallpox, malaria, and other complaints and, according to Plowden, was considered to possess "the greatest virtues." Much use of butter was also made by the Somalis of Lugh in dealing with sore eyes, according to Bottego. The fat of the sheep's tail was likewise highly regarded by the Somalis, who were said by Burton to have employed it for a wide range of complaints. Several types of beetle, as we have seen, were considered valuable in the treatment of rabies. The principal medicines drawn from the mineral kingdom consisted of dross (produced in the melting of iron), which, as Kirk noted, was often applied in the care of ulcers, and certain earths used in the treatment of syphilis, as earlier noted. Thermal waters, as shown in the following chapter, also played a major role in traditional treatment.

Counterirritation

The principle of counterirritation was extensively used. It was a "very favourite practice," according to Johnston, and often proved "very efficacious." In treating inflammation of the lungs, several small burns would be made on the chest either with a red-hot iron or a piece of burning charcoal. This treatment was also "widely employed" as a cure for rheumatism, which was common in the highlands of Shawa where people frequently displayed their scars to indicate the extent to which they had suffered from this complaint. The above cure for rheumatism was also recorded by both Kirk and the Earl of Mayo, who saw it carried out with either a piece of burning wood or a rag which was made to smoulder over the affected part, and by De Cosson, a British traveler of the 1870s, who stated that hollow reeds would be applied to the skin and then filled with boiling butter. Such practices were so widespread that at the end of the century the Russian physician Glinskii reported from Harar that almost all the patients his compatriots treated were "mottled with scars" resulting from burning of this kind.

Similar treatment was common in the Somali area. Burton, Revoil, and Robecchi-Bricchetti all described counterirritation by burning as one of the main nineteenth-century cures. Drake-Brockman, who confirmed that the principle seemed to be "the panacea for most internal complaints," likewise stated in the early twentieth century that it was "a rare sight" to find an adult whose body was not "decorated with an elaborate pattern of scar tissue." Jennings, his contemporary, went further, declaring that "one could often tell a man's medical history from the site and number of scars."

Counterirritation was also used in early nineteenth-century Tegré in cases of gangrenous amygdalitis, for which, according to Dr. Petit, pepper was sometimes applied.

Cautery

Cautery was widely practiced to disinfect skin and to prevent bleeding, as well as in the treatment of snake, scorpion, and other bites, as noted by Harrison Smith and De Castro.

An interesting use of cautery in the treatment of rupture was reported by Johnston, who witnessed it in early nineteenth-century Shawa. He related that he was taken to see a sixteen-year-old youth who was afflicted with a rupture of the groin. Being unable to do anything for lack of trusses, he merely recommended rest and the avoidance of violent exertion. The boy's family, however, decided upon the traditional treatment: the youth was laid on his back on the bed and held down by strong hands. The father then took a burning stick, and placed it on the diseased part, blowing vigorously all the time to keep it alight. The painful operation was over in less than a minute. The patient, who had previously been reminded that he was a man, bore the ordeal with great fortitude. Ruptures treated in this manner, it was popularly believed, did not recur, and Johnston considered this quite possible as the operation resulted in a great contraction of the muscles.

Bleeding and Cupping

Bleeding and cupping were both common traditional practices. The former was first mentioned in the eighteenth century by the Czech traveler Prutky, who recalled that the Ethiopians, "if urged by great necessity," would "make little knives of iron" with which they would "cut the middle veins on the leg—as they would cut the throat of a chicken," and then "sprinkle them with powder," presumably to arrest the flow of blood. A century later, Mansfield Parkyns recalled that bleeding was frequently carried out in cases of headache and similar complaints. The patient would be asked to place his hands one behind each ear whereupon a tourniquet made of a piece of rag would be wound around his neck and wrist and tightly compressed by means of a small stick. As soon as the veins of the forehead began to swell a razor would be filliped across the eyebrow, whereupon the blood would gush out in a stream to a distance of three or four feet. De Castro, describing similar operations in the early twentieth century, confirmed that the cut was usually made on the temple or nape of the neck, and that, where no better instrument was available, a sharp piece of broken bottle might be used.

The practice of cupping, which, according to Plowden, was considered useful in the treatment of rheumatism, was described by numerous writers. It was effected by means of a cow's horn perhaps four inches long with a hole at the end. The skin of the patient's forehead, according to Parkyns, would be held between the thumb and forefinger of the left hand of the practitioner, who then with his right hand would cut a gash a half-inch long with a razor. Johnston, who was himself operated upon, says that his hair was shaved off in a circle, whereupon his servant, who carried out the operation, gave three jerking cuts with a sharp razor, placed the horn on the skin and began to suck at the thin end of the horn. After a few minutes the ascending surface of blood, seen through the semitransparent horn, indicated that sufficient had been extracted, and the instrument was withdrawn, "the whole operation having been performed by these simple means as speedily and effectually as with the most expensive."

Such practices, according to Courbon, might result in the extraction of 100 to 150 grams of blood at a time.

Surgery

Simple and even advanced operations were practiced fairly extensively and with a certain amount of success. The nineteenth-century Italian missionary De Jacobis asserted that the Ethiopians "excelled in surgery" and gave proof of a "skill and courage" which was "truly amazing," while early in the following century Jennings wrote that the methods of traditional practitioners were "rude," but "sometimes ingenious."

Tonsilitis, according to Petit and Kirk, was treated by persons who allowed the nail of the index finger to grow long for the purpose; the inflamed tonsil was either scarified, or, if greatly swollen, extracted completely. The uvula, Harris and De Castro asserted, was likewise often removed, by means of a loop of thread or horse hair, which would be placed around it and tightened. More complicated apparatus was also sometimes used: De Castro reported that the organ was sometimes held in a metal hook and then cut off with a small knife; alternatively, two pieces of wood were sometimes fixed together to produce a kind of pincers.

Numerous operations on the intestines—many necessitated by spear wounds—were also reported. These procedures were often carried out with the aid of a gourd into which the intestines, Kirk stated, would be temporarily placed before being reintroduced into the stomach. A particularly remarkable operation in which a patient operated on himself was described by De Jacobis. He stated that the man "first filled a wooden bowl with butter, which he covered with a bladder, like a very fine net, of a cow recently killed. Then, sitting down on the ground, he opened the lower stomach with a razor, took out his intestines and placed them in the net, which was still hot, cleaned them, and placing them carefully back in their proper place. He then sewed up the wound, and lying down on his back, took as little food as possible till the wound was healed, and a complete cure effected."

Wounds, according to Kirk, would normally be stitched up with needle and thread, though alternatively the skin might be held together with thread tied to thorns pinned an inch or two apart.

Considerable skill was displayed in amputation, which was carried out not only for medicinal reasons but also as a punishment for severe crimes, including theft. Such operations, which were often performed with knives 18 centimeters long by 3 centimeters wide, were accomplished with dexterity, almost according to the rules of European surgery, Courbon states. First the skin would be cut, then the tendons, and finally the ligaments. The wound would then be either cauterized with hot irons or covered with leaves, cinders, or other powder. Boyes, one of the few eyewitnesses to leave an account of an amputation, stated that the traditional surgeon made "a good job of the operation," and exclaimed: "I was fascinated. I was rooted to the spot. I could not move until the job was finished. There was no excitement, they were all chatting as if nothing was happening. . . . As soon as the operation was over the stump was dipped in the pot of boiling fat to stop the bleeding."

Bone Setting

Bone setting was also performed, often with a high measure of success. Recent dislocations, according to Kirk, were corrected with the aid of a poultice made of the undigested contents of a sheep's stomach bound up in medicinal leaves. In more serious cases use was made of splints of wood or bone, tied with either cloth or leather, as reported by Kirk, Harris, Plowden, Glinskii, and others. Plates of copper, lead, and iron, according to Glinskii, were also in use in Harar. Even more difficult operations were mentioned by Kirk, who was told in Shawa that when a person's skull was fractured pieces of bone from sheep or goats were used as replacements. Practitioners in the Agamé area of Tegré were said by Plowden to have carried out trepanning, as well as Cesarean childbirth, and the enterostomy for removal of excess fat.

The Somalis were also reputedly excellent bone setters. Fractures when set were supported with twigs and reeds woven together, and some local surgeons, according to Jennings, were able to insert sheep's bones into the human frame.

Dentistry

Dentistry, doubtless because of the healthy character of Ethiopian teeth, was not as developed as other branches of medicine. Thus the typical dental instruments of early nineteenth-century Shawa, Harris stated, were more reminiscent of the blacksmith than of the English dentist's chair. In fact, according to Kirk, they consisted of little more than "blacksmith's pincers," and if these failed to extract an infected tooth it would be knocked out with a stone and nail. In some cases of toothache, however, the patient was often made to chew a small bag containing medicinal leaves.

Emphasis on the Supernatural

Great expectations were focused on the supernatural. There were innumerable prayers for the prevention or cure of disease. Some dealt with specific complaints, among them smallpox, epilepsy, dysentery, jaundice, rheumatism, malaria, colic, ulcers, pimples, and infection of wounds, while others focused on the parts of the body affected. A typical prayer was one imploring Christ in the widest possible terms to save the person who utters it from "the illness of man and woman, the illness of the liver and the loins, the illness of the hand and the foot, of the kidney, the bones and the fingers, the illness of the head, teeth and ears, the illness of the mouth, the nose, the throat, the teeth and the tongue, the illness of the body and the bones and intestines," etc.

Supernatural intervention was also sought in other ways. Emperor Zara Ya'qob (1434–1468), when faced with an epidemic, it will be recalled, was said to have built a church by his palace at Dabra Berhan, as it was believed that "there would be no plague, drought or death near a shrine." Three centuries later, as we have seen, Bruce told of a monk at Gondar who wrote on a tin plate holy words which where then washed off and given, to the patient to drink. An entirely different, but no more scientific, treatment was reported in the nineteenth century by Dr. Blanc, who stated that cholera victims were expected to eat seven grapes blessed by a priest who would at the same time pray for the patient's health.

Magical texts of all kinds enjoyed great popularity. The people of early nineteenth-century Shawa placed "more reliance" on the "efficacy of charms, spells and amulets", Kirk declared, than on actual medical treatment. Johnston, who concurred in this judgement, observed that the Ethiopians had great faith in "mysterious ceremonies" and "absurd formulae" inscribed on small pieces of parchment enclosed in red leather amulets worn around the left arm of a man or the neck of a woman. Such charms, according to Harris, were worn by "all ranks of both sexes," who were "loaded with amulets and talismans against every disease." Amulets, Kirk stated, were sometimes sold by *dabtaras* for as much as ten Maria Theresa thalers each. Red coral, sea shells, and the like were also carried on the wrist or the ankle, and were supposed to have protective powers against all sorts of complaints, including both rheumatism and possession by demons, according to Johnston. Almost a century later the French scholar Michel Leiris noted that the common people attributed most illnesses to "supernatural causes, evil eyes, spells, action of this or that spirit, etc." Magical remedies were "the most frequently used of all cures," and the sale of amulets consequently was one of the "most lucrative" professions.

Cures, it was generally believed, could also be effected by visits to religious centers or by immersion in holy water, which was found in the vicinity of most of the more important churches and monasteries. Among the most popular of such sites were those of Dabra Libanos and Mount Zeqwala in Shawa and Qeddus Mika'él in Tambén.

Magic, as indicated in earlier chapters, also played a considerable role in the traditional treatment of disease. Male creatures were not allowed in the vicinity of a smallpox patient, because, as we have seen, it was widely believed that the act of sexual intercourse even by animals and birds would cause the Devil to bring "the shadow of sin" upon the patient.

Often, prescriptions of an essentially medical character also incorporated appeals to the Almighty. The Entotto *dabtara*'s book, for example, contains a medical prescription for the treatment of syphilis, smallpox, and certain other diseases in which the reader, after being told which roots and plants to mix together, is exhorted to declare: "Glory to the heavens." An element of superstition was likewise embodied in one of the ritual methods of preparing *kosso* in which, as described in a previous chapter, a "naked sword" was placed on the ground and the practitioner walked around the taenicide three times reciting a prayer.

Surgery, though perhaps less influenced than medicine by nonscientific ideas, was not always entirely free of them. The case was thus reported by Pearce of a person with a swelling which was operated upon: the kernel was duly extracted—only to be ground into powder, and worn as a charm around the patient's neck.

Notwithstanding such admixtures of superstition, traditional Ethiopian medical and surgical practice was far from arbitrary. Many practices, on the contrary, were demonstrably successful and were based on more than a modicum of good sense.

XII

Thermal Baths

Thermal springs, which owing to the former volcanic activity are found in many parts of Ethiopia, were long recognized as of value in the treatment of rheumatism, skin disease, syphilis, leprosy, and other complaints.

The early history of Ethiopia's thermal baths is poorly documented, partly because they did not attract the attention of the Portuguese travelers of the sixteenth and seventeenth centuries and partly because they are not mentioned in the country's medicomagical writings. The first indication of a probably much older use of such baths is to be found in the eighteenth century writings of James Bruce, who told of several courtiers visiting the "hot wells" of Lebec, where a nobleman suffering from leprosy went "every year once, sometimes twice." The significance of the country's "numerous" thermal sources was later noted by many observers, among them the mid-nineteenth-century British consul Plowden, who observed that they were:

> generally supposed to be efficacious in cases of rheumatism, wounds, ague, the venereal disease, and of altogether salutary tendency, as after a fatiguing campaign and for delicate females.

Geographical Location and Temperature

Thermal springs, which Ethiopians sometimes referred to as *hammam* (the Arabic term for a steam bath), were found throughout the region. Some of the most important were in the north-west, between Lake Tana and Dabra Tabor. Four sites were particularly renowned: Wanzagay by the Gumara river in the district of Fogara; Guramba, a day's journey from Dabra Tabor; the lakeside town of Qorata; and May Cholot in the vicinity of Gondar. Gojjam and Wallo both also had several notable springs. The most patronized in Gojjam were at Achafer, Agitta, Dambacha, and Buré, and in Wallo at Barbaré Waha in the district of Ambasel, and in Warra Ilu. The Rift Valley was even more richly endowed. The most famous thermal sources in the north were at Aylet, 30 miles south of Massawa, and at nearby Ali Hasa. Springs further south included those at Felamba (which in Amharic signified "Boiling Mountain"), in the vicinity of Ankobar, and at Felwaha (or "Boiling Water"), also known as Finfini, later a suburb of Addis Ababa. Further south and east were the waters of Bilen in the Awash basin, several springs in the Afar lowlands, and at Artu (called after the Oromo word for "Smoke"), as well as others by the Gildessa river, and at Erer to the west of it. There were also a number of much frequented springs in the far west and south, which included one called Felwaha in Kambata, two within five kilometers of each other in Kaffa, and one at Mount Jannissa near Lake Stephanie and the Kenya frontier.

The temperature of these waters was "invariably high," frequently between 49° and 60° Centigrade. The spring at Aylet, which gushed forth at 60°, was "so warm," Wylde noted, that one could not "put one's hand in with comfort," while that in Kambata, according to Captain Wellby, produced so much steam that it seemed as if the surrounding grass "had been set on fire."

Curative Reputation

The curative value of such thermal springs, according to foreign travelers, was widely recognized. The waters of Aylet were reputed to have "wonderful effects," while those at Dabamata were considered a "marvellous panacea." The sources of Gojjam were supposed to be "very efficacious" and those of Wallo to possess the "maximum medical qualities," while those of Felamba were said to have the "highest sensitive virtues." The Afars likewise spoke with "absolute conviction" of the "infallible virtue" of thermal water in "curing all diseases," while the spring at Gildessa was "much resorted to by the natives" who had "great faith" in its "healing powers," and the "marvellous thermal waters" of Kaffa were "held in high estimation" by innumerable persons who flocked to them.

Diseases Treated

Thermal springs were reputed to be of value for a wide range of disorders, most notably rheumatism, skin diseases, syphilis, and leprosy. The source at Aylet was thus famed in the cure of "all skin diseases, rheumatism and many other complaints" and was frequently visited by patients suffering from venereal diseases, rheumatism, dysentery, and fever. The waters of Achefer were believed "very efficacious against rheumatic pains," while those by the Gumara river were used by people with skin complaints, syphilis, leprosy and other contagious diseases. The baths at Felamba, according to the early nineteenth-century British envoy Captain Harris were frequented by patients afflicted with "syphilis, the curse of Abyssinia" and with "cutaneous eruptions of the skin, green wounds, discharging ulcers and putrid sores." The waters of Artu served people with "rheumatism, arthritis and who knows what other complaints," and those of Haulle attracted sufferers of rheumatism and skin troubles of all kinds. The sources of Kaffa were similarly renowned for cure of a wide range of diseases, from articular complaints to leprosy. Persons afflicted with the latter disease were a common sight at many baths, such as those at Kambata, where Lord Hindlip saw "several lepers, chiefly women," whose appearance he found "hardly pleasant, for toes and fingers were conspicuous by their absence."

Thermal Cures

Thermal waters were traditionally employed both for immersion and for drinking. Bathers sought to spend "as long as possible in the water," and it was the custom to remain at the pools "either seven days or fourteen." People at the springs near the Red Sea coast declared that for the cure to be efficacious it was necessary to bathe every day for seven days and to enter the water seven times each day. After each immersion patients would take a light meal and drink a cup of coffee, and after the seventh they would dress and rest in the shade. Bathers by the Gumara river similarly would resort to the springs for exactly a week. It was widely held that after seven days the water's efficacy was neutralized and that anyone delaying his or her departure ran the risk of being visited by the Nedatitu, whom the Protestant missionary Stern described as "a race of graceless female Genii, who riot in carnage, and are reported to feast on human flesh."

Patients often spent the entire day submerged in thermal baths, with the water up to their necks, as noted at both Dabamata and Kambata, while at Gumara, the German traveler Stecker reported, it was normal practice to stay in the water for seven hours at a time. Bathing was so popular that the Italian scholar Cerulli's servant, who had been prescribed three immersions in one of the Kaffa pools, insisted on undergoing all three on a single day—and at the hottest possible temperature.

During their stay at the baths patients would also drink large quantities of thermal water, usually through a spout leading from the source, as at Guramba and Felamba. The water, which had "a very pleasant though peculiar flavour," was often taken with "copious draughts of honey, water and linseed." All this induced considerable perspiration.

Traditional Bathing Establishments

Thermal springs frequently were under the supervision of the local *shum* (or chief) of the area in which they were situated. Access to the water was free in most cases, though persons visiting the sources at Felamba in the early nineteenth century were obliged to pay a per capita fee of one *amolé* (or bar of salt).

Most pools were of natural origin, some having been formed "out of the rocky bed of the stream by the natural wearing away of the rock," as Wylde observed of those at Aylet. Others, however, were excavated by man. In some cases the thermal waters bubbled up directly into the pool, in others they were brought to it, often through a hollow bamboo. Water which was too hot at its source would usually be allowed to cool before it was utilized, though in some pools this was done by dilution with cold water from a nearby spring or river. Most bathing establishments consisted of two or three pools, usually reserved for different categories of patients.

Thermal pools chosen for bathing would often be covered with a hutlike structure, made of either straw or branches, which served both to protect patients from the sun and preserve the water's heat. This produced a steam-bath environment in which patients sweated profusely. Sudation (or sweating) in fact was an important feature of the cure—as in the *wesheba* (or Turkish baths), which, as we shall see, were also widely used for a time in the treatment of syphilis.

Many pools had an open space set aside for the bathers' possessions. At May Cholot for example there was an area where persons took off their clothes, as well as their *matab*s (or neck-cords worn by Ethiopian Christians), which would be placed on flat stones or in gourds or pot sherds before their owners entered the pool.

Perhaps the best account of an old-style Ethiopian bathing establishment was written by Plowden about his visit to the famous springs of Guramba in 1844 in the company of the French traveler Arnauld d'Abbadie. These springs had two bathing places, both covered. In the principal one the water flowed through a hollow bamboo into a pool ten feet in diameter and two or two and a half feet deep which was covered by an "elegant hut." The second pool was no more than "a ditch formed by the surplus waters of the upper basin." The structure over the main pool was the size of an ordinary hut and was "loosely built of grass and sticks." It was "a little doorway about three feet high" so that one side was "open to the rain, the wind and even to the gaze of spectators."

On entering this building Plowden at once found himself in the pool, and observed:

> the plunge from the cold air up to the knees in water of 127° Fahr. may be imagined. Had it not been for the very shame, I should have withdrawn my legs as rapidly as I had immersed them; but my cloth was already whipped off by an attendant, and I had only the choice between a desperate fire of laughter, and a cauldron of almost boiling water.

The inside of the hut into which the consul and his party were crowded "like herrings" was, according to d'Abbadie, "as dark as an oven." The consul, gritting his teeth on account of the heat, nevertheless succeeded in groping his way to a couch made of sticks, situated just above the level of the water. There he examined his limbs, which by then resembled "underdone beef." However, "by dipping in a finger and a toe at a time" he "gradually became used to the heat" so that in due course he was able to hold his entire body under the water for a minute at a time, and later even place his head under the spout through which the water poured into the pool. In this way he "remained stewing for nearly an hour." During this time he followed the well-established practice of drinking a considerable amount of thermal water through the spout. The resultant perspiration produced a "feeling of cleanliness, and also of languor" which was "pleasant enough," though he did not believe the experience "good for people in health."

The bath was used by persons of both sexes "promiscuously." The "greatest decorum" nevertheless prevailed. Husbands and wives lived entirely separated throughout the period of the cure, and it was "universally believed" that, should any "impure" person (i.e., one who had recently had sexual intercourse) enter the bath, a "large snake" would "issue from the spout."

The bathing establishment at Wanzagay, where the thermal water shot up in a jet "two or three metres from the ground," was essentially similar. There were two separate pools, each covered by "kennel-like structures," as Stern noted in the 1860s. At the main pool "large volumes" of water, brought from the source by means of a "hollow bamboo," were collected in a basin two feet deep, covered by "a small insignificant building." The other pool was "a little lower down." These twin baths, which reminded him of the biblical pool of Bethesda (John 5:1–9), were "continually surrounded" by "most haggard and ghastly" looking patients. Some "squatted on the bare soil, some lay at full length in the sun's fierce rays, and some leaned their aching frame for support against a rough stone or the trunk of a decayed tree." Though many of these "helpless creatures" were suffering from "incurable" maladies, they all watched with "cadaverous eyes" and "intense anguish" for a "vacancy" in the two "ever-filled" huts, the "objects of their longing desire." Stecker, who visited Wanzagay a generation later, drew a less lugubrious picture. Likening the establishment to those at Ostend or Trouville, he stated that "women and men, youths and girls" spent their time in "lively promiscuity" and "kept up an intercourse which was not always decorous." Quarrels often arose among the patients, "especially when some one had used the baths longer than is permitted to him." From early morning till late at night, therefore, one could hear the loud tones of the brawlers. Silence, added Stecker, did not return even with nightfall, for, because of the number of patients, the air resounded with the "devilish noise" of women singing and clapping, while the giant frogs in the Gumara river croaked loudly and many donkeys and mules added their own accompaniment to a hubbub which came to an end only well after midnight.

Similar establishments were found in the south. The people of Kambata, Hidlip reported, thus had "primitive steam baths" over a thermal rivulet, while near Lake Stephanie an American explorer, Donaldson Smith, saw "what appeared to be an enormous barnyard, with a solid stone floor, and in the centre a bubbling warm spring." Other springs, however, were entirely uncovered. At Aylet, for example, according to Wylde, there were no less than "seven or eight" pools, but patients had "no privacy" in any. They would merely enter the coolest water, furthest from the source, and proceed ever nearer to it, until they reached the uppermost pool, a small cavity which might "at a pinch hold three or four persons." Aylet also had a small graveyard nearby—for patients who failed to recover.

Segregation of the Sick

Almost invariably, persons suffering from different types of disease were segregated. The springs by the Gumara river thus consisted of two separate baths. The first, according to Stern, was occupied by "the lame, the blind and the halt," the second by persons with "scrofulous, scorbutic, leprous and other contagious diseasses" who "had to perform their lavations in an enclosed pool a little lower down" where "they enjoyed the double advantage of getting cool as well as already tested water." Segregation was likewise reported at Guramba, where there were two pools, the first for ordinary bathers and the second, according to Plowden, for "more miserable victims of disease."

The separation of patients sometimes went even further, as at Balidkeme in Wallo, where, according to the French scientific mission of the 1840s, there were three distinct pools. The first was reserved for patients with rheumatism, the second for those with skin diseases (who "entered pell-mell without fear of contagion"), while the third was occupied only by lepers. At Dabamata, in the north, Rohlfs, a later German traveler, likewise saw a large bathing hut used only by lepers. Segregation was practiced even where, as at Felamba, there was only a single pool which, according to Harris, was "partitioned" by a bar of wood into "two cells."

Supernatural Association

Thermal baths, like other forms of medical treatment in Ethiopia, were widely associated with the supernatural. Springs, both hot and cold, in many cases were believed to be of divine origin. The pools by the Gumara river thus were identified with Gannat, or Paradise, as well as with two Ethiopian Christian saints, Qirqos and Takla Haymanot. Local tradition, as recorded by Stern, held that Qirqos, having sprouted wings, was flying in the sky one day when he was attacked by eagles who consumed his body in the air, whereupon his bones fell by the Gumara river and wherever they landed warm healing water gushed forth as a memorial to his benevolence.

Thermal springs throughout the Christian highlands were often called after saints or other religious personalities. At May Cholot there were several separate sources, each of which was given a religious name, such as Madhané Alam (or Saviour of the World) and Kidana Mehret (or Pact of Mercy), as well as St. Michael and St. George. In the same way, the pools at Felamba were named after Selassé (or the Trinity), Maryam (or the Virgin Mary), and two saints, Aragawi and Abbo, while at least one in Kaffa was dedicated to St. Michael.

Thermal waters in non-Christian areas were also often given a religious connotation. A spring near Aleyu Amba was called after the Muslim holy city of Medina. Many people venerated it on account of a large mimosa tree that grew over it, while another source, in Kaffa, was worshipped by a population which paid homage to important rivers and lakes. Perhaps for this reason a spring in Ambasel was spoken of as Jaré, the Oromo word for an evil spirit.

Popularity and Attraction of the Baths

Ethiopia's thermal waters attracted considerable numbers of patients. At Guramba, according to Plowden, "the hum of contending bathers" could be heard "at some distance." There were at any one time about forty persons in the water, with "about a hundred" more awaiting their turn to enter. The source at Dabamata, Rohlfs reported, was attended by "hundreds of patients" and that at Barbaré Waha by "a great crowd of sick people," while at Felamba Harris saw "numbers of dreadfully diseased wretches" whose presence recalled "the scriptural account of the pool of Bethesda." The springs at Bilen, the British ethnographer Powell-Cotton stated, were similarly visited by groups of patients who "came down all day."

Notwithstanding the large number of springs, the populace often had to journey extensively in quest of thermal cures. The source at Aylet near the Red Sea coast was utilized by highlanders from Tegré, who according to Wylde, rode or walked "long distances" to reach it; similarly, the waters of Guramba were visited by people from Lasta, 170 kilometers away. Artu was frequented by patients from Shawa, Harar, and the Somali country, while the baths of Kecho in Kaffa, according to the French missionary Martial de Salviac, drew many persons "from far away in search of health."

The presence of thermal baths sometimes resulted in the emergence of small settlements. There were thus a number of huts in the vicinity of the springs of Guramba and Wanzagay. The latter, Stecker noted, was the only place in the country where he had seen "guest houses, or rather guest huts." A number of dwellings were also reported to be located near several pools in the south, while the springs of Kecho were the site of numerous tents—the abode, Cerulli said, of "an entire population of patients."

Court Life at the Springs

Thermal springs were a constant attraction to the country's rulers, who, when ill or otherwise indisposed, spent weeks at a time relaxing at the baths, with their families, their courtiers, and sometimes their entire army. Since the kings and chiefs were usually accompanied by a large number of relatives and favorites, as well as by innumerable soldiers and camp-followers, there were always many people desiring to take the waters on medical or other grounds. A significant proportion of patients at any one time would be sufferers from venereal diseases, which, as we have seen, were fairly common, particularly in aristocratic circles where chastity was far from the rule.

Early evidence of the custom of visiting thermal sources is found in an Ethiopian chronicle that records that Emperor Takla Giyorgis stopped at the springs of Labat in 1795, and that his successor, Egwala Tseyon, traveled there in 1806. This source was presumably that referred to by Bruce as Lebec, near the Gumara river.

The royal and princely practice of visiting the baths is well documented for the nineteenth century. Ras Ali Alula, the ruler of north-west Ethiopia in the first part of the century, patronized the springs of both Gumara and Guramba. The French travelers Combes and Tamisier reported that the chief and his mother, Empress Manan, traveled to Qorata on the shore of Lake Tana in the 1830s to bathe in a hot spring of Fogara, while Plowden told of the Ras spending a full week at Guramba. Ali's principal chiefs also often took the waters at Guramba, as well as at nearby Agitta. King Sahla Sellasé of Shawa similarly had recourse to the springs at Finfini and, according to the French scientific mission, he usually was accompanied by his entire court. Many nobles, whether ill or merely following their master's example, would drink the thermal water which "purged them immediately," while others washed their wounds and sores in the healing streams.

Emperor Téwodros II was also much interested in thermal baths. According to Stecker, he had a new bathing hut erected over the spring at Wanzagay and had two or three royal villas nearby. The Italian traveler Bianchi described the Emperor's bathing establishment as "quite commodious." A British visitor, Winstanley, was no less impressed. He stated that a space a hundred feet square by the Gumara was surrounded by a twelve foot fence, in the center of which, above the spring, was a "small circular house." The pool, "about thirty feet in circumference and four feet deep," was supplied by a jet of water which rushed up with "considerable force and the steam through an artificial spout, . . . emitting a powerful but not disagreeable odour."

Yohannes IV was not less enthusiastic about taking the waters. When visiting Wallo in 1877 he camped by the springs of Ambasel and returned there in the following year, accompanied by his then vassal King Menilek of Shawa. Yohannes also made use of the baths at Guramba and by the Gumara river. In 1879 he invited Colonel (later General) C.G. Gordon to accompany him to Guramba, where, Gordon recalled, there was "a hot spring coming up through a bamboo in an old hut." Yohannes also used Téwodros' bathing house at Wanzagay. He and his renowned commander Ras Alula were both devotees of the waters, in which they would crouch "for hours daily"—the sovereign because he was "afflicted with rheumatism," Alula for reasons of "court etiquette." The spring's sulphurous smell "permeated" both men, and was "easily perceptible" some yards away.

Menilek also often visited thermal baths. The Italian traveler Chiarini, who witnessed a visit by that emperor to Warru Ilu, recalled the "curious scene" of men and women, perfectly naked, paddling around in a bog formed by the hot water, and, on the monarch's arrival, singing his praises and clapping their hands to keep time.

The Founding of Addis Ababa

The hot springs of Finfini acquired enhanced popularity in the early 1880s when Menilek established his camp on the mountain of Entotto only an hour's ride away. He and his court were soon spending much of their time enjoying the nearby warm water and spoke of the area as Felwaha (literally "boiling water"). Borelli, a French traveler who visited the place a few years later, said it was frequented by courtiers in quest of relaxation as well as by sick persons seeking a cure for scrofula, syphilis, and leprosy.

Menilek's stay at Felwaha was also referred to by the chronicler Gabra Sellasé, who stated that the sovereign and his court relaxed in the warm waters and erected a "large number of tents". The site was so pleasant that Menilek's consort, Queen Taytu, "admiring from the gate of her tent the beauty of the countryside, and noting the softness of the climate, asked the King to give her a place to build a house"—to which her husband at once agreed.

Menilek and his courtiers later rode back to Entotto, but in the following year, 1887, Taytu once more left that settlement and "installed herself in the house which she had erected by the warm springs." The chiefs, in accordance with Ethiopian custom, were then allocated lands around those of their overlord. It was then—and there—that work began on the building of a new town, which, Borelli noted in his diary on November 4, was given the name Addis Ababa (literally "New Flower"). Ethiopia's new capital thus owed its location to the thermal waters of Felwaha.

Menilek's Baths at Felwaha

The hot springs at Felwaha prior to the establishment of Menilek's baths consisted of twelve or thirteen jets. These bubbled up through the mud and formed a number of small pools, which were dispersed over an area of about 100 yards and drained into a nearby stream. Access to the thermal water originally was difficult during the rainy season, when the springs were largely flooded by a neighboring cold rivulet. This, however, did not prevent patients from taking mud baths in the thermal area. The popularity of the springs struck one British visitor, Reginald Koettlitz, who noted in 1899 that they were "much used by the sick and diseased, especially those with rheumatism and skin eruptions." People of both sexes stripped themselves of all their clothing and sat "without any regard for decency in the small mud basins made by the water, choosing those in which the water was less hot, in full public view."

A minor crisis occurred shortly afterwards when Menilek's bathing shed was "swept away in the rains," as Hakim Warqnah noted in his diary on

October 23, 1900. Menilek soon afterwards took steps to divert the course of the cold-water streams and had an embankment built to prevent flooding. A new bathing establishment was then erected. The structure was designed and constructed by Menilek's Armenian craftsman, Sarkis Terzian, whose son recalled that it was of novel design and built with cement strengthened with the whites of hundreds of eggs. The hot water, which gushed forth at the rate of 160 liters a minute, was collected in two deep masonry tanks, each three meters square, built over the main source, about two meters above the ground. Cold spring water from Entotto was brought down by pipe to cool the thermal water, the flow of which was so regulated that the temperature was always "almost as hot as a man could bear."

The building itself was a modest affair, consisting of two rooms, each with a shallow bath and zinc-covered walls. There was also a third, much larger, open-air pool, the steam from which could be seen from a distance. The establishment thus had three sectons. First-class bathing, in the finer of the two rooms, was provided for the emperor and empress, members of their court, and such foreigners (mainly diplomats) as could afford a fee of one Maria Theresa thaler per week. Second-class accommodation was available— at a quarter of the price— in the other room, which might be crowded with as many as thirty men, women, and children. A third-class service was supplied to the poor in the open-air pool free of charge. Water was also conveyed by pipe to several troughs, where it was much sought after for the washing of laundry. An overflow tube led beyond the compound to a nearby field where, on cooling, it was drunk by cattle. The establishment was run on a concession basis, first by an Armenian and later by an Ethiopian nobleman, Tassama Eshaté, under whose management, Mérab stated, receipts rose from 500 or 600 to 2,000 thalers a year.

These baths were a source of great pleasure to the emperor, who, according to Dr. De Castro, visited them at least once a year. They were also frequented by many nobles, who, Mérab said, often erected their tents in the vicinity. The extent of such patronage is apparent from Hakim Warqnah's diary, which contains the following entries:

> *January 31, 1901.* Menilek and Taitu are at Felwaha camping.
> *October 17, 1909.* I went to the hot springs, Muleumebet (a prominent noble-woman) was there. Saw Fit. Habte Giyorgis (the Minister of Trade and Foreign Affairs). He still at Springs undergoing a cure.
> *October 26, 1909.* I went to the springs, Muleumebet there. Water very hot.
> *February 28, 1909.* Went to Felwaha. Saw Hayle Giyorgis there.

Visitors to the baths came, however, from every class. They included, according to Mérab, both the "bourgeoisie" and the poor, as well as peasants from the surrounding countryside who brought their livestock to drink. The bathers, who could be seen at the pools day and night, likewise comprised persons of both sexes and all ages, from infants to very elderly persons.

The establishment at Felwaha, like the Ethiopian baths of former times, was used by patients suffering from a wide range of disease, for its waters were considered effective against neuralgia, rheumatism, arthritis, syphilis, and leprosy. Patients suffering from such complaints were particularly interested in the sudation produced by the hot water and, in the case of fever, affirmed that "the illness went away with the sweat," according to Mérab. He claimed that the baths of Felwaha proved of value to many patients. Persons suffering from syphilis in particular obtained considerable relief, though, he felt, this resulted not from the sulphuric content of the water, as was often thought, but from the sudation produced by its heat and steam.

Menilek's baths, though modern in design and technology, were, it must be emphasized, the expression of an old Ethiopian medical tradition. Patients at Felwaha thus followed essentially the same practice as at the baths of earlier times, and, as Mérab described, would immerse themselves up to the neck, inhale the vapors, and drink the warm thermal water, while invoking the aid of their favorite saint—as their ancestors had done since time immemorial.

The early years of the twentieth century, as we shall see, also witnessed one other development in this field: the establishment of a swimming pool with bathing huts at Ambo, to the west of the capital. Its water, according to a contemporary report, was likewise "very efficacious" for rheumatism and for stomach and liver complaints.

XIII

Wesheba or Steam Baths

◊ ◊ ◊

Despite its relative isolation, Ethiopia was significantly influenced by foreign medical practices, as we shall see. One of the most important areas of innovation was in the treatment of syphilis. Sudorifics, principally sarsaparilla and compounds of mercury, which had revolutionized European medicine during the Renaissance, seem to have reached Ethiopia within, at most, a century of their appearance in Europe. These medicines were largely administered in the form of vapor baths, and were referred to by the generic term *wesheba*, a corruption of the Arabic *khashaba* or *ishaba* (literally, "wood" or "shrub"), the term used for sarsaparilla in the Sudan and elsewhere.

Vapor baths, intended mainly for the treatment of syphilis, seem to have acquired great reputation at Gondar, the Ethiopian capital founded in the early seventeenth century. Bruce, describing the popularity of such treatment, observed: "The common and total regimen in this country has been to keep their patient from feeling the smallest breath of air; hot drink, a fire, and a quantity of covering are added . . . and the doors shut so close as even to keep the room in darkness whilst this heat is further augmented by the constant burning of candles."

Numerous *wesheba* were constructed in the seventeenth and eighteenth centuries at Gondar in the vicinity of its palaces and other imperial structures. One bath lay immediately to the east of the great castle of Emperor Fasilidas (1632–1667), where the ruin of a small stone edifice consisting of three interconnected windowless cubicles, each about two meters square, can still be seen. Beneath one of the cubicles a fireplace and underground flue may still be discerned, while in the roof of another, five small holes some ten centimeters in diameter have been cut into which earthenware tubes were fixed for ventilation. Beside the "lion house" (in which lions are said to have been kept), there is a considerably larger bath comprising one long narrow chamber and half a dozen small interconnected cubicles each about two meters square and devoid of windows. Two rooms have a couple of ventilation holes and tubes in their roof. A third large *wesheba* lies next to the palace of Empress Mentewwab (1730-1775) and consists of five interconnected chambers with a dozen holes in its roof. The ruins of a fourth and still larger *wesheba* stand between the latter edifice and the "lion house." Three further complexes of baths are found near the "bath of Fasilidas," just off the road to the present-day College of Medicine. Each of these *weshebas*, one of which curiously enough was referred to during the Italian fascist occupation as a "chicken house," comprises half a dozen small interconnected windowless chambers, some of them as much as three meters square, each with between one and six ventilation holes in their roof. Several rooms show signs of having been heated from beneath by means of ovens, while others were supplied by a surface trench with water from the nearby Kaha river. In one of the ruined buildings are the remains of a bath about two meters long.

Vapor baths, which served primarily for the treatment of syphilis, continued to be constructed into later times, and the term *wesheba* served as the standard Amharic name for a "medical vapor bath." Early in the century, King Sahla Sellasé of Shawa had one built at his capital, Ankobar. Another royal *wesheba* appears to have been erected towards the end of the century at Emperor Menilek's then capital, Entotto, where its ruins may still be seen. A small building of rough-hewn stones, it had two concentric circular walls, forming an inner chamber two and one-half meters in diameter, and an outer corridor a meter wide. Such buildings primarily served the rulers, their families, and courtiers, among whom there was a high incidence of syphilis; the common people had recourse to simpler alternatives.

Sarsaparilla, the root of the smilax plant from Central America had been introduced in Europe, it may be recalled, as a cure for syphilis in the early sixteenth century; it rapidly gained acceptance also in Ethiopia, as in other parts of the Middle East, and provided one of the main medicaments for the vapor baths.

By the early nineteenth century sarsaparilla was widely used. It was imported into the port of Massawa from the Arabian port of Jeddah and was used by such as could afford it. Many Ethiopians knew the use of sarsaparilla, and many who made the journey to Massawa were careful to obtain a supply. An amount equal to the weight of six Maria Theresa thalers cost one thaler at Massawa, and as the quantity required to complete the cure cost at least twenty thalers, its use was restricted to the wealthy classes.

The physical appearance of sarsaparilla and the manner in which it was administered were described by Pearce. He stated that the drug resembles small brown sticks, or dried stalks of a plant, which, being pounded and made into boluses, the patient swallows six at a time, morning and evening, and is then put into a dark place, where he is laid between two large fires, allowed to eat nothing but cake made of wheat flour without salt, and obliged to drink several large horns of honey and water every day. The sudorific effect of this mode of treatment is beyond conception. After the seven first days the patient leaves off taking the boluses, but still continues to inhale the steam through a hollow cane from a pot on the fire in which some of the medicine is boiling. At the expiration of fourteen days, he is allowed a little meat, and his diet is increased by degrees for forty days, after which he is allowed the air, and gradually goes about until he has entirely recovered his strenth.

Sarsaparilla treatment, though soon abandoned in Europe, continued in Ethiopia throughout the nineteenth century and was still in vogue in the early twentieth. The drug was on sale in Menilek's day in many Addis Ababa stores where 56 grams (or the weight of two Maria Theresa thalers) sold for one thaler, an entire cure costing five or six thalers.

The term *wesheba*, to judge from the Entotto *dabtara*'s textbook, was then used also for the drug itself as well as for the vapor bath. Treatment was often formulated in terms of the magic number seven. The patient thus was advised to grind the *wesheba* sticks into powder, and to mix one *waqét* (or ounce) with two *waqéts* of *qundo barbaré* (or black pepper) and an unspecified amount of honey, the resultant mixture being molded into seven balls. He had to boil one ball each day in milk and *berz*, or in honey and water, and drink this concoction warm, eating only *qita*, or unleavened bread. After seven days he was permitted to see people if he covered his nose, ears, and head, but for the subsequent seven days had to subsist on pepper and ginger stew, and drink only warm *berz* and milk. Fumigation was likewise based on the number seven: the text in question recommended that the leaves and roots of *azza* (?) and *araq resa* (*Clematis simensis*) and the bark of *keya* (?) should be obtained in seven different places and be pounded together. The mixture had to be divided into seven parts, each being boiled daily in a large earthenware jar while the patient inhaled the steam.

The manner of operating a vapor bath was explained in another early twentieth-century medical text written by Grazmach Gabra Wald Aragahagn, who stated that the person responsible for bringing the patient to the *wesheba* should not stay inside with him, but there should be two nurses so that "when one of them is asleep, one of them watches." This was important, for a fire had to be kept burning night and day. It had to be made from wood which burned slowly.

Mercury Treatment

Mercury preparations, which the medical historian Garrison described as "the great sheet-anchor" of syphilis treatment in fifteenth- and sixteenth-century Europe, were also used in vapor baths in Ethiopia. At the close of the seventeenth century, the French physician Charles Poncet reported that "sublimate"—presumably, corrosive sublimate or mercury chloride ($HgCl_2$)— was imported from Sennar and had "a good vent" (or sale). By the early nineteenth century, mercury treatment was extensively practiced. Sublimate, locally referred to as *bohur*, was imported from Jeddah. It was employed, as the German traveler Rüppell reported, in vapor baths, which had much in common with the sarsaparilla fumigations already described.

Two distinct forms of *wesheba* treatment based on cinnabar, or red mercuric sulphide (HgS), were reported from Tegré in the 1880s. In the first, the medicine was made into pills with bread or flour, and taken orally until the patient showed signs of salivation and mercury poisoning. In the second, he was warmly dressed, his head and feet covered, and placed in a closed hut in which the pills were burned on a charcoal fire every day for many days, during which period he consumed only light food and milk. He was made to inhale the mercury vapor at times, though at other times he would remain in the nude with his head sticking out of the roof of his hut so that he could breathe fresh air while the vapor worked on his body.

Part II

Modern Medicine

XIV

The Coming of the First Foreign Medical Practitioners

Though the Ethiopians had their own ages-old traditional methods of treating disease, they also displayed great interest in foreign medicine. They took full advantage of overseas contacts to obtain foreign cures and revealed greater readiness to accept innovation in the medical field than in almost any other.

João Bermudes
The first foreign practitioner on record is João Bermudes, a barber-surgeon from Portugal, who arrived with the Portuguese embassy of 1520-1526. His services were considered so valuable that he was not allowed to leave the country until 1535, when he was dispatched to Portugal on an important diplomatic mission. The then Ethiopian ruler, Emperor Lebna Dengel, who was much interested in importing foreign medical skills, had already written to King João III of Portugal (in 1521), asking him to send various foreigners, including "men who make medicines, and physicians, and surgeons to cure illnesses."

Peter Heiling
A century later a German Lutheran missionary, Peter Heiling, practiced medicine at the then new city of Gondar. According to Ludolf he "took up his abode in a Church, not far from the Court," in 1636, and "as soon as he was settled in his new mansion, he began to practice Physick." Heiling, who also taught the children of the nobility, soon won the favor of the Emperor Fasiladas (1632-1667) and was given a "delightful Apartment" and a large revenue.

Charles Poncet

Emperor Iyasu I (1682-1706) also was very eager to make use of foreign medical skills. In 1698 he sent an agent, Haji Ali, to Cairo, with instructions to procure medical aid, as Iyasu and his son both were suffering from a troublesome skin complaint. As a result of this request the French consul in Cairo arranged for Charles Jacques Poncet, a local French physician, to set forth for Ethiopia. Dr. Poncet, who reached Gondar on July 11, 1699, was well received by the Emperor. "An apartment," he recorded, "was prepared for me, near to that of one of the Emperor's children. I had the honour the next day to see His Majesty, who gave me several marks of his goodness. . . . He came almost every day to visit me, thro' a little gallery which had communicated with his apartment."

Poncet, who did not describe Iyasu's illness, confined himself to saying that the emperor and his son "began their course of physic" and "both observ'd exactly the dyet (*regime*) I prescrib'd, which was so successful that in a little time they were perfectly cur'd." James Bruce, who visited Gondar almost three quarters of a century later, claims that Poncet's two royal patients were suffering from "a scorbutic habit, which threatened to turn into leprosy."

Iyasu was deeply interested in Poncet's medical knowledge, for the Frenchman reported:

> I had carried with me into Aethiopia a little chest of chemical medicines, which had cost me the labour of six or seven years. The Emperor inform'd himself exactly after what manner those remedies were prepar'd, and how they were to be applied: what effects they produced: for what distempers they were proper. He was not satisfied with only a verbal account of these things, but he ordered it to be taken in writing. But what I most admir'd (i.e., wondered at) was that he seem'd to be extremely pleas'd with the physical reasons I gave him of everything. I taught him the composition of a kind of bezoar, which I always made use of with great success in intermitting fevers, as the Emperor and two of the princes his sons experienc'd. He was also curious to see after what manner I extracted essences. Upon this project he sent me to Tsemba, a monastery situated upon the Reb, half a league from Gondar. The Abbot . . . receiv'd me with a great deal of civility. There I set up my stoves, and prepar'd all that was necessary. The Emperor came thither incognito. I made several experiments in his presence, and communicated to him many secrets, which he was wonderfully curious to know.

Poncet also treated the emperor's consort, Malakotawit, and other prominent personalities. He related that "Her Majesty consulted me about some of her ailments of which she complained." Describing another consultation and his personal belief in prayer, he elsewhere declared:

> They desir'd me to visit a person that was sick. One of the standers by said to me in my ear 'Mich.' that is to say 'he is struck by the evil spirit'. At the time I was at Gondar I heard them often speak of that illness; and the Emperor himself more than once ask'd my opinion concerning it. I answer'd that God did not permit those obsessions, but either to punish our sins or to discover his power, that we had an

infallible remedy in the sign of the cross; and that the Devil had no power over a true Christian.

The Frenchman set forth from Gondar on April 22, 1700, leaving the emperor in possession of some familiarity with foreign treatments and a box of medicine, but no doctor. Determined to remedy this deficiency, Iyasu wrote on September 24, 1701, to the French consul in Cairo, M. de Maillet, for a good physican or surgeon. Nothing came of this request, but shortly afterwards Iyasu took into his service a Greek physican called Demetrius. Several other Greeks were later employed in medical work in Ethiopia, and Bruce related that at the time of his own visit (1768–1773) he found one of their number, a certain Abba Christophorus, acting at Gondar as a physican as well as a priest.

James Bruce

James Bruce of Kinnaird, author of the classic *Travels to Discover the Source of the Nile*, was himself an amateur physician. His knowledge of medicine, not inconsiderable by late eighteenth-century standards, con-tributed significantly to his success in penetrating unknown lands. He used his medical skills extensively throughout his travels, and claimed that he treated the rulers, or members of their families, in most places he visited. His memoirs, which were dictated almost twenty years later, are anecdotal, and in some places demonstrably misleading, but nevertheless contain a remarkable store of information on diseases and traditional treatments as well as on the cures he himself attempted and sought to popularize with later travelers.

Bruce, who was appointed British consul-general in Algiers in 1763, was there befriended by the Bey's surgeon, an Englishman named Ball. The latter, a man "of considerable merit in his profession," proved a valuable source of medical knowledge, for, Bruce recalled, he "did not grudge his time or pain in the instructions he gave me, . . . I . . . made myself master of the art of bleeding, which I found consisted only in a little attention, and in overcoming that diffidence which the ignorance how the parts lie occasions." From the surgeon he also learned how to dress sores and wounds and apply bandages.

At the conclusion of his stay in Algiers in 1765 Bruce sailed to Aleppo, where he made friends with the British community's physician, Dr. Patrick Russell, who supplied him with "some books and much instruction." These lessons, he claimed, "greatly enhanced" his "knowledge of physic and surgery." While at Aleppo he conceived the idea of the enterprise for which he will always be remembered—a journey to discover the source of the Nile. Profoundly aware of the value of medical expertise on so difficult an expedition, he obtained "a small chest of the most efficacious medicines," a book to teach him how to make up others, and "some short treatises" on tropical diseases. He then set forth, confident of his ability to treat the maladies of the East. Considering himself virtually a member of the medical profession, he was later to write:

> I flatter myself, no offence I hope, I did not occasion a greater mortality among the Mahometans and Pagans abroad, than may be attributed to some of my brother physicians among their fellow Christians at home.

Such pomposity was to infuse much of his writing as well as his reports of the speeches he claimed to have made to the potentates he visited. The authenticity of such utterances, it should be emphasized, rests entirely on his own word, and it is impossible to tell with how much proverbial salt they should be taken. There is, however, little gainsaying that his medical knowledge greatly assisted him on his journey, as his first biographer, Alexander Murray, testified.

Bruce landed at Massawa, then an island port just off the Ethiopian coast, on Septmber 19, 1769. The town, he recalled, was suffering from an epidemic of smallpox, which, according to the *naib* (or local ruler), had carried off "above 1,000 people" there and at the nearby mainland port of Arkiko. Mortality was so great that it was feared "the living would not be sufficient to bury the dead. The whole island was filled with shrieks and lamentations both night and day." The death rate was so high that the inhabitants "at last began to throw the bodies into the sea, which deprived us of our great support, fish." Despite his vaunted medical skill, he had no wish to become involved in an epidemic which might have prevented his journey inland. He therefore "suppressed" his "character of physician," lest he were "detained by reason of the multitude of sick." He did, however, treat the *naib*'s nephew, Ahmad, who was "in bed, ill of a fever." The young man believed he had been "poisoned or bewitched" and had "tried many charms without good effect", but in the Scotsman's opinion he actually was "ill of an intermitting" (i.e., recurrent) fever. Bruce prescribed "proper medicines" to ease the pains, and the next morning began with "the bark" (i.e., cinchona bark, or quinine, as it was later called). This cure, which had then recently been popularized by John Sydenham, worked particularly quickly, Bruce thought, because of the heat, and caused the fever soon to depart.

Bruce, who was detained at Massawa for almost two months on account of the *naib*'s reluctance to allow him to leave, was the first traveler to describe the place from a medical point of view. He stated that the port was "very unwholesome," for it suffered from "violent fevers," locally known as *nedad* (i.e., the Tigrinya and Amharic word for fever). Drawing a gruesome account of what was presumably falciparum, or malignant malaria, he declared that the disease "generally" terminated "the third day in death," after which "black spots were frequently found on the breast and belly" and three hours later the stench became "insufferable," though, often, if the patient survived until the fifth day, he recovered. The usual local treatment was to give him nothing but water and to throw cold water onto, or even into, his bed. Though Bruce himself had not dared to practice so uncomfortable a cure, he was convinced that it was "frequently of great use." For his part he relied on cinchona bark (i.e., quinine) and believed that in Massawa's torrid climate there was "no remedy so sovereign." Emphasizing the need in that temperature to dispense with the preliminary purging then customary in Britain, he attacked both bleeding and the use of ipecacuanha, which the Dutch physician Helvetius had popularized half a century earlier. Writing with an eye to future foreign travelers, many of whom doubtless followed his advice, he urged that "the bark" must be given in "very different times and manners" than in Europe, for:

> Were a physician to take time to prepare his patient for the bark, by giving him purgatives, he would be dead of the fever before his preparation was completed. Immediately upon a nausea or aversion to eat, frequent fits of yawning, straitness about the eyes, and an unusual, but not painful sensation along the spine, comes on, no time then is to be lost; small doses of the bark must be frequently repeated, and perfect abstinence observed, unless from copious draughts of cold water. . . . The second or third dose of the bark, if any quantity is swallowed, never fails to purge; and, if this evacuation is copious, the patient rarely dies, but, on the contrary, his recovery is generally rapid.

He recognized that the foregoing was "contrary to the practice" of European physicians, but he maintained that he was simply reporting what he had observed and left "everybody afterwards to follow their own way at their peril."

Another disease common at Massawa, as well as in the lowlands throughout Ethiopia, was "tertian fever," (so called because it was said to recur every three days), which presumably was nonmalignant malaria. Its symptoms included headache, frequent yawning, a moderate pain in the nape of the neck, shivering which quickly disappeared, coldness down the spine, and "a more than ordinary cowardliness and inactivity." This complaint, he explained, was never fatal, so that time could be allowed for diagnosis, though it was "safest" to begin with "the bark" which should be "infused in water," and the patient should refuse "every sort of food."

Dysentery, Bruce believed, was rarely cured if it began in the rainy season, but at other times it responded well to ipecacuanha or (if the condition developed into an intermittent fever) to "the bark."

The Scotsman, who was much interested in preventative medicine, recommended that anyone following in his footsteps should eat the local food, even if it was spicy. Visitors from other climes, he argued, could not "act more wisely than to follow implicitly the regimen of sober, healthy people of the country." Referring specifically to pepper and other condiments he observed: "I lay down . . . as a positive rule in health, that the warmest dishes the natives delight in, are the most wholesome strangers can use."

News of Bruce's presence at Massawa—and his delay in advancing inland— duly reached the Ethiopian interior where, he claimed, it evoked some anger.

Early in November 1769, messages arrived from Ras Mika'él Sehul, the powerful governor of Tegré, and from Janni, a Greek in charge of customs at Adwa. Ras Mika'él's letter stated that the emperor at Gondar who was suffering from "bad" health, "wondered" at hearing that the physician had not been "forwarded to him instantly" and ordered the *naib* to furnish Bruce with all necessities for travel without delay. Janni's communication likewise expressed the "great necessity the king had for a physician, and how impatiently he had waited for his arrival."

Faced with such pressure, the *naib* agreed to permit Bruce to continue his journey. This involved difficulties with various local customs officials, but these were speedily overcome by the Scotsman's imperious claim that he was a physician. When stopped, he said, he adopted "a high tone" as someone who had been "sent for by the King," and was

> going to Ras Michael. . . . I affected to laugh when they talked of detaining me; and declared peremptorily to them, that I would leave all my baggage to them with great pleasure, rather than that the King's life should be in danger by my stay.

The persons who had sought to obstruct him were so "staggered" by this that they allowed him to proceed inland without further ado.

He thus made his way from sweltering Massawa to the cool highlands of Tegré. Though the highlands were generally healthy, he learned that in the lowlands of Sheré "putrid fevers, of the very worst kind", were "almost constant" and carried away "a number of people daily" while "violent fevers" reigned "perpetually" in the lowlands of Waldebba. On entering the former area he found the inhabitants unfriendly, so making no attempt to treat them, he "left the fever and them to settle accounts together."

On reaching Adwa, on December 6, 1769, he claimed to have found that the smallpox was raging there too. Abandoning his earlier feigned ignorance of medicine, he devoted himself to the sick and "saved many young people's lives" by "a new manner of treating them." This method, which Bruce later followed at the Ethiopian capital, was no doubt much influenced by Sydenham's teachings.

From Adwa Bruce journeyed to Gondar where he arrived on February 15, 1770, only to learn that the epidemic had already struck there. He found—or so he claimed—that news of his cures at Adwa had preceded him, so that on the very evening that he took up his abode he received an urgent summons to the palace. The courtier who brought it, Ato Haylu (or, as Bruce rendered, "Ayto Aylo"), rode up with great speed, and, uncovering his head "as if he had been approaching a person of distinction," explained that Walda Hawaryat, the son of Ras Mika'él, was "ill of a fever, and that they were afraid it was the smallpox." The cures Bruce had achieved at Adwa being known, the *etegé* (or dowager empress) Mentewwab desired him to come up to her palace at Qwesqwam on the following morning.

Bruce, whose accounts of these events, as we shall see, is open to some doubts, stated that on arriving at the palace he was informed that Walda Hawaryat was "much better," alledgedly because a holy man from a monastery in Waldebba had given him a concoction consisting of "some characters written with common ink upon a tin plate" and "washed off by a medicinal liquor." Bruce, a vigorous opponent of any kind of superstition, believed that the patient was actually suffering from the smallpox and that his apparent recovery was only temporary, produced by a hearty meal of raw beef, before which he had been famished and had "called perpetually for drink."

By afternoon, however, it was admitted that Walda Hawaryat's condition was again "very bad." Haylu informed him that the empress, her daughter Wayzaro Astér (who was married to Ras Mika'él), and the patient's wife, Wayzaro Altash, all three desired that he should visit the sick man on the morrow. Walda Hawaryat's daughter, Wallata Sellasé, had also been ill for "some time" and was "thought in great danger." The Scotsman, who had definite ideas on the treatment of smallpox and was not one to suffer fools gladly, replied:

> Look . . . Ayto Aylo, the smallpox is a disease that will have its course . . . if people feed them and treat them according to their ignorant prejudices, my seeing him, or advising him, is in vain. This morning you said a man had cured him by writing upon a tin plate; and to try if he was well, they crammed him with raw beef; I do not think the letters he swallowed will do him any harm, neither will they do him any good; but I shall not be surprised if the raw beef kills him, and his daughter, Welleta Selassé, too, before I see him tomorrow.

Returning to the palace on the following day, Bruce was just entering its gate when he saw "a large procession of monks, with the priests of Koscam at their head, a large cross and a picture carried with them." Haylu and another nobleman informed him that "three great saints from Waldubba, one of whom had neither ate nor drunk for twenty years of his life, had promised to come and cure Welled Hawaryat by laying a picture of the Virgin Mary and the cross upon him, and therefore they would not wish me to be seen, or meddle in the affair". Supposedly unruffled by this withdrawal of the request for his assistance, the traveler replied ironically:

> I assure you, Ayto Aylo . . . I shall strictly obey you. There is no sort of reason for my meddling in this affair with such associates. If they can cure him by a miracle, I am sure it is the easiest kind of cure of any, and will not do his constitution the least harm afterwards, which is more than I will promise for medicines in general; but, remember what I say to you, it will, indeed, be a miracle, if both the father and the daughter are not dead before tomorrow night.

Bruce and the two courtiers accordingly agreed, as he brutally put it, that it was better that the patient "should die, than I trouble by interfering." He nevertheless treated some inhabitants of the Muslim quarter where he resided, but, being less interested in describing his relations with the common people than with the great, he referred to this only in passing.

Meanwhile, according to Bruce, report of his conversation with the courtiers soon reached the empress, who summoned him to her presence. After the customary exchange of compliments she inquired why he did "not believe in miracles," to which he answered that he "did not believe laying a picture upon Welled Hawaryat would recover him when delirious in a fever." The *etegé* piously commented that "there was nothing impossible with God," to which he "made a bow of assent".

On returning to his house that afternoon, Bruce claimed, he learned that his prophecy was being fulfilled: Wallata Selassé was dead and her father, Walda Hawaryat, passed away the same night. "The contagion from Masuah (i.e., Massawa) and Adowa," he observed, "spread it self all over Gondar." Emphasizing the extent of the calamity,

> I professed my intention of doing my utmost, although the disease was much more serious and fatal in this country than in mine, but I insisted one condition should be granted to me, which was, that no directions as to regimen or management, even of the most trifling kind, as they might think, should be suffered, without my permission and superintendence, otherwise I washed my hands of the consequence, which I told before them would be fatal. They all assented to this, and Armaxikos declared those excommunicated that broke this promise; and I saw that, the more scrupulous and particular I was, the more the confidence of the ladies increased. Armaxikos promised me the assistance of his prayers, and those of the whole monks, morning and evening; and Aylo said lowly to me, "You'll have no objection to this saint, I assure you he eats and drinks heartily, as I shall shew you when once these troubles are over!"

Having ensured himself exclusive supervision, Bruce "set the servants all to work." Adhering "strictly" to the rules of Dr. Russell of Aleppo, he ordered the palace doors and windows to be opened, fumigated the building with incense and myrrh, and had it washed with warm water and vinegar. This insistence on ventilation and cleanliness must have struck the courtiers as strange, for, as the Scotsman noted, "the common and fatal regimen" in Ethiopia, as we also have seen in an earlier chapter, was

> to keep their patient from feeling the smallest breath of air; hot drink, a fire, and a quantity of covering are added . . . and the doors shut so close as even to keep the room in darkness, whilst this heat is further augmented by the constant burning of candles.

His action, though novel, won him immediate favor and he received "many promises of Michael's favour, of richness, greatness and protection." The treatment, moreover, proved a great success, by Bruce's account. Wayzaro Altash's daughter Ayabdar and Wayzaro Astér's son Kenfu and two later victims, also sons of Astér, one of them by Ras Mika'él, all recovered, though the first two were "very much" pock-marked. Another of his patients, however, a daughter of a nobleman called Beru, died. Nonetheless, Bruce claimed, medical achievement won him "remarkable attention and favour" at court, while the Muslims were also "very grateful for the successful attention" he had shown their children.

Bruce's account, however, cannot be accepted wholly without comment. In the first place, his dating of the epidemic is open to question. He gives the impression, as we have seen, that when he reached the city in the middle of February 1770 the disease was still in its infancy, and that it was only after the death of Ras Mika'él's son Walda Hawaryat that it "spread itself all over Gondar." The chronicle for the reign of Emperor Iy'oas states, on the other hand, that the epidemic had broken out in the capital a year and a half earlier, in Genbot (i.e., May-June 1768), and mentions a nobleman dying of the disease early in January 1769. There is no reference to any later deaths from smallpox in the subsequent, admittedly fragmentary, chronicle for the time of Bruce's visit. This would suggest that he arrived not at the beginning of the epidemic but in its later stages and that he may have played a less important role in combatting it than he claimed. His statement that the contagion came, like him, "from Masuah and Adowa" is likewise unproven, and indeed far from probable since smallpox was traditionally endemic in Ethiopia and, unlike cholera, did not usually enter the country along the trade routes from the coast.

Doubts as to the accuracy of Bruce's report are reinforced by his account of the death of Ras Mika'él's son Walda Hawaryat, who according to the chronicle, had died almost a decade earlier, on May 22, 1760. An additional element of confusion is provided by Bruce's claim, in the subsequent volume of his *Travels*, that the young man recoverd, supposedly as a result of his treatment, and that subsequently Ras Mika'él took Bruce by the hand "and said, 'Welleta Hawaryat . . . is well, you are very kind' ".

Corroboration of Bruce's claim to have treated the royal family is nevertheless provided by the memories of Abram, a learned Ethiopian who thirteen years later informed the orientalist Sir William James in Calcutta that he had seen the Scotsman in Gondar. Referring to Bruce as Yacob (Amharic for James), he stated, significantly, that the traveler was "a physician." Abram's account, however, differed considerably from Bruce's and made no reference to any smallpox epidemic. The Ethiopian was quoted as recalling merely that the traveler "attended the King's brother, who was also a Vazir, in his last illness; the prince died; yet the King loved Ya'ku'b, and, indeed all the court loved him."

Another version of Bruce's medical activities was later published by the British traveler Henry Salt, who said he obtained it from Dabtara Astér, an old Ethiopian ecclesiastic who had known the Scotsman at Gondar forty years earlier. Salt stated, almost in Bruce's own words, that the latter cured "one of Ras Michael's children and Ayto Confu, who were then ill of the smallpox" and thereby gained "great reputation," so that the *etegé* took the Scotsman "under her protection" and Wayzaro Astér "became much attached to him." Salt's testimony, however, cannot be accepted as fully trustworthy either, for it was written after the appearance of Bruce's memoirs, and may be drawn from them as much as from the *dabtara*'s by then possibly hazy reflections.

There is thus insufficient evidence to come to any firm conclusion as to the accuracy of Bruce's account. However, in view of his reliability in most (but by no means all) verifiable matters, it may be assumed that his visit coincided with an epidemic of smallpox, but that this was probably in its last rather than its initial stage. It is clear, moreover, that he was confused as to the names of one or more of the participants in the event, may well have embroidered the story, either for the sake of effect or to emphasize his own medical prowess.

Bruce, like later visitors to Ethiopia, was expected to treat all the diseases that flesh is heir to. His most important patient was Ras Mika'él, then an old man suffering from rheumatism and bad eyes. The author recorded in his diary—a more reliable source than his *Travels*—that on March 11, 1770, the chief complained of pain in his knee and called for Bruce's assistance. This was a notable compliment, Bruce claimed, in that the *ras* "seemed averse to using all remedies, and refused taking any, except those which I tasted before him." The "physician" then administered a typical eighteenth-century cure, and embrocation of spirits of wine and camphor, after which the patient felt better for two days. On March 15, however, the *ras* complained of "a pain in his side" which continued until March 18, when "he proposed to be cupped, but changed his mind; he looked ill, but had no fever." On March 19, he was again "very ill, but would take no remedies." On the following day he was "visibly worse," though, as reported two days later, he would "take no medicines" except melted butter. The chief's indisposition is confirmed in the royal chronicle, which stated that God, knowing that Mika'él had "fallen sick of a slight illness" while in the provinces, made him return to Gondar so that "this illness would not seize him away from home."

Another personage Bruce claimed to have cured was an officer of state, Shalaqa Walda Amlak, whose case illustrates the kind of difficulty faced by foreign doctors unable to rely on their patient's understanding or cooperation. The *shalaqa* and one of his servants were both suffering from intermittent fever. The servant, "a poor, timid wretch, exceedingly afraid of dying . . . adhered strictly to his regimen. . . . and very soon recovered"; his master, however, secretly arranged to be given raw meat, mead, and spirits, which "more than once threw him into a fever and violent delirium." Luckily, Bruce was "early informed of this by the servant . . . who did not doubt but this was to end in his master's death, and it very probably might have done." The man who brought in the forbidden food and drink was thereupon banished and the *shalaqa*, "after several weeks illness," was cured.

Other persons treated included the chief of the Banja Agaws, Nana Giyorgis, who was "very ill of the low-country fever" (presumably malaria), and a courtier suffering from "a cancer" (or growth of some kind) on the lip. Bruce gave the courtier a preparation of hemlock of circuta (i.e., *Conium maculatum*), which had been recommended by the Viennese physican Dr. Anton von Storck and which he had obtained from France. He ordered the patient to "keep a milk diet," to "avoid eating raw meat," and to "drink plentifully."

Bruce on several occasions traveled to the provinces, where he also practiced his medical arts. One of his journeys took him to Emfaz, east of Lake Tana, where he suffered an attack of ague. He resorted to "the bark" (i.e., quinine) and kept a strict diet of boiled rice, with abundant draughts of cold water. Subsequently, on reaching the source of the Blue Nile, he once more served as a doctor and for three days "practiced medicine gratis" for the local Agaws.

The return journey gave Bruce further evidence of the extent of fever in the malaria-infested lowlands. At one village he found the inhabitants all "sick of the fever." Perhaps for that reason, the villagers were markedly unfriendly and quartered him and his companions in a house in which two families had just died of the disease. On learning this disquieting fact, he at once infused a dose of "the bark" in a glass of aqua vitae, and, after drinking it, he and his party, following the practice employed in Massawa and Arabia, fumigated themselves with frankincense and myrrh. "Whether the bark prevented the disease or not," Bruce commented, "the aqua vitae certainly strengthened the spirits, and was a medicine to the imagination." The villagers, seeing the "eagerness and confidence" with which their visitors swallowed this medicine, flocked round to demand assistance, but, as Bruce brusquely recounted,

> I was so exasperated with their treatment of us, and especially that of lodging us in the infected house, that I constantly refused them their request, leaving them a prey to their distemper, to teach them another time more hospitality to strangers.

In 1770, Bruce accompanied Emperor Takla Haymanot, Ras Mika'él, and their army to Sarbakusa, site of three battles in a civil war then raging. On one occasion during the hostilities, the Scotsman allegedly advised the monarch, who was unwell, to take warm water to make him vomit, while on another (crossing the battle line in his capacity as "physician"), he was asked by one of the great lords, Ras Goshu, governor of Amhara, to bleed him. Bruce replied, however, that he would "by no means agree" to this, for,

> if he was well, as I saw he was, the unnecessary bleeding might occasion sickness; and, if he was dangerously ill, he might die, when the blame would be laid on me, and expose me to mischief afterwards.

He nevertheless treated Goshu's family, who were all "ill of the fever," by giving them ipecacuanha and "the bark." When one of Goshu's nephews succumbed to the smallpox Bruce warned the uncle "seriously of the danger to which he exposed all his army if that disease broke out among them"; on another occasion he won acclaim by treated a wounded courtier.

During his residence in Ethiopia, Bruce acquired a fair understanding of the country's diseases and was indeed the first writer to report on them and their traditional treatment in detail. He devoted a long description to "fever" (i.e., malaria). He described its symptoms and course as follows:

> This fever is called Nedad, or burning; it always begins with a shivering and headache, a heavy eye, and inclination to vomit; a violent heat follows, which leaves little intermission, and ends generally in death the third day. In the last stage of the distemper the belly swells to an enormous size, or sometimes immediately after death, and the body within smells most insupportably; to prevent which they bury the corpse immediately after the breath is out, and often within the hour. The face has a remarkably yellow appearance, with a blackish cast, as in the last stage of a dropsy or the atrophy.

Though unaware that the disease was spread by the mosquito (a fact which was not discovered until over a century later), he realized that outbreaks were related to the seasons (and hence, as we now know, to the vector's life cycle) and observed:

> . . . fever begins immediately with the sun-shine; it ceases upon the earth being thoroughly soaked in July and August, and begins again in September; but . . . at the beginning of November, it finally ceases everywhere.

Writing specifically of Dambeya, the low-lying province on the northern shores of Lake Tana, he noted that "a mortal fever" raged from March to November, after which "gentle showers" fell and the "dangerous fever" immediately stopped.

He was likewise aware that the disease was not encountered in regions of higher elevation (where the mosquito could not exist). Elaborating on these geographical variations, he remarked:

> fever prevailed . . . in all low grounds and plains, in the neighbourhood of all rivers which run in valleys. . . . It is not in all places equally dangerous, but on the banks of the Tacazze it is particulary fatal. The valley where that river runs is very low and sultry, being full of large trees. In Kuara, too, it is very mortal; in Belessen and Dembea less so; in Walkayt it is dangerous; but not so much in Tzegadè, Woggora, and Waldubba. It does not prevail in high grounds or mountains, or in places much exposed to the air.

Understanding the importance, if not the cause, of this unequal distribution he noted the significance it had on the location of Ethiopian settlements, and observed that it was the reason why the seventeenth-century capital had been at Gorgora, which, though by Lake Tana, stood on elevated land, and was thus "one of the healthiest" of places, entirely free from "malignant fevers."

Much concerned with smallpox, Bruce made a number of inquiries about it. He learned that the Shanqella, or black people near the Sudan frontier, had been "greatly reduced" by the disease: "whole tribes" had been "extinguished, to a man" and the malady, by "greatly diminishing their numbers," had reduced "their power of troubling their neighbours." The Mecha Galla by the Nile, however, were so terrified of the illness (which seldom appeared "more frequently than every fifteen or twenty years") that they had developed the previously mentioned draconian method (see chapter III) of setting fire to the (still inhabited) houses of smallpox victims.

Perhaps because of his limited medical experience, Bruce had nothing explicit to say about venereal diseases, the high incidence of which was to so impress later foreign visitors. He may, however, have seen some cases of yaws, or conceivably postcutaneous leishmaniasis, for he reported noticing patients with "small tubercules or swellings . . . all over the body, but thickest in the thighs, arms and legs," and in some instances with ulcers in their nose and mouth. This complaint, though of "a very terrible appearance," was, he believed, "not dangerous" and was "completely and speedily cured by antimonials."

Another disease he mentioned was called *hanzeer* (i.e., "hogs" or "swine") and was characterized by "a swelling of the glands, and under the arms." This was no doubt a severe laryngopharyngitis, also found in the Levant (where it is referred to as *halzoun*). Persons suffering from such inflammations, he stated, usually endeavored to bring them "to suppuration, but in vain" and would then open them in several places, thereby producing running sores. His own experience was that they could be treated with mercury, though this was a "slow" and often "imperfect cure."

Bruce also interested himself in elephantiasis, which, being still little known in Europe, tended to be confused with leprosy. For that reason he referred to it as "the most terrible" disease that can "fall to the lot of man." Though using the two terms almost interchangeably, he was aware that elephantiasis, characterized by leg-swelling such as he witnessed in Gondar, was quite different from the "leprosy of Palestine" (i.e., true leprosy). He admitted that he had "never" seen "the beginning" of the disease, but claimed to have been familiar with several advanced cases. In a vivid description of the symptoms he remarked:

> The chief seat of this disease is from the bending of the knee downwards to the ankle; the leg is swelled to a great degree, becoming one size from bottom to top, and gathered into circular wrinkles, like small hoops or plaits; between every one of which there is an opening that separates it from the one above, and which is all raw flesh, or perfectly excoriated. From between these circular divisions a great quantity of lymph constantly oozes. The swelling of the leg reached over a foot, so as to leave about an inch or little more of it seen. It should seem that the black colour of the skin, the thickness of the leg, its shapeless form, and the rough tubercles, or excrescences, very like those seen upon the elephant, gave the name to this disease, and form a striking resemblance between the distempered legs of this unfortunate individual of the human species, and those of the noble quadruped.

The Ethiopians, he reported, considered this disease "not infectious," and in support of this he stated that he had observed that wives of men suffering from it gave birth to healthy children.

Having discussed the complaint with Dr. Russell of Aleppo, who advised him to experiment with Dr. Storck's hemlock or cicuta, he obtained permission from the emperor, Ras Mika'él, and the chief justice, Azaj Takla Haymanot, to maintain a man suffering from elephantiasis in quarters near his own house in order to supervise his treatment. The judge was particularly sympathetic, and declared:

> no harm that may accidentally befall one individual, now already cut off by society, should hinder the trial (the only one we shall have an opportunity of making) of a medicine which may save multitudes hereafter from a disease so much worse than death.

The patient remained under Bruce's inspection for "nearly two years," during which he was subjected to "every sort of regimen" that could be devised. Anxious to inform the medical profession of his findings, the Scotsman reported that "nothing was to be expected" from cicuta, and that mercury and tar-water had "no better effect." If anything had produced "any seeming advantage" it was whey, of which the man was "exceedingly fond" and which the king ordered him to be furnished with in any quantity he pleased. This treatment was beneficial, Bruce felt, as elephantiasis patients experienced "constant thirst" because "the lymph, which constantly ouzed from their wounds, demanded to be replaced."

Dysentery, and one of the traditional means of treating it, Bruce learned about at first hand. On the point of leaving Gondar to return home, he himself was attacked by this disease and tried in vain to cure it, both by "hot medicines and stringents" and by "the contrary method of diluting." Doses of ipecacuanha and quinine produced temporary relief, but relapses soon followed. He nevertheless began his journey, but, on reaching Hor Cacamoot, near the borders of Sennar, his condition "grew worse." He chanced, however, to meet "Sheba," chief of the Ganjar Shanqella, who, hearing of his illness and his fear of traveling through the desert in that condition, made "very light of both," for he saw by the door of the hut where they were seated the *waginos* shrub, a well-established local specific that figured in several traditional Ethiopian medical texts. Under the chief's directions the root was at once dug up, cleaned, dried in the sun, and ground into powder. Bruce was then given two doses, each consisting of a heaped teaspoonful in camel's milk. The second day he began to feel better, stopped taking laudanum and ipecacuanha, and by the sixth or seventh day was entirely recovered. On returning to Britain he showed a sample of the shrub to Dr. Daniel Solander of the British Museum and published an engraving of it in his *Travels*. The plant was later named *Brucea antidysenterica* in Bruce's honor.

Bruce's knowledge of the Guinea worm (*Dracunculus medinensis*), which was also partly acquired at personal cost, was valuable, for the parasite, though long familiar to Arab medicine, was but rarely seen by European practitioners. He stated that this "extraordinary animal" was spoken of at Massawa and elsewhere as *farenteit* and thought that this meant "worm of Pharaoh." Both statements, however, are dubious. The worm, he learned, afflicted persons who drank stagnant water (the abode, as we now know, of the intermediate host, the small insect Cyclops), and appeared "indiscriminately" in any part of the human body, though unusually in the leg and arms. On the first appearance of the parasite, its "small black head" was "extremely visible, with a hooked beak of whitish colour" and its body "seemingly of a white silky texture". The traditional treatment was to seize it "gently by the head", and "wrap it round a thin piece of silk or small bird's feather." After this,

> every day, or several times a day, they tried to wind it up upon the quill as far as it comes readily; and, upon the smallest resistance, they give over for fear of breaking it. I have seen five feet, or something more, of this extraordinary animal, winded out with invincible patience in the course of three weeks. No inflammation then remained, and scarcely any redness round the edges of the aperture, only a small quantity of lymph in the hole or puncture, which scarcely issued out upon pressing. In three days it was commonly well, and left no scar or dimple implying loss of substance.

On arriving in Cairo he himself was afflicted with this worm, which appeared seven inches below his knee and produced itching. He was given various medicines which proved useless, and was obliged to resort to the above method of extraction. Three inches of the parasite were successfully removed in a week, but it was then broken through carelessness, after which

> a violent inflammation followed; the leg swelled so as to scarce leave appearance of knee or ankle; the skin, red and distended seemed glazed like a mirror.

The experience cost him 35 days of "the greatest agony" before his leg eventually suppurated. During this time he was obliged to make "constant use of bark, both in fomentations and inwardly" and, on reaching Marseilles, was actually advised to have his leg amputated. The inflammation, however, later subsided, but he did not regain his strength for nearly a year.

Bruce also turned his attention to the famous Ethiopian taenicide *kosso*, which he was the first writer to describe in detail. He recalled that many people in Ethiopia took it every month or so, and that the infestation for which the drug was used resulted, as we have seen, from the widespread Ethiopian habit of eating raw meat. Describing *kosso* as "one of the most beautiful" as well as "the most useful" trees, Bruce stated that a handful of its dried flowers would be infused all night in about two quarts of beer and that the patient, while taking this treatment, made "a point of being invisible to all his friends, and continued at home from morning to night." On his eventual return home, Bruce published a drawing of a branch of the tree and its flowers, and named it *Banksia abissinica* after Sir Joseph Banks, president of the Royal Society. The term *Banksia*, however, was appropriated for another plant, with the consequence that Bruce's nomenclature was not adopted.

XV

Foreign Medicine in the Early Nineteenth Century

The impact of Western medicine expanded substantially in the first decades of the nineteenth century, which witnessed the arrival of increasing numbers of foreign travelers. Most of them—whether missionaries, sportsmen, scholars, or diplomats—dabbled to a greater or lesser extent in medicine.

Foreign Travelers

Not untypical was the case of the French traveler Arnauld d'Abbadie, who while visiting Gondar treated the consort of Emperor Sahla Dengel (1832–1840) and, according to a contemporary British report, generally "practised medicine with considerable success," raising himself "to a high place in the eyes of the ignorant populace by professing chiromancy."

The Swiss missionary Samuel Gobat, another sometime resident at Gondar, also treated numerous patients. On May 3, 1830, he was summoned by Wayzaro Wallata Teklit, the "first lady of Gondar," who requested him to see her brother Gajar Haylu, who had "gone mad" and failed to respond to the prayers of the local priests. The missionary, following the European practice of the time, thereupon bled him. "I took from him," Gobat recorded, "three or four pounds of blood; and when he was on the point of fainting, I made him lie down on the bed, recommending his people to let him rest." The treatment appeared to have been successful, for on the following day Wallata Teklit called Gobat and declared, "I have sent for you to testify my gratitude for the good you have done to my brother. Since you saw him yesterday, he is as reasonable, in what he says to me, as if he had never lost his sense". Gobat, who was a modest man, refused to claim all the success for himself. He replied to the good lady: "I think that the quantity of blood was the cause of his malady; but I assure you that I did not bleed him without prayer, and especially not without asking of God that he would cause you to see that the word of the priests is not always the truth."

Gobat's success was so great that he was soon besieged by hordes of prospective patients. "I can hardly get across the city any more," he wrote on May 4. "Everybody stops me, begging me to go and see the sick. The more I tell them that I am not a physician, the more they are persuaded that what I advise them is the best remedy. There are some persons who believe that it is sufficient for me to look on the sick to affect a cure." He had constant visitors. On May 25 he noted, "Today I had to deal only with sick people," while on the following day he wrote: "I had hardly risen this morning, when suddenly my house was filled with people." On May 27 he wrote, "I passed the forenoon in visiting the sick," and on the next day, "From sun-rise, till ten o'clock, my house was full of people."

The French Saint Simonian travelers, Edmond Combes and Maurice Tamisier, also testified to popular interest in European medicine. While in the Gondar area, they reported:

> Everyone was persuaded that in our capacity as whites we must be profoundly versed in the study of the medicinal sciences; also each person is anxious to come to consult us, to ask us for remedies or amulets with the conviction that we could cure the ill with which they were afflicted. . . . Important men appealed to us to give them aphrodisiacs and sterile women thought that we could procure for them the means of becoming fertile. A priest came to present to us his son who was afflicted by a disease considered in Europe as incurable.

Belief in foreign medicine, they commented, was often based on supersition, as exemplified by the villagers of Danqaz who:

> begged us, with the most lively insistence, to make them an amulet to preserve them from the terrible storms which ruined them, and we feared for a moment that we would be held by force if we refused to subscribe to their wish. 'We know,' they said to us, 'that a white man enters into direct communication with heavenly bodies and spirits, and that he can, by his own power, drive away the hail and the illnesses of a country which he protects; remain therefore in our midst the time that is necessary for this beneficent work; we will treat you like princes, you will lack nothing, and when you leave, we will pray for you so that God will bestow his favours upon you.

Though critical of this attitude, Combes and Tamisier sometimes felt obliged to pander to it. Pressed by a young woman for an amulet to cure her sterility, they therefore consented. Justifying their action they declared: "We might be blamed in Europe perhaps for having by this compliance contributed to maintaining or even propagating such a ridiculous belief; we reply, firstly, that we have never denied the power of moral influence which can alone, in certain cases, cure illness often existing merely in the imagination of those who believe themselves afflicted, and we will add that we have always held the principle of never destroying a useful or agreeable error when we have nothing to propose with which to replace the charm of a lost illusion." Putting their argument in another way, the Saint Simonians added, "In a country deprived of remedies and of men knowing how to administrate them, the essential thing is not to undeceive the inhabitants as to the powers of amulets, but rather to procure for them medicines and doctors."

The German Protestant missionary Johann Ludwig Krapf was also actively involved in medical work in this period. On visiting Shawa, he wrote to the British political agent in Aden in 1841 requesting five or six ounces of calomel (i.e., mercurous chloride [Hg_2Cl_2]). His letter stated that this medicine had proved a "very useful" remedy for venereal disease, which was "so prevailing" that "you cannot but furnish asking people with a remedy against it."

Calomel was likewise used at this time by the Englishman Mansfield Parkyns, a sometime resident in Tegré, who recorded that he treated "many cases" of venereal disease "with much success" by means of this substance when administered in time.

A no less interesting visitor was Charles Johnston, a British naval surgeon who resided at Ankobar, Aleyu Amba, and Anglolalah in 1841. He subsequently wrote a two-volume account entitled *Travels in Abyssinia*, but, though devoting many paragraphs to traditional treatments, mentioned only in passing that he supplied "professional services."

Popular interest in foreign medicine was so great that it contributed on one occasion to the willingness of some inhabitants of the coast to sell their land to the Europeans. Peluchenau, a Frenchman, who landed at the port of Edd in 1840, was asked by a local elder for medicines for his child who was covered with sores. The visitor replied "that many months would be required to cure the illness." " 'Well then,' the chief replied, 'stay with us.' " "It was thus," Combes explains, "that the negotiations began. 'Friend,' resumed M. Peluchenau, 'will you give us houses and a small piece of land if we wish to establish ourselves among you?' 'Without any doubt,' replied the African. 'And if we ask you to sell the land, will you agree to sell it?' 'Certainly.' 'Very well,' said M. Peluchenau."

Resident Practitioners

Besides such foreign travelers, there were several resident "doctors" who dispensed medicine. They included a Turkish veterinary assistant who had deserted from the Egyptian cavalry and settled in the Muslim quarter of Gondar in the 1830s, and a Bashibazook at Massawa a decade or so later who had received a small stock of medicine from various visiting travelers, but was "not acquainted with their properties or doses." In Tegré in the 1840s there was likewise an Armenian, called Gorgorius, who supplied sufferers from venereal disease with what he claimed to be a "certain cure." According to Parkyns, this "cure" consisted of "a dozen or two pills containing corrosive sublimate . . . no doubt obtained from some quack." This mercury preparation, if properly administered, might have been beneficial, but the practitioner never troubled either to examine his patients or to inquire how long they had been afflicted. He merely received his fee and told his patients to take so many pills per day until the box was finished so that it was "a case of kill perhaps, oftener than of cure." The public, moreover, being unaccustomed to this type of treatment, could not easily be made to understand that "where one dose will do them good, two may be injurious."

Such "physicians" tended to discredit foreign medicine. D'Abbadie reported that, though the people of Tegré had formerly had great belief in European doctors, ever since one had practiced among them this had disappeared and they had returned to the methods of their forefathers.

French and British Scientific and Diplomatic Missions

The advent of formal French and British scientific and diplomatic missions to Ethiopia in the late 1830s and early 1840s was significant in that it brought modern medicine to a sizeable section of the population, at least in the capitals and more important towns of Tegré and Shawa.

The members of the French scientific mission of 1839–1843 included two physicians, Petit and Quartin-Dillon, who contributed substantially to its success. Petit has left an account of some of the treatments they employed, particularly at Adwa and elsewhere in Tegré. He used emetics with ipecacuana and saline purgatives in treating persons suffering from influenza, astringent lotions and calomel insufflations in cases of ophthalmia, and emetocathartic treatment for gastric and intestinal complaints. In the treatment of light abrasions and wounds he used compresses imbued with a solution of opiated acetate of lead, though where complications set in he cut open or enlarged the fistular passage and injected astringent and opiated solutions. He applied poultices in cases of acute inflammations, destroyed fungosity in wounds by sprinkling them with pulverized acetate of lead, removed many bullets "to the great admiration" of the populace, and cauterized scorpion stings with ammoniac. He also imported vaccine from France and Egypt and carried out a "large number of inoculations," but the serum was spoiled in transit, presumably by the heat, with the result that, despite the "good will" and "blind confidence" of the inhabitants, almost all his inoculations proved ineffective. The mission later traveled to Shawa, where Petit prescribed for King Sahla Sellasé's sister Wayzaro Tekule.

Sahla Sellasé was also visited, in 1839, by a French mission headed by Rochet d'Héricourt. The latter, though not actually a physician, was a member of the Société Royale de Médecine de Marseille, and fancied himself an expert on medicine. He was warmly welcomed by the king, who declared, "You belong to a very enlightened nation: no doubt you understand the art of curing diseases." The Frenchman claimed that he answered with modesty, saying that he had not made any "special study" of medicine, but nevertheless brought with him "remedies which in certain cases brought good effects."

Rochet treated the king, as well as the latter's consort, Queen Bezabesh, who was suffering from toothache. He gave her a piece of cotton soaked in muriatic acid, which caused the pain to disappear "as if by magic." This cure, he recalled, "assured me a high place in the esteem of the princess," who later had two other occasions to obtain treatment from him.

Rochet d'Héricourt visited Shawa again in 1842, when Sahla Sellasé was suffering from an attack of rheumatism to which he was prone. "Haven't you brought a remedy which can cure me of this ill?", the king asked. Apparently unable to treat him, Rochet resorted to a trick. Seeking to obtain a hippopotamus fetus for a French museum, he told the king that the only cure for his complaint lay in the body of that animal and in this way encouraged him to organize a hunt.

The British diplomatic mission to Shawa, which was led by Captain W.C. Harris and remained in the country from 1841 to 1842, was medically far more important than the French. It too treated a number of prominent personalities, including both Sahla Sellasé and Queen Bezabesh, the heir to the throne Sayfa Sellasé (whose eyes were in a "high state of inflammation"), and a princess called Warq Feré.

Harris, whose reports to the British East India Company contain a wealth of material not published in his three-volume *Highlands of Aethiopia*, recalled that the monarch was on one occasion indisposed and desirous of trying some Seidlitz powders, of which the mission had a supply. The British were duly summoned to the palace. In accordance with the custom of the country they would normally have been expected to take the medicine themselves to prove that it was not poison, but the king "laughingly observed, 'There is no necessity for that. I am not afraid of you.' "

The treatment of the royal women, however, presented problems, for a message arrived "to the effect that Queen Bezabesh was extremely indisposed and in need of medical aid, but it being contrary to court etiquette that the king's consort should be seen by strangers, the physician could not be accorded an interview." Kirk, one of the mission's two surgeons, accordingly visited her on the morrow, but she was "concealed behind a small coloured tent" and merely passed her hand out through a small hole. On another visit a noblewoman hid behind the basket pedestal of a wicker table whence her feet were thrust forth for inspection.

Sahla Sellasé, who had a palace-full of courtiers and others to look after, was keenly interested in obtaining medical supplies from abroad. By the mid-1830s, he had acquired a "mass of European medicines from India by way of Zeila," according to Combes and Tamisier. He was, however, always asking for more. Harris noted, for example, that in May 1842, "the King's attention" was "solely engrossed in amassing medicines" and, finding that the mission's stock of calomel was exhausted, "sent constantly" to request every other drug in the British stores. He asked for explicit directions on their use and "expressed much disappointment" that the mission's store "contained neither the horn of a serpent which he believed to possess the most valuable virtues, nor any cure for those who go mad from looking at a black dog." Six weeks later the envoy reported that the royal stock of imported medicines had been "brought down to be labelled by the mission," although "very ample directions" on their use had already been given some time earlier.

The Shawan public was no less responsive to modern medicines. Barker, a member of the British mission, reported that the populace, despite its original "asserted contempt for the white strangers," had been obliged to confess that the latter's medicine was in many respects "superior" to theirs. He had in consequence received "many" visits from "persons residing at great distances who came to be cured for their real or imaginary diseases or to procure medicines for their relatives." Elaborating, he recalled:

> One man begged earnestly for medicine for his daughter residing at Angolalla (32 miles distant) upon whom the evil eye had fallen, another on behalf of his brother who had his skull fractured by a fall from his mule, . . . another also on behalf of his brother, a man in the downhill of life, or to use a more common expression, on the wrong side of forty.

The mission was thus kept busy on the medical front. Surgeon Kirk reported in March, 1842, that since their arrival in August of the previous year they had "afforded medical assistance to at least 1,000 individuals, two-thirds of them being common cases of syphilis," and had "found mercury combined with opium a mild and certain remedy for every form of the disease." Considerable use was made of blue pills known as the *pilula hydrargyri*.

Harris, who must have realized that the medical side of his mission was at least as important as the political, reported to the British East India Company that for a population "so scourged with syphilis" the work accomplished by his doctors was "no ordinary blessing" and was "appreciated by all from the King to the mendicant." He proposed to Sahla Sellasé a scheme whereby a preparation of mercury (the principal cure for syphilis) would be distributed "throughout the kingdom" by "natives instructed in its use." In accordance with this offer he asked the British government to supply a "large" quantity of "blue pills," as well as some 40 other items, including a lancet.

The British government failed to respond to this request, and the mission was soon obliged to leave the country. Before its departure, however, Harris and his colleagues struck upon the idea of converting fourteen pounds of mercury intended for fuze-horizons into blue pills. This enabled them to treat several hundred more syphilitic patients. The cure which earned the "most universal amazement," however, according to Harris, was that of one of the king's pages who had been seized by a fit of apoplexy but was "suddenly revived by venesection after having lain for several hours in a state of such total insensibility that he was believed to be dead."

During its stay in Shawa the mission treated between 2,000 and 3,000 patients. Records, however, were kept of only 717 cases seen at Ankobar between December 1841 and April 1842. According to those records, 317 (or 40%) of that number were suffering from syphilis. The breakdown of cases by disease is given in the following table. The mission thus treated a sizeable number of cases, though Harris surely exaggerated when he claimed that his compatriots "rescued three thousand patients from the jaws of death."

Medical cases treated by the British diplomatic mission of 1841-1842, arranged by disease category.

Complaint	Number of Persons
Syphilis	317
Cutaneous affections	63
Ophthalmia	36
Rheumatism	33
Scrofula	26
Leprosy	26
Cephalagia	24
Ulcers	21
Intermittent fevers	10
Gonorrhea	10
Hepatitis	9
Opacity of cornea	9
Pulmonary affections	9
Ear inflammations	8
Epilepsy	7
Dyspepsia	7
Bronchocele	7
Wounds	6
Elephantiasis	6
Catarrh	6
Dysentery	5
Hydrocephalus	5
Abscesses	5
Heart diseases	5
Chronic enlargement of knee joint	5
Cracked integument of sole of foot	4
Nyctolopia	4
Aneurism of aorta	3
Arasarca	3
Steatomatous tumours	3
Fevers chronic	2
Diarrhoea	2

Continued

Medical cases treated . . . *continued.*

Complaint	Number of Persons
Phthisis	2
Hysteria	2
Chorea St. Viti	2
Paralysis	2
Stone in bladder	2
Hernia	2
Amaurosis	2
Chronic enlargement Bursa	2
Hypopium	2
Inflammation of testicle	2
Fractures (recent)	2
Dislocations (old)	2
Bronchitis	1
Ascites	1
Exostotis	1
Gastritis	1
Abscess antrum maxillare	1
Threatened abortion	1
Total	*717*

Imported Medicines for Syphilis

The early nineteenth century, as indicated above, witnessed considerable use of imported medicines, particularly in the treatment of syphilis.

Sarsaparilla enjoyed great popularity. Combes and Tamisier reported in the 1830s that Ethiopians were aware of its value, and that those who traveled to Massawa made extensive use of it. It was, according to Kirk, also known in Shawa, where, however, it was far from cheap, for a complete cure (which weighed about six ounces) cost 20 Maria Theresa thalers, though it could be obtained for only one thaler at the coast. The drug continued to be used for many decades, and was mentioned by Dr. Blanc in the 1860s as still a popular cure.

Pills containing mercury preparations (i.e., either calomel or corrosive sublimate) were also dispensed, as we have seen, by a number of foreign travelers. Muslim traders who visited the coast, according to Plowden, were also "pretty generally acquainted with the use of mercury" and took "doses that would astonish a European practitioner," for they appeared to think that "the sooner salivation is produced, the quicker must be the cure." The use of mercury ointment was likewise reported elsewhere, notably by d'Abbadie, who stated that in Gojjam it was mixed with lemon juice.

XVI

Developments During the Reigns of Téwodros and Yohannes

◇ ◇ ◇

Foreign medicine made further advances in the second half of the nineteenth century, during the reigns of Emperors Téwodros II (1855-1868) and Yohannes IV (1872–1889).

Téwodros

Téwodros, a notable innovator, was fully receptive to Western medical ideas. Consul Plowden, who spoke to him about European-type vaccination in June 1856 (a year after the emperor's coronation), reported that the monarch had declared himself "happy to see it introduced." A few years later Téwodros received, and honored, a French physician, Dr. Legard, sent to his court by Emperor Napoleon III. Téwodros also sought, and followed, the medical advice of Europeans resident at his camp. When epidemics of cholera, smallpox and typhus broke out in June 1866, as we have seen, he inquired what was done in Europe in such circumstances. On being advised to move to higher land and to leave the sick at some distance from his capital at Debra Tabor, he followed this recommendation, and, according to Blanc, "before long had the satisfaction" of seeing the epidemics "lose their virulence, and, before many weeks, disappear entirely."

The Ethiopian public also displayed itself responsive to foreign medicine, often indeed annoyingly so. Dr. Blanc related that soon after entering the country from Matamma his "troubles began," for

> I was at all hours of the day surrounded by an importuning crowd, of all ages and sexes, afflicted by the many ills that flesh is heir to. I had no more privacy, and no

more rest. Did I leave our camp with my gun in search of game, a clamorous crowd followed me. On the march, at every halt from Wali Dabba to Theodore's camp in Damot, I heard nothing else from sunrise to sunset but the incessant cries of *Abiet abiet medanite medanite* (Help, help, medicine, medicine)! I did my best; I attended at any hour of the day those who would benefit from a few doses of medicine. But this did not satisfy the great majority, composed of old syphilitic cases, nor the leper, nor those suffering from elephantiasis, the epileptic, the scrofulous or those who had been mutiliated. . . . Day after day crowds of patients increased; those who had met with refusal remained in the hope that on another day the 'Hakeem's' boxes of unheard-of medicine might be opened for them also. New ones daily poured in. The many cures of simple cases that I had been able to accomplish spread my fame far and wide, and even reached my countrymen at Magdala, who heard that an English Hakeem had arrived, who could break bones and instantly set them, so that the individual operated upon walked away like the paralytic in Holy Writ. At last the nuisance became intolerable, and I was obliged to keep my tent closed all day long; whenever I left it I was surrounded by an admiring crowd. The officers of the escort were obliged to place an escort round my tent and only allowed their relatives and friends to approach.

Elsewhere, in a report in the French *Gazette Hebdomadaire de Médecine et de Chirurgie*, he recorded that out of every 100 cases he treated 90 were cases of syphilis. The other most common diseases were scabies, leprosy (particularly around Lake Tana), and taenia.

Blanc was unable to carry out any vaccinations for lack of serum. While at Massawa he had obtained vaccine and carried out inoculations with it, but "in no case did it take," owing, he thought, to the "extreme heat." During the cold season he applied again for serum, but could not obtain any.

Téwodros's British captives—whose detention had led to the monarch's famous dispute with Britain—also played a modest medical role during their enforced residence at Magdala. Consul Cameron, in a humorous report on May 28, 1865, called all his party "doctors," declaring:

> In the afternoon we resolve ourselves into a dispensary. Every one has been in the school, and has a doctor's degree; Dr. Kerans, my Secretary, son of the well-known physician of that name in County Galway—arrah! by St. Patrick, but he shows the family talent still in drawing teeth and cutting up tumours like oranges. M. le Docteur, my head man, blinds those who can see, and finishes off the entirely blind as our optician. There is plenty of ophthalmia here, so he has enough to do; for all diseases above the waist emetics, all diseases below the waist purgatives. It must be a discovery in medicine. I have not lost a patient, we do an immense deal of good with our handful of medicine, especially as regard eye diseases. We have cured perhaps 300 cases. The patients are either prisoners or guardians of the mountain. This has ensured . . . our being better treated than we were at first.

Many missionaries of this period were also medically active, and thereby won a degree of popular respect which otherwise would not have been shown them. Mrs. Flad, wife of one of the leading missionaries, was, according to her colleague Waldmeier, "like a mother to our mission station; to the missionaries as well as the Abyssinians, among whom her medical knowledge opened the door to the hearts of many thousands." Even more important was the Italian missionary Massaia, who deserves special notice for his work against smallpox. During his 35 years of missionary activity he traveled widely in Shawa, Wallaga, and Kaffa, and sometimes inoculated as many as a hundred persons a day. He became known, as already noted, as the "doctor of smallpox" because the disease disappeared from the areas in which he operated. He also made extensive use of mercury pills in the treatment of syphilis, and declared that they were so popular that he could have become rich if he had sold them.

Yohannes

Emperor Yohannes IV, though regarded as a traditionalist, shared his predecessor's acceptance of Western medical practices. He had his own physician, the Greek Dr. Nicholas Parisis, who was sent to him by King George I of the Hellenes, and resided in the country in 1885-1886. Parisis, as already noted, was particularly successful in introducing smallpox vaccination. Though the practice was unknown in Tegré at the time of his arrival, it became so popular—above all during the smallpox epidemic of 1886—that Emperor Yohannes, his commander, Ras Alula, the *abun* (or head of the Church), King Menilek of Shawa, and King Takla Haymanot of Gojjam all agreed to be vaccinated, as were "many other generals, officials, soldiers and numerous children." The emperor, according to Parisis, was so convinced of the superiority of variolation that he issued a decree forbidding his subjects from employing the old practice, which, according to the British envoy Harrison Smith, thereafter was declared a "heinous" offense. European vaccination became remarkably popular. This caused A.B. Wylde, a sometime British consul, to observe:

> The Abyssinian is not nearly such a fool as regards vaccination as some of the British fanatics; he has had experience of many epidemics, and has seen the terrible ravages caused by this loathsome complaint among those that have never had the chance of being vaccinated, when perhaps ninety percent of those that have not been operated on die, and the majority of those that recover are marked for life or sightless; while those that have been to the sea coast and have been fortunate enough to have been vaccinated escape altogether, or perhaps only three or four per cent of those taken with it die. I do not believe there is any nation that are more willing to put themselves under the doctor's care.

Parisis has left a record of his stay in Ethiopia in a Greek autobiographical work *Aethiopica*, which was later translated into Italian, as well as in a *Rapport sur la Médecine en Abyssinie*, which was presented to the Egyptian Medical Congress. He relates that he used sulphate of quinine extensively both in the treatment of and as a prophylactic against malaria. On one occasion, while traveling in the lowlands, he gave Emperor Yohannes and his courtiers 20 to 25 centigrams of quinine every morning, apparently with complete success. In cases of taenia, he prescribed one gram of calomel followed by one gram of sulphate of quinine, after which the tapeworm would usually be ejected on the following day, and he also achieved the same result with Indian coco nuts. He believed that Ethiopians were sensitive to the action of medicaments, above all of mercury, iodide of potassium, digitalis, and morphine, medicines to which they were not yet habituated.

Parisis cured many syphilitic ulcers by sprinkling them with iodoform or calomel. For one chief suffering from a syphilitic tumor he prescribed a month's course of three centigrams of mercury biiodide and 50 centigrams of potassium iodide per day. Many soldiers with blennorrhea were cured in a week by injecting a light solution of chloride of iron into the urethra. Numerous dermic ulcers were likewise cured by making the patients take hot mineral baths, as well as by cutting open the ulcers and sprinkling iodoform or applying a poultice soaked in a light solution of phenic acid.

Another foreigner engaged in medical work at this time was a Hungarian called André who specialized in the manufacture and repair of weapons, but also made artificial arms and legs for the bandits and thieves whom Emperor Yohannes ordered amputation as a punishment. André charged 10 thalers per limb, and often was also given presents of grain, honey, meat, and the like. The French traveler Girard reported that when the emperor first saw these artificial limbs he "could not believe his eyes."

Foreign missionaries were excluded by Emperor Yohannes from working in Ethiopia proper, but played a significant role on the periphery of the realm. In the 1880s the Roman Catholic order, Filles de la Charité, thus ran dispensaries at both Karan and Massawa. At the former station, treatment was given to an average of 60 patients a day.

The advance of foreign medicine in this period resulted in a further increase in the use of imported drugs, particularly of mercury preparations which were replacing both traditional medicine and sarsaparilla in the treatment of syphilis. Dr. Blanc in the 1860s noted that mercury was a favorite cure, and that copper sulphate was also sometimes used, while Gerhard Rohlfs reported in 1883 that the use of mercury was becoming common throughout the northern provinces. Parisis, who confirmed the popularity of this medicine, said that in cases of secondary or tertiary syphilis patients would be subjected to 40 or 50 days of mercury fumigation, while syphilitic ulcers would be sprinkled with calomel or cauterized with silver nitrate or copper sulphate, all of them imported from abroad. Mercury sulphate and other mercury preparations, he felt, were particularly successful in Ethiopia where the inhabitants, accustomed to strong purges, did not suffer like Europeans from the excessive laxative effect of this type of medicine.

The Coming of the Italians to Eritrea

The Italian occupation of Massawa in February 1885 was followed by the introduction of Italian doctors and medicine into what was soon to become the colony of Eritrea. The British traveler Theodore Bent shortly afterwards reported: "The Italian doctors say that the amount of diseases of a syphilitic nature is appalling among the Christian population." Smallpox was also rampant as the country was in the grip of one of the worst epidemics on record. Compulsory vaccination was therefore decreed on February 21, 1889, a year or so before the establishment of the colony, and widespread injections took place in the highlands in 1890.

XVII

Menilek's Era of Innovation

◊ ◊ ◊

Though many earlier Ethiopian rulers had made use of Western medicine, its introduction entered an important new phase during the long reign of Menilek, a keen friend of science who reigned as King of Shawa from 1865 to 1889 and as emperor from 1889 until 1913.

Menilek and the Palace Pharmacy

Menilek, like his grandfather Sahla Sellasé, had at his palace a combined pharmacy and clinic which was constantly expanded and which was the repository of many foreign gifts. In 1885, for example, a set of surgical instruments from a visiting Italian physician, Dr. Leopold Traversi, were donated. A decade or so later, a Russian mission reported that the "court pharmacy" was "fairly extensive," and that each medicine was carefully labeled with its Latin name transcribed into Amharic characters. This is confirmed by the Italian physician De Castro, who noted in 1915 that this establishment was by then supplied by the foreign legations with "every kind" of drug. Each bottle or container had a label in Amharic, stating its contents and medical composition as well as its use, and everything was "jealously guarded by the officials in charge."

Menilek took a keen interest in medical and other innovations of all kinds. The British envoy Rennell Rodd reported that, on visiting the court in 1897, he informed the emperor that he had in his inventory some X-ray equipment but feared to present it because of possible opposition from the clergy. The emperor characteristically replied, "You should have brought it." Dr. R. Wurtz, a French physician who arrived in the capital the following year, likewise wrote of the Ethiopian ruler with admiration, remarking that it was the "high intelligence" of the emperor above all else which enabled him successfully to introduce mass vaccination into the country. A decade or so later the Georgian doctor, Mérab, observed that Menilek had a "remarkable spirit of inquiry" and did not see a surgical instrument—be it a spatula of unusual shape, a stethoscope, a sphygmometer or a percussion hammer—without immediately asking what it was and for what it was used.

The First Italian Medical Mission

Menilek's first important foreign contacts were with the Italians. Four Italian doctors visited the country between 1885 and 1889. They were Vicenzo Ragazzi, Leopoldo Traversi, and Raffaele Alfieri (who were established at the Italian Geographical Society's station at Let Marefia in Shawa), and Cesare Nerazinni (who took up residence at Harar). Traversi also accompanied Menilek on an expedition to Arussi in 1886, while Alfieri, who had travelled to that province with Ras Dargé, joined Menilek's expedition to Harar in 1887. Ragazzi, Traversi and Nerazinni all wrote extensively on their travels, but their reports, in the *Bulletin of the Italian Geographical Society*, had little to say on medical matters. Some idea of the treatment they employed, however, may be surmised from the writings of their colleague, Antonio Cecchi, who stated that his compatriots cured fevers with emetics and sulphate of quinine. He believed that, though seven to eight centigrams were sufficient for the average European, Ethiopians should be given 20 because they had been so hardened by taking *kosso*.

The work of the Italian doctors was of short duration, for it was suspended as a result of the Italo-Ethiopian dispute which culminated in the war of 1895–1896. An Italian physician, Dr. Alfredo Zarich (actually a Slav from Dalmatia), was, however, later attached to the Russian Red Cross mission which arrived shortly afterwards.

The Russian Red Cross Mission

The advent of the Russian Red Cross mission, which was a major event in the medical history of the Menilek era, was a direct result of the 1895–1896 war. The Russians, as Orthodox Christians, sympathized with Ethiopia in the conflict and accordingly dispatched a medical mission, which arrived in Addis Ababa in July 1896, four months after Menilek's victory at Adwa that effectively ended hostilities. The mission was led by an army general and consisted of four staff members, six cavalry officers, eleven artillery officers, seven noncommissioned officers (NCOs), four doctors, thirteen Medical Corps NCOs, and a chaplain.

The Russians, who entered the country by way of Jibuti, remained in Harar from May 15 to June 18, before traveling to Addis Ababa, where they served from July 26 to October 5, while a small contingent left behind in Harar provided treatment there from June 25 until November 8, when they began their return journey. During this time the mission gave 26,419 outpatient consultations (15,955 of them in Harar and 8,919 in Addis Ababa); the total number of outpatients actually treated was 13,056 (7,819 in Harar and 5,237 in Addis Ababa). Ninety patients, moreover, were admitted to hospital, 75 of them in the capital and 15 in Harar. A detailed breakdown of the characteristics of these patients is given in the tables at the end of this chapter.

The Russian mission was much impressed at the strength of tradition displayed by the Ethiopian public in its approach to medicine. Glinskii, one of the Russian doctors, stated that when his colleagues decided to cauterize— and thus to follow an age-old Ethiopian practice—the patients expressed "not only complete agreement but even special pleasure. None of our other instruments," he added, "made as much impression on them as those for cauterization."

A Russian Amharic Textbook of Medicine

Besides its medical work, the Russian mission—at Menilek's personal request—produced the first modern medical textbook in the Amharic language. It was written by Petr Schusev, a Russian medical student attached to the mission, and was translated by the mission's interpreter, who is referred to as "Elias, Ato Bezzabeh." This work contained 22 pages of text and discussed ten main types of disease, their causes, and possible cures on the basis of the medicines readily at hand.

The first section was devoted to scabies, a parasitic complaint which, the text explained, resulted from dirty clothes and unclean bodies. Three remedies were mentioned: (1) the removal of the parasites by squeezing the affected parts, a cure which "hurts a great deal and is also difficult"; (2) a hot bath every eight days with plenty of soap, frequent washing of clothing with soap or *endod* (the Ethiopian soap plant, *Phytolacca dodecandra*), and the use of clean bedding; and (3) the application of an unspecified medicine to be left on the skin for two days and repeated until all the parasites are killed.

The second section, on trachoma and other eye diseases, explained the dangers of touching the eye with dirty hands and stated that a person suffering from gonorrhea could easily infect that organ. The need for special care in the case of children's eyes was urged. In cases of inflammation the textbook recommended that a handkerchief or piece of cloth be soaked in cold water and placed on the eye. Another treatment was based on a certain medicine that was to be applied to the eye five times a day, or twice in the case of children.

The third section, on lice, explained that people were infested "because they do not wash." The cure recommended was the shaving of the head, followed by daily washing with soap and repeated application of a medicine called *berqe* (?).

The fourth section, on wounds, stated that they should be washed with clean water and kept free from dirt and contamination. Two medicines, phenic acid and *dofor* (?), were recommended. Bandages or pieces of clean cloth were to be applied and changed every seven hours. Bleeding was to be prevented by a tight bandage and by sewing the wound with a strong white thread. Needle and thread both had to be boiled before use.

The fifth section, on tapeworms, stated that Ethiopians suffered from them because they ate raw meat and drank impure water. The textbook declared that it was not good to take *kosso*, the traditional cure, with the traditional frequency, and urged people instead to eat cooked meat and drink boiled water.

The sixth section, on complaints of the stomach, stated that these were often due to the excessive eating of *barbaré*, or red pepper. The reader was informed that, "When one has stomach pain one must eat very little. Also drink boiled milk. Do not sleep on the ground; sleep if possible on a bed, otherwise on a well carpeted floor. Massage the stomach, then put on a new belt."

The seventh section, on malaria, gave unconditional support to the use of quinine, which it described as the "best" medicine for this condition. The patient was instructed to take half a gram in the evening.

The eighth section, on syphilis, emphasized its infectious character and explained that a person with an open cut could easily catch the disease if in close contact with an infected person. The cure recommended was to apply medicinal ointment to the whole body, starting with the feet. This treatment had to be continued for a month, the patient being washed with soap and hot water every five days.

The nineth section dealt with fractures and dislocations. In the case of dislocation of the shoulder it recommended that the shoulder should be pushed down while the arm was first raised and then bound to the chest with a piece of cloth tied round the neck, and kept in that position for three or four days. In the case of dislocation of the fingers, one person had to hold the patient's hand while another held the finger in one hand and pushed down the joint with the other. To discover whether a fracture had occurred, the reader was instructed to hold the bone with two hands and endeavor to move it. If it moved, the supposition was that there was indeed a fracture. The bones in such a case had to be put together and bandaged with splints for 50 to 60 days.

The tenth and last section, on gonorrhea, recommended that the affected parts be washed for 15 days with 6 drops of permangenate solution.

The book also contained nine pages of illustrations, comprising 33 diagrams, including a representation of the human skeleton and drawings showing how to make bandages, splints and stretchers, how to stop bleeding, and so forth.

The Russian Red Cross Hospital

The original Red Cross mission of 1896 was replaced in the following year by a second group of doctors who established Ethiopia's first hospital. It was erected in the capital between the Russian legation and the palace. This hospital, which cost the Russian government £7,000 a year to run, had a staff of five doctors as well as several nurses and pharmacists. The establishment contained twenty beds in addition to an outpatient department and pharmacy and gave absolutely free service. By August 1897, some 31,000 Ethiopians and 188 Italians had been treated, and a few years later Mérab stated that 100 to 150 patients flocked to the hospital every day.

The hospital, though a notable landmark in the history of Ethiopian medicine, evoked considerable hostility from many foreigners, particularly from the British. Powell-Cotton snidely remarked that the Russians wore "gorgeous but dingy uniforms" with Ethiopian decorations, but lived together in "wretched looking tuculs and tents, in a very untidy compound." The doctors, he claimed, did not have "a very high reputation for medical skill," though they had done "much useful surgical work for the natives," especially for those wounded in the then recent war with Italy. For Russia, he declared, the hospital was thus "a means of ingratiating herself with the natives, and showing how dear is their welfare to the Czar." Vivian likewise described the establishment as "an ingenious short cut to popularity with the people," and Wylde, also looking at it from a purely British standpoint, observed that the Russians, who had "so kindly and disinterestedly come to the aid of the Abyssinians" with pills and bandages, had thus made their "first footsteps" in Africa, "opening, perhaps, under the cloak of charity and humanity what may become a foundation to build a right to interfere in the politics of Abyssinia and the north-east of Africa and also on our line of commerce to the east."

Italian, French and British Medical Diplomacy

Notwithstanding such criticism, or, more correctly, because of the fears which underlay it, the other Great Powers soon followed the Russians into the medical field. The Italians, French, and British all added medicine to their diplomatic activity, which became intense in 1897, the year following the Battle of Adwa. The Germans arrived on the scene somewhat later, in the early twentieth century.

Italian medical endeavors, which were the most significant after those of the Russians, started even before the end of hostilities. During the Ethiopian siege of Maqalé, which took place from December 20, 1895, to January 7, 1896 (two months before the clash of arms at Adwa), the Ethiopians requested that an Italian doctor treat Ras Mangasha Atikim, who had been injured by a fall from his horse. Eliseo Mozzeti, the only doctor at Maqalé, therefore crossed the lines on December 30 and visited the Ethiopian camp.

Not long afterwards, the Italian government sent a medical mission under Dr. Angelo de Martini to treat the prisoners captured by the Ethiopians. It established itself in Harar, where it remained five months and catered to members of the public as well as to prisoners; 3,432 people were treated between January and May, 1897.

A few years later, after the establishment of peace, the Italians set up a clinic in their legation compound in Addis Ababa, under the direction of Dr.

Dominico Brielli. Between September 1901 and April 1911, it gave 59,695 consultations which were classified as follows: eye (12.0%), surgical (30.5%), venereal (21.0%), skin (9.5%), and medical or internal (27.0%).

The clinic, a busy place, was attended, according to Mérab, by more than fifty patients a day. Photographs of the establishment, which was a building of traditional type, are found in two contemporary works: Lincoln de Castro's *Nella terra dei Galla* and Cipolla's *Nell'impero di Menelik*. Both works also contain an Ethiopian painting depicting the doctors at work.

Some impression of how pleased Menilek, his consort Queen Taytu, and members of the court were with the Italian doctors can be obtained from the letters which De Castro received. Some were entirely matter-of-fact requests for medical assistance while others were messages of greeting, enquiring after the doctor's health or thanking him for favors received. In the traditional Ethiopian manner, such communications were often accompanied by gifts of livestock. A not untypical appeal for help was one that came in a letter from the emperor himself. Addressed, on March 25, 1902, to "the Italian *hakim* (i.e. doctor) Dekastro," it declared, "I have sent this servant because his tongue is sick (i.e. infected). Look (i.e. examine) his illness and cure him."

A no less characteristic letter of May 7, 1910, from the then regent, Ras Bitwadad Tassama, declared:

> The wife of my son Fitawrari Kabbada is expecting, but she is now seriously ill. It has become impossible for her to come to you. It would be my pleasure if you were to come and see her briefly.

Another epistle revealing its author's motives with disarming frankness was from the minister of foreign affairs and commerce, Nagadras Hayla Giyorgis. Written on June 7, 1910, to "the honourable *doktor*" it recalled that the chief had previously sent his brother for examination, but that

> Since his illness has become worse I have sent him to you (again) today. The reason I am always troubling you is (that) instead of me being troubled by what I do not know I feel you should be troubled on my behalf in matters that are possible for you.

The medical efforts of France in Ethiopia were also notable. The French attached a physician, Dr. Rousseau, to their legation staff and in 1898 dispatched a medical mission under Dr. R. Wurtz, chief of the laboratory of experimental pathology at the Paris Faculty of Medicine, to study the rinderpest epidemic of the late 1880s and early 1890s that had led to the Great Famine, and to introduce vaccination among a population suffering acutely from a smallpox epidemic of major proportions.

The British also entered the field of medical diplomacy. At the turn of the century they too appointed a medical officer to their legation staff. He was a Eurasion surgeon, W.A.M. Wakeman, who spoke Amharic "like a native," and came into "intimate contact," as Jennings put it, "with a great many persons of both low and high stations." He was soon dispensing 5,000 capsules of male fern extract a year as a cure for tapeworm and was visited by "many patients" who came "long distances" to obtain it.

This diplomatic entry into the medical field was much appreciated by the Ethiopian public, who, in the opinion of one of the Italian physicians, Dr. Annaratone, liked being treated by foreigners, and, as Dr. De Castro observed, were already accustomed to free treatment for which it did not have to pay a single centime, kopek, or penny.

Visiting Doctors

The diplomatic missions of course had no monopoly on medicine, for foreign travelers of all kinds were also active in the medical field.

Perhaps the most important nongovernmental group to visit the country was the French Duchesne-Fournet mission of 1901–1903, which included a physician, Dr. Goffin, who treated many patients, among them Empress Taytu's mother Wayzaro Wubdar, whom they found at Ibaba, a village in Gojjam.

Mention may also be made of the Englishman Arthur Hayes, a medical officer of the Suez Quarantine Office, who traveled in the Lake Tana area. He recalled that he then for the first time in his life found his reputation as a doctor embarrassing, for "patients poured in." Most of them were suffering from syphilis, leprosy, ophthalmia, malaria, itch, or tapeworm, and he remarked that, had they possessed any money and had he wished to establish a practice, he would have "done very well."

Besides the qualified doctors, there were many other foreigners who dispensed medicine, for the Ethiopian public, according to Annaratone, would go to any European in quest of treatment. As previously, any visitor from abroad was popularly considered to be a doctor. As Mérab was later to warn would-be foreign visitors, "From the moment you are a *Faranj* you become a *Hakim*."

One of the most interesting foreign travelers to practice medicine was the Frenchman Jules Borelli, who treated Gartiti, daughter of the former king of Kaffa, to whom he gave opium on January 19, 1888, shortly after childbirth. On January 30 of the following year, he was asked by a nearby chief to treat one of his wives, who had a double nose. "I resigned myself," Borelli noted, "and a doctor despite myself, tried to be inoffensive. I assumed a grave air and gave my client a small piece of soap: 'Rub,' I said to her, 'rub your nose daily with this medicament dipped in water. If it is used up before you obtain the desired result, all hope of cure is lost.' " Borelli archly concluded: "For this beautiful consultation I received a magnificent ox. I was ashamed to accept such an honorarium, but could I refuse? My client would have been offended and I would have incurred his displeasure."

No less important was the British game-hunter Powell-Cotton, who, describing his travels in Gojjam, recalled:

> Besides shooting for a few hours every day, I filled up my time . . . doctoring the natives, who, I found, came in ever increasing numbers as my name as a great 'medicine man' spread, till my little stock of drugs was being rapidly exhausted, and I was reduced to all sorts of expedients in order to give them something that would do no harm, and, by the exercise of faith, might even do good.

Evidence of popular interest in foreign medicine is provided by numerous other travelers, including Jennings in the eastern provinces, Bottego in the south, and Austin in the west. The "superiority of European medicine," Jennings claims, was thus "freely admitted," and whenever available was "readily sought."

Some opposition to foreign medicine was occasionally expressed, however, notably, according to Herzbruch, by some of the clergy, who remained faithful to traditional medical lore.

Balambaras Giyorgis

Some medical treatment in Addis Ababa was also given at the turn of the century by Balambaras Giyorgis, an old Greek who ran a curio shop and acted both as a doctor and a pharmacist. De Castro maliciously observed that this practice was of "undoubted benefit" to the practitioner but an "uncertain" one for his clients. Giyorgis, however, in his own way was a man of science, who also drew up a geographical treatise in Amharic.

Vaccination

Substantial advances in vaccination were made during the reign of Menilek, who, as we have seen, had been inoculated for smallpox prior to his coronation as emperor and was keen that his people should follow his example.

Vaccination at this time, however, was far from easy, for most serum failed to survive the journey through the hot surrounding lowlands. Dr. Wurtz, who arrived in Addis Ababa in 1898, reported that European-type inoculation was still unknown then and that local foreigners had been obliged *faute de mieux* to resort to the traditional Ethiopian treatment, variolation. Monseigneur Taurin, head of the Apostolic Mission at Harar, stated that he had often employed it in the Ogaden as well as in highland Ethiopia without a single death. Alfred Ilg, Menilek's Swiss adviser, had similarly variolized 114 persons, of whom only one had a confluent eruption, the others having only a few pimples. Wurtz explained this success by the fact that, unlike traditional Ethiopian practitioners, he had not used the smallpox scab but used instead the product of the scraped pimple just as it was turning into a pustule.

Wurtz, on his arrival, was shocked by the prevalence of smallpox, as well as by its serious effects. He noted that secondary ocular lesions were as common as in eighteenth century Europe and that he he often met with people who because of smallpox were one-eyed or even entirely blind.

The Frenchman's first vaccinations were carried out in the presence of the emperor. Some forty persons, adults and children alike, were inoculated. "On the fifth day," he wrote, "I asked for news, and was told there was none, no inoculation pustules at all. It was (happily for me) a false report. All the children and the greater part of the adults—I could not learn the exact proportion—had the typical vaccine eruptions. The thing having taken place in front of the eyes of the Emperor he could see its success, and from that moment I obtained from him the power to organise a proper vaccination service."

Menilek was so impressed by Dr. Wurtz's work that he issued a decree, on May 12, 1898, for compulsory vaccination in Addis Ababa. This edict declared, "We have found in the town of Addis Ababa a new remedy against *fantata* (smallpox). Go on the eve of St George's day to be vaccinated at the house of Dr Wurtz, but if you have already got smallpox do not go." This proclamation was read out in the marketplace by heralds, and from the following day onwards, Wurtz recalled,

> hundreds of men, women and children, led by their chiefs, came to be vaccinated. One could not believe that they were led by force. Their eagerness was so great that I was obliged to have guards at the gate of my compound to prevent the invasion and I can testify to much hustling and many battles with the guards.

Wurtz was deeply impressed by the ease with which vaccination was accepted by the populace, and, like Wylde before him, explained it by the great fear with which the disease was regarded. He observed:

> The eagerness of the people, adults as well as children to be vaccinated, exceeded all my expectation; it was unbelievable. I have seen Galla peasants make a journey of three, four, five and six days' march from their village to Addis Ababa to be vaccinated by me, camping outside my house. Gilbert Fenski (the doctor's assistant), in his camp at Ankobar, found about 250 people waiting for him for three days by the road.

The result was that between February and August, 1898, Wurtz and Fenski vaccinated no less than 20,700 people, mainly at Addis Ababa and Ankobar. These vaccinations were said to have been very successful. Wurtz claimed 90% to 98% (among some families, 100%) efficacy. He left during the rains of 1898, when the swelling of the rivers prevented further patients from traveling to the capital. Sufficient vaccine was then handed over to the Ethiopian authorities for 250,000 more inoculations, to be carried out by two Ethiopians specially appointed by the emperor for the purpose.

Wurtz, not surprisingly, was proud of his achievement. He claimed, probably with little exaggeration as far as Shawa was concerned, that he had the "good fortune" of being the first to introduce vaccination, all earlier attempts—whether by Italians, such as Ragazzi and Traversi, by Ilg, or later by other doctors—having failed, as the vaccine had been spoiled during transit.

Vaccination edicts continued to be issued from time to time in early twentieth-century Addis Ababa. They were written in simple but forceful language full of persuasion and exhortation. One, signed by Nagadras Hayla Giyorgis on March 11, 1904, observed:

> You see how the smallpox having entered the town is destroying the people. To exterminate this evil disease from the country, let the people who are in town— adults and children— go and be vaccinated. No charge is required and it does not cause loss of time; it does not detain one more than five minutes.
>
> Now all of you who think for yourselves and for your children, if you fail to have the vaccination done and anyone dies, know that it is owing to your laziness.

Later, during the smallpox epidemic of 1905, an even more imperative proclamation was issued, under the seal of the Minister of Agriculture, and read as follows:

> Advice re Smallpox
>
> We have before this given notice that the veterinary stations at Gulelé have a new medicine for all persons who will be vaccinated. But because many have failed to be vaccinated during the present smallpox epidemic, many have died. So now let everyone who has not had smallpox go to the veterinary surgeons and be vaccinated. If they have not already contracted the infection, vaccination will prevent it. But if they are vaccinated after having caught the disease, vaccination will have no effect. Therefore everyone should be vaccinated at once before he visits his neighbour, or goes home.
>
> Moreover, if anyone suddenly falls ill, the others in the house should be vaccinated before they are attacked.
>
> The smallpox which is the result of vaccination will not damage the body and spoil the face like the smallpox of our country. It has no bad effects. It is not necessary to die; it does not stop work.
>
> Children can be vaccinated two months after birth and this protects them up to fifteen years. Again, being vaccinated at 15 suffices for a life's span.
>
> Let people whose country is far away come and buy the medicine and take it away. The doctors show how vaccination should be done. The price of the vaccine for one person is 2 piastres. The doctors vaccinate every day except Sundays, from early morning until 5 o'clock (i.e., 11 AM, European style).
>
> After we have brought this advice to your notice if you fail to get your family vaccinated, when smallpox kills your children you will greatly repent.

Vaccination was likewise carried out at the Italian legation, by Dr. De Castro, who gave 6,000 shots between September 1901 and April 1901. He also traveled on several occasions in the provinces, notably in 1901 when he was asked by Menilek to vaccinate his grandson Lej Iyasu, who was then at the village of Temka near Ankobar, and took advantage of the occasion to inoculate all the villagers.

Menilek and his courtiers often sent crowds of men, women, and children to De Castro for vaccination. The doctor once received a letter from the emperor's daughter Zawditu, asking him to send "smallpox vaccine" for five children in her care. Such requests were usually made, however, during periods of epidemics, for at other times, the doctor complained, people tended to forget their fear of the disease.

Hakim Warqnah, The First Ethiopian Doctor

While diplomats, doctors, and other foreigners had been introducing modern medicine to ever wider sections of the public, the first Ethiopian doctor, quite unknown to Menilek or anyone else in the country, had been obtaining his training abroad.

The story of this physician, variously known as Dr. Martin and Hakim Warqnah, is most romantic. Born in October 1865 of a good family, he was not yet three years of age when his parents, along with other prominent people of Gondar, were seized by Emperor Téwodros and taken with their families to his fortress at Magdala. On the arrival of the Napier expedition not long afterwards, the child was found wandering away from his parents, and was assumed by the British to be lost. He was therefore annexed by Colonel Charles Chamberlain, of the 23rd Indian Pioneer Regiment, who took him back with him to India and kept him at his home in Rawalpindi. The colonel died in 1871, after which the boy was dispatched to the mission school at Amritsar, the expense of his education being met by one of their number, Colonel Martin. The missionaries christened the boy Charles after the colonel who had brought him to India and Martin after the one who paid for his education.

Charles Martin, as he was now called, was sent in due course to a boarding school at Batala and thence to the Lahore Medical College, where he graduated as a licentiate in Medicine and Surgery in 1882, standing third in the final examination. He was then appointed, at the age of 22, as an assistant surgeon in the British medical service in India. He resigned his appointment in 1889, and, having saved enough to pay his passage, traveled to Scotland where Dr. Russell, the Glasgow medical officer of health, gave him hospitality during his studies for the Edinburgh and Glasgow degree, and nine months' attendance at the Glasgow Western Infirmary. In 1890 he secured the diploma of L.R.C.P., L.R.C.S. of Edinburgh and the F.P. and S. of Glasgow and returned to India, after which he was appointed district medical officer and civil surgeon at Tongwa in Burma and later held a number of appointments in that country.

In 1986, hearing that the Italians had invaded his native land, he obtained three months' leave and rushed off to Aden, thence to Zeila in British Somaliland, only to be stopped by the British district officer, J.L. Harrington, who told him that on account of the war he would not be allowed to proceed, and in any case it would take six weeks to reach Addis Ababa. Dr. Martin was sadly obliged to return to Burma. His effort, however, was not wasted, for

Harrington, who was subsequently appointed British agent in Addis Ababa, duly informed Menilek about the young Ethiopian doctor. The emperor was most anxious to meet his compatriot and asked Harrington to arrange this. The result was that Martin in 1898 received a letter from the envoy telling him that if he could obtain leave, arrangements would be made to convey him from Aden to Addis Ababa.

Dr. Martin in due course arrived in the Ethiopian capital. In his diary (which, although unpublished, provides the basis for the present account), he recorded that after being presented to the emperor he secured an interpreter (for he had long forgotten the few words of Amharic which he knew as a child), pitched his tent in the center of the town, and began to treat patients free of charge.

He was soon surprised to see an old lady, accompanied by attendants, going back and forth in front of his tent and regarding him with obvious attention. He sent his interpreter to inquire what she desired. She replied that she wished to examine his arms and legs, as she believed him to be her grandson who had been lost at Magdala as a child. He cordially invited her to examine him, but stipulated that she must first tell him what she expected to find. She replied, "a long scar on the left arm and another on the right leg."

Sure enough, the scars were there. His grandmother then told him that his name was Warqnah, that his mother had died of grief a few days after he had been carried away, and that his father had not long survived her. His uncle, who was the principal customs officer in Addis Ababa, and other relatives soon made themselves known to him, his aunt apologizing for having deserted him in panic over thirty years earlier.

The emperor meanwhile arranged with the British government for Warqnah to obtain leave of absence for a year, and informed them that he himself would pay the young man's services. Warqnah, who now set about learning Amharic, urged the emperor to open schools. Menilek agreed, but so much opposition was encountered from the Church that no progress was made. The young man therefore asked the emperor's permission to depart, but Menilek refused to let him go, promising him to put down the opposition. Warqnah meanwhile was working continuously as a physician and surgeon. He was, however, by no means in a satisfactory financial position. He found it difficult to obtain any remuneration, and although the emperor finally agreed for him to be given a salary of £200 a year, £45 of it went towards his Burma pension. Moreover, the French and Russians, who were very jealous of him, intrigued, claiming that he was a British spy. He nevertheless remained in Addis Ababa till February, 1901, before setting forth for Burma.

On the journey back he met Ras Makonnen, the governor of Harar, from whom he learned that the British government, at Menilek's request, had extended his leave for another year, without pay. He had finished his service with the emperor, which had left him almost penniless, but agreed to serve with a British expedition then being dispatched against the "Mad Mullah" of

Somaliland and was appointed medical officer for the campaign. At the end of the expedition he went to Harar, where he treated Ras Makonnen and worked for six months, in return for which he was given some 70 acres of land.

In February, 1902, Dr. Martin at length returned to Burma, taking with him five Ethiopian boys, to secure their education. (One of them, Tedla Abebiyeu, later became a doctor.) A year later the British government requested him to join another expedition against the mullah, and at the close of his service he took another four boys to educate.

Shortly afterwards he obtained study leave to attend King's College and the Skin Hospital, both in London, and in 1908 was appointed temporary medical officer to the British legation in Addis Ababa, where he was assisted by one of the young men he had educated in Burma. Warqnah stayed in the country five years, until June 1913, during which period he treated the emperor as well as many other patients and did much to popularize modern medicine.

The Dispatch of Students Abroad

The first Ethiopians to be sent abroad for medical studies left during the Menilek period. They were Gezew of Tegulat and Dagne of Allobarat, both of whom were dispatched to Russia.

The First Leprosarium

Ethiopia's first leprosarium was founded at Harar by the local governor, Ras Makonnen, in 1901. On the advice of a local French Capuchin missionary, Monseigneur Jarosseau, he entrusted the institution to the latter's order. The establishment, which was named after St. Anthony, was run by two priests, Fathers Marie Bernard and Bernadin, assisted by a friar, Brother Thiotin, and three women missionaries, Mother Gervasie and Sisters Gertrude and Zoe. Ras Makonnen, who provided the leprosarium with ample land, took a keen interest in its work, and frequently visited it with his retinue.

The institution consisted of 49 huts and a "large building with stone-and-plaster walls and a thatched roof." The patients, who came mainly from the local Oromo population, suffered from the anaesthetic more than from the tuberculated variety of the disease. They were treated free of charge and attended voluntarily, being allowed to come and go as they wished and to mix "more or less indiscriminately with the healthy," though, as a rule, they remained in the home until they had noticeably improved.

Treatment was based mainly on the Indian specific chaulmoogra oil, though the priests, Jennings learned, were also "experimenting with some new remedy" but were "not at liberty to disclose the nature of it." Jennings, who noted that their management was "most excellent," declared that they "appeared to have no doubt as to the contagiousness of leprosy," for they saw that husband and wife "transmitted it to one another, and union between two leprous patients produced a doubly severe form of the disease." The missionaries were "very uncertain as to its hereditary transmission," however, for "healthy patients sometimes had leprous children, and leprous patients healthy children." Leprosy moreover "sometimes developed early in infancy," but in those cases "they felt sure that contagion was commonly present."

Despite the missionaries' success, no other leprosaria were set up for several decades. This delay was partly due to considerations of cost, but also to the widespread Ethiopian belief that leprosy was a God-given inherited disease, and not contagious. Menilek, in particular, was said to have been opposed to the founding of further leprosaria. When it was proposed to him that lepers should be segregated, he is said to have objected to the idea, which he considered unnecessarily cruel, and declared, "Have I not enough other things on my conscience?"

Ras Makonnen's Hospital in Harar and the Railway Hospital at Dire Dawa

One of Ras Makonnen's ambitions was to establish a modern hospital. At first he sought to do this with British help. After attending the coronation of King Edward VII of England in 1901, he traveled to Edinburgh in an attempt to arrange for a British medical mission to visit Harar. An English physician, Dr. John C. Young, of Aden, duly traveled to the city to explore possibilities, but the idea of British assistance was soon abandoned. Ras Makonnen therefore established the proposed hospital in 1903 at his own expense.

The hospital was at first run by Dr. Vitalien, a coloured physician from the French island of Guadeloupe, who had studied medicine in Paris, and was known in Ethiopia as the *tikwur hakim* or "black doctor." He left Ras Makonnen's service, however, in 1904, and was succeeded by an Italian, Dr. Brunati.

Ras Makonnen's hospital was built of stone. Jennings, who left an account of it early in the century, described it as follows:

> It consists of six wards on the ground floor facing the front, and three double wards on the first floor facing the back. The floors are concrete, and the walls are whitewashed on the inside. The ordinary spring, wire and hair mattresses, sheets, blankets, iron bedsteads and bedside tables are in use. The latrines and urinals are in a separate out-building in the back, with a modified cesspool; on the left side is the dispensary; on the right are the operating theatre and offices, while the cookhouse is at the back to the left. Utensils and drugs are supplied to the patients, but with the exception of milk they find their own food; and laundry work is done outside.

Not long after its establishment, the hospital was purchased by the French government, which wanted a medical establishment in the cool highlands for its personnel in its low-lying Somaliland protectorate. The hospital was thereafter run as a French institution, though it agreed that it would attend to the local Ethiopian population as well as to patients from the French protectorate.

The country's second provincial hospital was founded a few years later, in 1911, when the Franco-Ethiopian railway company set up a small medical institution at Dire Dawa.

Closing of the Russian Hospital

The advance of modern medicine suffered a reverse in 1906 when the Russian Red Cross mission was withdrawn and its Addis Ababa hospital closed. The Russians, who had become introspective in the aftermath of their abortive revolution of 1905, were said to have taken umbrage when the Ethiopian customs officials sought to impose a high tax on the 6,000 roubles' worth of medicaments sent annually by the Russian Red Cross. The Russian ambassador, General Lichine, refused to pay, and telegraphed to his government in St. Petersburg informing them of his action. Three days later he received orders to close the hospital.

Early Resident Foreign Doctors

Though the departure of the Russians left the capital without a hospital, several new doctors arrived in subsequent years. This influx resulted in part from an attempt to succeed the Russians and in part from Menilek's prolonged illness, which attracted a number of foreign practitioners who hoped to achieve an imperial cure.

One of the first to arrive was Menilek's personal physician, Dr. Vitalien, who was appointed to the post in 1904 at a monthly salary of 400 Maria Theresa thalers. He was highly esteemed by the emperor, who in 1907 contemplated appointing him minister of health in his first cabinet, but was dissuaded by the Great Powers, who regarded the doctor with jealousy. Vitalien remained in Menilek's service until 1908, when he was replaced by a French military physician, Dr. L'Hermenier, but stayed in the country until his expulsion by the then Ethiopian regent, Ras Tassama, in 1910-1911.

Vitalien, who treated the emperor in the early stage of his long illness, reported in April, 1908, that Menilek was suffering from arrhythmias resulting from chronic nephritis and inflammation of the kidneys. Within a few months, however, the monarch suffered his first attack of hemiplegia, or partial paralysis, after which he could no longer walk. Despite his acceptance of modern medicine, the reforming ruler agreed to the entreaties of his spouse Queen Taytu and the patriarch that he should go to the monastery of Dabra Libanos to take holy water in accordance with traditional practice. He left for the site on December 1 and stayed there for two months, subjected to a treatment of very cold holy water which L'Herminier felt unable to oppose for fear of going contrary to the traditions of the country. The result, the French traveler Rémond related, was that "each morning at the break of day the Emperor went to the baths, and, naked, bathed himself, while the chiefs, their clothes extended to stop the passage of evil spirits and malignant glances made a curtain." Despite this solicitude, the weather was "violent" and the water icy. Menilek suffered greatly, and at last called the French doctor, and said to him, "They are killing me. Prohibit me from going into the water, or, in two days, if you do not pull me out of their hands, I will be finished." L'Herminier took immediate action, and forbade the treatment to continue, thereby, as Remond put it, at last assuming full responsibility for his patient's life. The doctor's decision was justified, for the royal patient recovered, as far as could be expected.

Menilek's illness meanwhile was drawing other foreign doctors to the capital. The emperor was anxious to receive any physician who might be able to help him, and the Great Powers were desirous of winning his friendship by giving him medical aid. As De Castro later observed, all the Powers interested in Ethiopia—save the Italians (who were perhaps not fully trusted)—sought through their nationals the glory of saving the Ethiopian sovereign.

Perhaps the astutest appointment was made by the British, who, as we have seen, attached Dr. Martin, the first foreign-trained Ethiopian doctor, to their legation in Addis Ababa in 1908.

Menilek and Taytu also took steps on their own to import foreign practitioners. The empress in 1907 arranged for the coming of the country's first dentist, Dr. Caracatsanis, a Greek who had earlier worked in Egypt. In the following year, her husband brought in a physician often referred to in these pages, Dr. Mérab, a young Georgian of French nationality who had previously practiced at Constantinople, where he had treated an Ethiopian delegation led by Ras Mangasha Warqé. Mérab, who was appointed a physician to the emperor, also ran a dispensary at the palace that cared for over 50 patients a day. Remaining in the capital for over a decade, he acquired a considerable knowledge of the Ethiopian medical scene, which enabled him to write two important works, *Médecins et Médecine en Ethiopie* and *Impressions d'Ethiopie*, the latter running to three volumes.

Another doctor who arrived at about this time was a Syrian who gave electrical treatment to the by then partially paralyzed emperor in 1908. Not long afterwards, in 1909, there came a German, Dr. Steinkuhler, who also treated the royal patient with electricity. This physician was attached to the German legation and soon afterwards created a sensation by claiming that Menilek had been poisoned. Another German, Dr. Zintgraff, arrived to treat the sovereign in the same year, and was appointed an Ethiopian counselor of state. The two Germans, however, meddled unduly in local politics and made powerful enemies. Things came to a head when the doctors claimed that the poisoning had been carried out by two courtiers, Bajerond Mulugéta and Azaj Metaferya, who were connected with the empress. The Germans were thereupon thanked for their services—and dismissed. These events were subsequently made the subject of a pamphlet, *Le docteur nouvellement venu*, which was published by the Ethiopian government in both French and Amharic.

Other doctors in the capital in this period included a Greek, Dr. Jacob Zervos (who treated the young Tafari Makonnen after the boat in which he was traveling sank in Lake Aramaya near Harar), Dr. d'Antoine de Taillas (a Frenchman who had served as physician to the railway company and later set up private practice), and an Armenian, Dr. Emm Terzian (who opened a clinic in 1910).

The Menilek Hospital

A major development of the latter phase of Menilek's reign was the founding by the emperor himself of the Menilek II Hospital, the first government institution of its kind. It was erected in 1909 on the site of the old Russian hospital, and opened in May of the following year. The hospital, which at its inception was under the direction of Dr. Vitalien, was in the next few years directed successfully by Dr. Rousseau, Dr. Ganier, and Dr. L'Herminier. Its staff also included Gezew and Dagne, the two young Ethiopians who had studied medicine in Russia. The institution, according to Mérab, operated only on a modest scale and was staffed solely by nurses. It attracted only ten or so patients a day, or a tenth of the number that has previously flocked to the Russian hospital. The provision by the hospital of free medicines was nonetheless a popular feature—and one which, as we shall see, incurred the disgust of the early pharmacist "Hakim" Zahn.

Retail Stores and Pharmacies

The penetration of foreign medicine was facilitated by the founding of Addis Ababa in the late 1880s and by the subsequent establishment of retail stores and pharmacies.

The latter years of the century witnessed the advent of a score or so of French, Indian, and other shops which dealt in the most popular types of medicine. Articles generally stocked, according to Mérab, included iodide of potassium, Ricord's pills, quinine, castor oil, Epsom salts, laudanum, phenic acid, various balms, and antiseptic cotton. Such medicaments, however, tended to be sold in a haphazard way, without expert advice.

The need for a proper pharmacy was met a few years later by Dr. Mérab, who founded Addis Ababa's first such establishment, on December 1, 1910. Named the Pharmacie la Géorgie after Mérab's original homeland, it was situated next to his Policlinique la Géorgie on Ras Makonnen Avenue on land rented from a Greek called Cherassimos.

Mérab's pharmacy was remarkable in that it stayed open night and day. The Georgian, who wrote about it with pride, contrasted it with the private pharmacies of doctors who dispensed only their own prescriptions, as well as with those of the foreign legations, which, he argued, were primarily interested in politics. The Pharmacie la Géorgie had thus "liberated the Ethiopians," he claimed, from the "interested tutelage of the Legations," and added: "The founder considers that he rendered service to the country in contributing in a way to its true civilisation which consists more in raising human dignity than in the chemical industry and material progress." A no less practical advantage of the pharmacy was that it struck a blow at the less responsible trade in medicaments carried on by merchants, for the most part Indian and Armenian, who lacked any kind of medical training.

Mérab's pharmacy was a valuable and well-stocked establishment. According to its proprietor, it supplied medicines for a wide range of ailments, which, if tapeworm was excluded, consisted mainly of syphilis and gonorrhea—which were almost equally widespread—followed by bronchitis, gastritis, malaria (among merchants and other travelers to the lowlands), diarrhoea, influenza, pneumonia, angina, nervous diseases, and tuberculosis. Medicaments at the pharmacy, as in other shops, were sold mainly by weight, often against the Maria Theresa thaler, which weighed 28 grams or about an ounce. A contemporary advertisement stated that in Mérab's shop "more than 700 medicines, all of the first quality" were "on sale at a reasonable price." They included *kosso*, and various "remedies for taenia, syphilis, gonorrhoea, fever, and wounds, iodide, iodoform, and medicines for all other diseases" as well as "good perfumes." Iodide of potassium and iodoform sold for a thaler an ounce, sulphate of quinine for a thaler and a half if in powder, or two thalers if in pills, and sarsaparilla roots for half a dollar, while aloes, opium, cynanide of potassium, and strychinine were dispensed ad lib for a thaler, and bottles of Santy Midy were two thalers.

Some idea of the medicines most in vogue can be gathered from Mérab's advice to travelers to carry sulphate of quinine for the treatment of malaria, as "everyone" would ask for it on the journey; ipecacuanha for cases of gastritis, bronchitis, and pneumonia; and emetics, which were always popular as their use accorded with traditional Ethiopian ideas of medicine. He also advocated, perhaps for the same reason, the use of sodium sulphate and castor oil, but added that excessive purging cured less people than it killed. A sublimate solution of tincture of iodine of 1 in 2,000, however, was useful for the removal of ascarides as well as for the cleaning of wounds, though he thought it more convenient to use a 5-centigram mercury bichloride pill dissolved in a liter of water. Wounds could also be disinfected by tincture of iodine carried in liquid form or prepared by dissolving one gram of iodine in 20 grams of alcohol diluted with water. This medicine, he added, was very popular with the Ethiopian public, which also favored iodoform. Chloroformed water he recommended against vomiting, as well as for gastric pains, while laudanum—with caution—or nitrate of bismuth could be used for intestinal colic and diarrhea. Antiseptic cotton and antiseptic gauze, he concluded, should also be carried by all travelers for dressings.

Dr. Mérab's pharmacy closed in 1914 when its owner, loyal subject of France that he was, went to fight in World War I.

The capital's second pharmacy was opened at about the same time by a German actor, Walter Zahn, who in 1914 arrived in the company of a German physician with whom he soon quarreled. Zahn started in business by selling off supplies previously sent for by the then defunct Russian hospital. His first establishment was on the outskirts of the capital where he had few customers, but even after moving nearer to the center he still found trade slack—largely, he felt, because he could not compete against the Menilek Hospital with its free medicines. Later, however, he transferred his activities to a commercially strategic site on the junction of streets leading the Post Office and Railway Station.

The Pharmacy St. Georges, as the new establishment was called, proved much more successful than its predecessors. Zahn, who afterwards wrote a popular autobiography entitled *Adami Tullu*, states that the number of his clients steadily increased. He soon had an income of two to four Maria Theresa thalers a day, which, since he paid only 45 a month, enabled him to begin showing a profit. His finances were later much improved when he was appointed chemist to the Ethiopian Alcohol Monopoly. He was subsequently able to employ, at a salary of 30 thalers a month, a German-speaking Ethiopian interpreter, Gabra Kidan, who had lived in Germany as a youth.

The outbreak of World War I placed Zahn in serious difficulties, as his supplies of medicine—which had come from Germany—soon ran out. He ordered supplies from a Belgian in France, but they were long in coming. In the meantime he managed to purchase some medicaments from local Greek, Indian, and Armenian shops, and received help also from the Russian and Italian legations. The transaction with the Russians, who were officially obliged to regard him as an enemy alien, was curious. He was introduced to the Russian commercial attaché, who, even though unable to deal with him because he was a German, nevertheless asked Zahn to visit him a few days later in his overcoat. On the appointed day the pharmacist arrived as instructed, was shown into a room well stocked with medical supplies, and was allowed to fill his pockets, while the Russian conveniently looked out of the window. The attaché, though smiling, maintained his official propriety throughout the visit. Soon afterwards the Italians also came to Zahn's assistance. The German legation, however, gave him no help, and in fact seems to have been consistently hostile.

Zahn, whose memoirs contain many glimpses of the early pharmacy trade, stated that it was not unusual for his shop to be visited by an Ethiopian noble who would enter with all his followers, among them his gun-bearer, shield-bearer and briefcase-bearer. If the room was crowded, and the chief was wearing the traditional curved sword, the tip of which stuck far out behind him, other customers would occasionally be poked, thereby creating some confusion.

One of Zahn's recurrent fears was that a client would die while under his treatment. To obviate such an eventuality, he took care to send all his extreme cases to the Menilek Hospital. Another difficulty arose from the fact that many customers had little acquaintance with commercial medicine and were often reluctant to pay for medicaments, particularly when uncertain as to whether or not these would prove efficacious. Some customers declared that they would pay only when the cure was achieved. On one occasion, a peasant who ordered a cough medicine refused to pay for it. Zahn's servants therefore seized him, took off his trousers and thus prevented him from leaving the shop until a friend paid up on the patient's behalf. Another recurrent problem was the shortage of materials for wrapping medicines, in particular the absence of small bottles for eye drops and jars for ointment. Zahn was obliged to purchase all sorts of containers and even had to resort to using matchboxes.

Further troubles befell Zahn—always an impetuous figure—when, during the disorders that marked the end of Lej Iyasu's reign in 1916, he was arrested for shooting a man. His pharmacy, however, was by then so popular, he claimed, that the public insisted on his release; it was arranged therefore that, pending his trial, he should attend to his shop each morning between 10 AM and noon.

A large part of Zahn's business, as might be expected, was concerned with the sale of medicines for syphilis and tapeworm. Observing that the former disease was very prevalent, he noted that it seemed less serious than in Europe and therefore easier to cure. He usually supplied *jodur* (a solution of potassium iodide with a mercury preparation) to drink, as well as a red ointment for external application. This treatment, he claimed, improved the patient's condition for a year or so, and thus ensured a tribe of satisfied customers who nonetheless conveniently returned in due course for further treatment. Mistakes, however, sometimes occurred. On one occasion an old man purchased medicaments for a slave who was suffering from syphilis only to return with the news that he had given the slave to drink a sublimate solution—intended for external application to wounds—instead of the *jodur*. The patient, naturally, had collapsed, but after three days begun to recover. In the treatment of tapeworm the German used croton oil which he found both efficacious and popular. Since Ethiopians liked strong medicines, he made up twice the normal dose and sold it in yellow capsules which, he claimed, in some quarters were referred to as dynamite.

As a result of the activities of Mérab, Zahn, and others, the import of foreign medicines greatly increased. In 1918 a United States consular report observed: "The Abyssinians use a lot of drugs and medicines, and foreign patent remedies have met with considerable favor."

Provincial Clinics

The later Menilek period also witnesses some medical developments in the provinces, notably at Gondar and Dasé where the Italians set up commercial agencies with clinics shortly before World War I.

The Gondar agency was manned first by Dr. Vittorio Calo, who gave 11,006 consultations between July 1, 1909, and November 30, 1910, and later by Dr. Amleto Bevilacqua who provided a further 9,078 between July 10, 1911, and

October 31, 1912. These 20,084 consultations were classified by type of disease and number (and percentage) of cases as follows: medical (general), 5,699 (28.38%); surgical, 7,944 (39.55%); eye, 2,492 (12.40%); venereal, 1,931 (9.61%); skin, 1,441 (7.17%); and gynecological, 77 (0.04%).

Medical activity at Dasé began in May, 1911, when Dr. Domenico Brielli, a former assistant to Dr. Lincoln de Castro at the Italian Legation in Addis Ababa, was appointed. Dr. Carlo Annaratone, another Italian physician, reported treating 5,700 patients and classified the cases as follows: medical, 45.04%; surgical, 28.38%; ophthalmic, 13.42%; venereal, 11.56%; and skin, 1.64%.

Cures for Syphilis

Imported medicines continued to be widely used in the treatment of syphilis. Mercury preparations remained the most popular. Medicines such as *Mercuricum sulfuratum rubrum* were sold, according to Dr. Annaratone, by Arab merchants in Addis Ababa, while the inhalation of cinnabar, or sulphuret of mercury, De Castro reported, was common. Such medicaments were generally designated by the time-honored term *wesheba*, which was applied to mercury and iodide-of-potassium pills made up by local *farange* (or foreigners) as well as to what Mérab called a "charlatan mercurial ointment" composed of mercury, powdered roots, and butter. One such ointment contained the ground roots of *waginos* (*Brucea antidysenterica*), which had earlier been used in the sarsaparilla cure. Treatment of this kind continued up to the time of the Italian invasion of 1935–1936. The German pharmacist, Zahn, recorded that a large part of his business was based on medicines for syphilis, notably *jodur*, a sublimate solution for the cleansing of syphilitic sores, and a red ointment also for external application, the effects of which, he claimed, lasted for a year.

The late nineteenth century also witnessed the adoption of other foreign treatments for syphilis. The Italian geographical mission which visited Shawa in the 1870s cauterized syphilitic ulcers with silver nitrate and made use of saltpeter, or potassium nitrate, three tablespoons of which were dissolved in a liter and a half of water and a third of this dose taken three times a day for two months.

A subsequent innovation, of the early twentieth century, was salvarsan, or Medicine 606, which was discovered by the German P. Erlich, and first tried out by his Japanese assistant Hata in 1910. This drug reached Addis Ababa with remarkable rapidity, for Mérab stated in 1912 that he was already in possession of samples and was planning to introduce the medicine more extensively. It did not gain much popularity, however, for, as Zahn noted it proved too expensive for general use.

Despite their popularity, such foreign cures were available only to the richer classes. The mass of the population, particularly in the remoter areas, continued to rely on traditional forms of treatment, based on herbal medicines, many of them purgatives, used in combination with magical incantations.

Sanitary Innovations and Hygiene in Addis Ababa

The establishment of Addis Ababa in the late 1880s had significant sanitary and hygienic consequences. Situated on abundant and relatively well watered land, the new capital was probably healthier, at least in its early days, than many of the older and more crowded settlements of former times. The city in the opening years of the twentieth century was said by Pease to have had "no slums or overcrowding," for each hut had its own garden, and the wind "circulated freely" around them, thus keeping the place "fresh and wholesome." The houses of the nobility constructed in this period, moreover, were finer than those of the past, and were equipped with lavatories and cesspits. Ras Makonnen, for example, was said to have had a modern-style bathroom.

The capital's first water pipes, which were laid in 1894, supplied only the emperor's palace. Their installation was conceived and executed by Menilek's Swiss adviser and craftsman, Alfred Ilg, and created a sensation. When the palace was first erected it had no water supply. Ilg, as his biographer Keller explained, therefore proposed that water be brought from a spring on a neighboring hill by a system of pipes. Many courtiers considered this impossible. They argued that water could be brought to the bottom of the hill, but never run uphill, and that the scheme was surely a financial swindle. Menilek was nevertheless convinced, and the pipes were duly laid according to Ilg's plan. There was, however, one unpleasant incident. The water did not flow; the Swiss had to go all along the pipe tapping it to find the fault. He at length discovered that it had been stopped up with cotton seeds, apparently by a European "friend" who often visited his house. After the stoppage was removed the water flowed as required, and the system was popularly regarded as a marvel.

Contemporary admiration for the water system may be seen in the following pair of Amharic poems:

1)   We have seen wonders in Addis Ababa,
     Water worships Emperor Menilek.
     O Dagnew (i.e., Menilek), what more wisdom will you bring?
     You already make water soar into the air!

2)   King Abba Dagnew, how great he is becoming!
     He makes the water rise into the air through a window,
     While the dirty can be washed and the thirsty drink.
     See what wonders have already come in our times.
     No wonder that some day he will even outdo the *faranje* (foreigners).

Menilek's chronicler, Gabra Sellasé, who devoted many lines to the installation, recorded that when the water reached the Addis Ababa plain a large reservoir was dug and coated with lime, sand, and cement, so that its water was never muddy. Beside it was placed equipment brought from "the country of the *faranje*" (i.e., Europe), at a cost of 7,000 Maria Theresa thalers. Revealing the sanitary significance of the innovation, he continued, "Drinking water and water for washing was separated. The clothes of Atsé Menilek, those of Etegé Taytu, and those of their favourites and the guards of the *elfegn* (part of the palace) were washed in special laundries. From that time onwards people were no longer seen going to the river to wash their clothes."

Well-digging for the rest of the citizens began shortly afer 1902, when Menilek decided against moving from Addis Ababa to an alternative site at nearly Addis Alam. Good water in the capital was, however, by no means plentiful. There was often a dearth, Mérab stated, in April, May and June. In the summer of 1910, for example, two-thirds of the wells were dry, and half a dozen canals which by then had been dug to draw water from the springs of Entotto entirely depleted the town's three rivers for half the year.

In view of the water shortage, it was decided to construct reservoirs at Gulelé on high land north-west of the capital. The first, on the Ambo road, was built during the Lej Iyasu period (1913–1916) by an Armenian engineer, Krikor Howayan. An Anglo-Egyptian technical mission of 1920–1921 never-theless reported that "the provision of a really adequate supply" was "a very difficult problem," as the city was built "at a considerable altitude" and the springs above it were "only enough to supply the needs of a few of the better-class inhabitants."

Another innovation, as we have seen in an earlier chapter, was the establishment by Menilek of a bathing establishment at Felwaha, which was visited by persons suffering from syphilis and leprosy.

The Use of Soap

The use of soap in the capital became significant in the first years of the twentieth century, but made slow progress. By 1912 Mérab reported that locally produced soap could by then be obtained, but was of poor quality. Twelve pieces, weighing three kilograms, sold for a Maria Theresa thaler. Marseilles soap was also imported. Neither the local nor the French article was widely used, however, in part because it was thought that they caused clothing to wear out faster than when washed with the traditional washing agent, *endod.*

The first local manufacturer of soap was a Frenchman, Trouillet, whose initiative was soon followed by three Greeks, Polydoros Zecou, N. Halcoussis and N. Petratos, and by the Indian firm of G.M. Mohammedally. An Ethiopian, Fitawrari Daressa, also subsequently set up a soap factory, which, according to Rey, competed "strongly" with the cheaper imported article.

Provincial Developments, the Ambo Baths, and Modern Towns

Though Addis Ababa was the site of most of the country's innovations, a few were also reported from the provinces.

Water pipes were laid in Harrar in 1908.

Modern thermal installations were established around 1914 at Ambo, to the west of the capital, where Lej Iyasu built a swimming bath with bathing huts. The composition of the mineral water in parts per 100,000 was later analyzed by H. Silvester, a London public analyst, in 1930 as follows: alkaline solids states as sodium chloride, 5.6; sodium sulphates, 10.97; sodium bicarbonate, 95.24; calcium, 20.25; magnesium, 20.37; nitrates, absent; iron, trace amounts; silica, 6.0; sulphuretted hydrogen, absent; for a total mineral content of 158.43 with hardness (parts of carbonate of lime) 26.45.

"The water," the analyst concluded, "would be very efficacious for rheumatism, stomach and liver complaints."

Three modern towns, Dire Dawa, Gambela, and Jigjiga also came into existence in this period. Dire Dawa was planned, and largely constructed, in the first years of the century by the French engineers responsible for the Jibuti-Addis Ababa railway. The settlement was described in 1903 by Wolynsky, an Italian author, as a "systematic and elegant" town which had within a year "taken on the aspect of a gracious city," while a generation later Rey called it the most "progressive" and "advanced" urban center in the country, and one which rejoiced in roads, piped water, and electric light. Most of the local population, however, lived in a nearby traditional-type village which, as Barrois, a French observer, noted in 1908, was "growing every day."

Gambela, which was situated in an Anglo-Egyptian enclave in the far west of the country, likewise consisted of two settlements—a small modern town concieved and partly built by the Anglo-Egyptian authorities, and a nearby fairly typical Ethiopian village.

Jigjiga was planned in 1916 by Fitawrari Takla Hawaryat, an Ethiopian nobleman who had studied in Russia. Steer, who visited it two decades later, described it as a "methodical town," with houses laid down systematically in square streets.

These three settlements, though inhabited by no more than a few thousand persons, were significant as "model towns," with better sanitary conditions than prevailed in the country at large.

Sick and wounded treated by the Russian Red Cross Mission of 1896.

Place and Date Of Admission	Total No. of Out-patients	No. Treated Once	No. Treated More Than Once	No. Wounded	No. Visited at Home	No. Admitted to Hospital	No. Discharged from Hospital	No. of Operations Performed	
								On Out-patients	On In-patients
On journey from Jibouti to Harar	49	46	3	–	–	–	–	–	–
Harar, May 15 to June 18, 1896	1,196	978	218	28	28	–	–	51	–
Harar section of the mission June 25 to November 8, 1896	15,955	6,831	9,124	170	105	15	15	483	13
On journey from Harar to Addis Ababa	300	293	7	8	–	–	–	7	–
Addis Ababa section of the mission July 26 to October 5, 1896	8,919	4,908	4,011	358	70	75	45	217	68
Total	26,419	13,056	13,363	564	203	90	60	758	81
									839

Number of cases treated by the Russian Red Cross mission of 1896, categorized by type of disease or injury.

	Harar	Addis Ababa	Total
I. Mechanical injuries			
In the 1896 war			
By firearms			
Flesh	45	81	126
Bones and joints	143	257	400
Internal organs and larger blood vessels	2	7	9
Internal organs and bones and joints	5	21	26
By other weapons	1	2	3
In peacetime			
By firearms			
Flesh	9	2	11
Bones and joints	4	2	6
Bones and internal organs	1	1	2
By other weapons			
Flesh	5	4	9
Bones and joints	5	3	8
Internal organs and larger blood vessels	1	–	1
Other injuries			
Bone fractures	9	5	14
Dislocations and strains	21	16	37
Injuries	359	19	378
Other wounds	32	67	99
Bites of wild animals (hyenas, leopards, lions)	9	11	20
Total	*651*	*498*	*1,149*

II. Burns and related injuries			
Burns	21	9	30
Sun and heat stroke	1	1	2
Total	*22*	*10*	*32*
		(0.2% of all cases)	
III. Infectious or communicable diseases			
Relapsing fever	247	193	440
Influenza	–	3	3
Whooping cough	1	–	1
Mumps	2	2	4
Typhoid fever	9	–	9
Dysentery	12	13	25
Bites of poisonous snakes, etc.	3	–	3
Venereal diseases			
Salpingitis	165	127	292
Primary syphilis	17	14	31
Secondary, tertiary and congenital syphilis	630	703	1,333
Total	*1,086*	*1,055*	*2,141*
IV. Disorders of nutrition and associated conditions			
Anaemia	31	9	40
Diabetes	2	2	4
Tuberculous adenitis	348	302	605
Senility	9	8	17
Total	*390*	*321*	*711*

Continued

Number of cases treated . . . *continued.*

	Harar	Addis Ababa	Total
V. Diseases of the digestive and related organs			
Stomatitis and pharyngitis	13	19	32
Chronic stomatitis and pharyngitis	–	2	2
Gastroenteritis	53	73	126
Colitis	2	3	5
Proctitis	10	13	23
Chronic gastroenteritis intestines	643	421	1,064
Chronic colitis	–	21	21
Prolapsus recti and haemorrhoids	5	22	27
Acute peritonitis	2	–	2
Chronic liver disease	6	12	18
Intestinal worms or helminths	25	23	48
Tumours of the stomach, intestinal canal, liver, and pancreatic gland	–	4	4
Hernia	16	8	24
Dental diseases	79	26	105
Total	*854*	*26*	*105*
VI. Disease of the circulation			
Heart disease	6	7	13
Chronic inflammation of the joints, endarteritis and aneurysm of the arteries	6	3	9
Phlebitis, lymphangitis, lymphadenitis	5	6	11
Varicose veins	6	–	6
Total	*23*	*16*	*39*

VII. Diseases of the respiratory organs

Rhinitis	24	12	36
Laryngitis	–	10	10
Chronic rhinitis	1	6	7
Acute bronchitis	10	21	31
Chronic bronchitis	76	105	181
Bronchopneumonia	4	–	4
Chronic bronchopneumonia	112	33	145
Emphysema of the lung	2	1	3
Acute and chronic pleurisy	40	9	49
Asthma	2	–	2
Total	*271*	*197*	*468*

VIII. Genitourinary diseases

Acute nephritis	–	1	1
Chronic nephritis	11	4	15
Cystitis and urethritis	10	22	32
Dysuria and calculosis of kidney and gall bladder	12	4	16
Vesical calculus	4	1	5
Acute and chronic diseases of testes, epididymis, and seminary channels	32	19	51
Women's diseases	17	30	47
Total	*86*	*81*	*167*

IX. Diseases of the nervous system

Encephalitis and meningitis	3	–	3
Chronic encephalitis	5	15	20
Chronic myelitis	11	43	54
Epilepsy	25	30	55
St. Vitus' dance, hysteria	23	4	27

Continued

Number of cases treated . . . *continued.*

	Harar	Addis Ababa	Total
Neuritis	–	3	3
Neuralgia	204	144	348
Peripheral paralysis and partial paralysis	7	22	29
Mental derangement	2	9	11
Total	*280*	*270*	*550*
X. Diseases of the musculoskeletal system			
Rheumatic fever, chronic rheumatism	302	267	569
Chronic and acute inflammation of the joints	36	66	102
Acute inflammation of the bones and periostitis	9	8	17
Periosteum, chronic diseases of the bones and marrow	122	148	270
Chronic diseases of the joints and tendons	21	34	55
Total	*499*	*523*	*1,013*
XI. Diseases of the sensory organs			
Diseases of the eye muscles and eyelids	102	23	125
Inflammation of the eye membrane, conjunctivitis, catharalis, flictena	436	178	614
Blennorrhea in inflammation of the tear glands and tear ducts	113	23	136
Trachoma	596	78	674
Diseases of the lenses	318	191	509
Retinitis	114	9	123
Diseases of the optical nerve	90	3	93
Atrophy of the eyes	79	–	79
Chronic otitis	514	121	635
Total	*2,380*	*630*	*3,012*

XII. Skin diseases			
Inflammation of the skin and subcutaneous tissue	49	24	73
Various inflammations of the subcutis	68	56	124
Cellulitis	117	80	197
Ulcers	368	213	581
Tropical ulcers	143	–	143
Acute and chronic noninfectious rashes	133	214	347
Parasitic diseases of the skin	26	10	36
Fungus	158	85	243
Nonmalignant tumours	50	59	109
Malignant tumours	7	25	32
Lupus	35	21	56
Elephantiasis	25	23	48
Leprosy	143	233	376
Total	*1,205*	*963*	*2,168*
XIII. Diseases not falling within the other categories			
Goitre	3	16	19
Foreign bodies (not bullets)	2	8	10
Other diseases	76	–	76
Total	*81*	*24*	*105*
Total (Categories I–XIII)	*7,819*	*5,237*	*13,056*
Repeated Visits	9,342	4,021	13,363
Grand Total	*17,161*	*9,258*	*26,419*

Summary of relative number and incidence (%) of cases treated by the Russian Red Cross mission of 1896.

Category	Number of Cases			% of All Cases
	Harar	Addis Ababa	Total	
I. Mechanical injuries	651	498	1,149	8.8
War casualties	196	368	564	4.3
II. Burns and related injuries	22	10	32	0.2
III. Infectious diseases	1,086	1,055	2,141	16.2
Secondary, tertiary, or congenital syphilis	630	703	1,333	10.2
IV. Disorders of nutrition	390	321	711	5.4
V. Diseases of the digestive organs	854	647	1,501	11.5
VI. Diseases of circulation	23	16	39	0.3
VII. Diseases of the respiratory organs	271	197	468	3.6
VIII. Genitourinary diseases	86	81	167	1.2
IX. Diseases of the nervous system	280	270	550	4.2
X. Diseases of the musculoskeletal system	490	523	1,013	7.7
XI. Diseases of the sensory organs	2,380	632	3,301	23.0
Eye diseases	1,848	505	2,353	18.0
XII. Skin diseases	1,205	963	2,168	16.6
XIII. Other diseases	81	24	105	

Duration, location, and type of medical treatment given by the Russian Red Cross mission of 1896.

	Harar	Addis Ababa	Total
No. of hospital days of treatment	313	1,634	1,947
No. of patients bandaged	2,500	3,357	5,857
No. of patients given medicine	3,978	4,936	8,914
No. of operations			
Hysterectomy and oophorectomy	4		
Dilatation and curettage	1		
Cholicystectomy	1		
Resection of shoulder	1		
Resection of knee	2		
Resection of elbow	4		
Resection of collar bone	1		
Arthrotomy of knee joint	2		
Osteotomy, sequestreitomy, trepanation, and other bone operations	123		
Orchidectomy	6		
Removal of tumour of glands	67		
Extraction of bullets and shell splinters	29		
Extraction of cataracts	7		
Iridectomy	8		
Enucleation of eye	2		
Other eye operations	106		
Incision of the stricture of the urethra	2		

Continued

Duration, location, and type of medical treatment given . . . *continued.*

	Harar	Addis Ababa	Total
Various other operations, plastic, correction of dislocations, abortions, cauterization, etc.	471		
Hernia	2		
Total	*839*		
No. of anesthetics administered			
Chloroform	66		
Local	95		

Number of sick and wounded treated by the Russian Red Cross mission of 1896, categorized by age, sex, and ethnic group.

	Harar	Addis Ababa	Total
Age (years)			
<1	78	18	96
1–10	–	217	217
10–20	1,382	652	2,044
20–30	2,598	1,724	4,322
30–40	1,817	1,563	3,380
40–50	769	672	1,441
50–60	320	302	622
60–70	170	71	241
70–80	44	11	55
80–90	–	6	6
>90	1	1	2
Total	*7,819*	*5,237*	*13,056*
Repeated visits	9,342	4,021	13,363
Total	*17,161*	*9,258*	*26,419*
Sex			
Male	5,682	3,938	9,620
Female	2,137	1,299	3,436
Total	*7,819*	*5,237*	*13,056*
Repeated visits	9,342	4,021	13,363
Total	*17,161*	*9,258*	*26,419*
Ethnic group			
Amharas		7,634	
Gallas		2,990	
Hararis		1,204	
Somalis		832	
Dankalis		170	
Arabs		132	
Italians		40*	
Greeks		25	
Turks		15	
Indians		9	
Frenchmen		5	
Total		*13,056*	
Repeated visits		13,363	
Total		*26,419*	

*Prior to December 10, 1896, the number of Italian sick and wounded was 133.

<h1 style="text-align:center">XVIII</h1>

The Tafari Makonnen–Hayla Selassé Period

The process of modernization initiated by Menilek was consolidated and accelerated during the regency of Ras Tafari Makonnen (1916–1930) and the latter's subsequent pre–World War II reign as Emperor Hayla Sellasé (1930–1935). This period of almost twenty years witnessed significant developments in the governmental, missionary, and commercial fields, resulting in the increasing popularization and availability of foreign medical cures.

The Menilek Hospital

The old Menilek Hospital, which, as we have seen, had originally been staffed only by nurses, was now reorganized and expanded. It was administered by a succession of directors, mainly French or French-trained, namely Germain (who died in 1932), Mozert, Renauld, Mayenberg (a Swiss surgeon), Sassard, and J.E. Martinie, who was in charge at the time of Mussolini's invasion. Rey, who visited the hospital in the 1920s, complained that it was "in a perpetual state of re-building" and suffered from "lack of equipment," but Zervos later described it in 1935 as a "well organised institution with a modern operation theatre, laboratory and pharmacy." The establishment by then had 100 beds and charged 3 Ethiopian dollars* a day for first-class and 75 cents for third-class patients.

One of Renauld's achievements as director was the importation from Norway of a large barrel of cod liver oil, which he prescribed for children suffering from rickets. This oil was particularly appreciated as it arrived in

---

*The Ethiopian dollar was by now replacing the Maria Theresa thaler—but was the equivalent of the latter in value.

205

Lent when the consumption of animal products was forbidden. Though the oil had a "definite flavour of fish" no one objected; on the contrary, people flocked with bottles to buy it for cooking, as it seemed specially designed for the Lenten fast.

The Bét Sayda Hospital

A much finer and better run institution, the Bét Sayda Hospital, was established in 1924. Unlike the Menilek, whose directors were constantly coming and going, it was run from the first day until the Italian occupation by a single director, Dr. Kurt Hanner, a Swede, who arrived with two nurses. They were later joined by another Swede, Dr. Harold Nystrom, a missionary's son born in Ethiopia, and by a German engineer and electrician, Herr Stift.

The hospital was well equipped, with radiography, diathermy, and ultraviolet-ray units. It was originally built to hold 30 beds, but plans were later drawn up to increase them to 120. Farago, a Hungarian journalist, stated that on the eve of the Italian invasion the hospital had its own electricity and water supply and was "well fitted and scrupulously clean." He described an operation for appendicitis, which he witnessed, as follows: "The doors were closed, and the anaesthetic mask applied; the patient counted in Amharic and dropped off into unconsciousness. The white doctor and his black assistants then worked together in perfect harmony. The theatre sister handed the instruments to the doctor with precision; everything proceeded as smoothly as in a European hospital." Hanner was quoted as declaring, "There is no better hospital in Africa." Charges, however, were relatively high: 10, 5 and 3 Ethiopian dollars per day for the first, second, and third classes respectively, though the poor were treated free of charge.

Missionary Hospitals

Foreign missionaries in this period proved of considerably greater assistance than in the past, for they were responsible for the establishment of three hospitals and a leprosarium in the capital as well as other institutions in the non-Christian provinces, where they were largely confined by government policy.

The most important missionary work was carried out by the United Presbyterian Church of North America, which had long operated in the Sudan but did not become involved in Ethiopia until the great influenza epidemic of 1918. "At that time," Rey recalled, "a chief living near the Sudanese frontier petitioned for medical help to be sent from the Sudan." The request was transmitted by a British official in western Ethiopia, Major James McEnery, to Dr. Tom A, Lambie, a missionary in the Sudan. Lambie at once cabled his board, "British official in Abyssinia telegraphs inviting me to go there to open medical work with Abyssinian sanction. Consider it a wonderful opportunity." The board on January 15, 1919, agreed to Lambie's request, but no action could be taken for several months until the opening of the boat season between Khartoum and Gambela. On June 11 an investigation committee consisting of Dr. and Mrs. Lambie and two other missionary couples duly sailed to Gambela, where they received "a very hearty welcome" from the local Ethiopian officials. Dr. Lambie was given a stretch of land at Dambidolo. Medical work in the town was instituted by two American missionaries, Dr. and Mrs. Paul E. Gilmor, who were assisted by a nurse. The Gilmors subsequently left on account of ill health, but were replaced by two Swedish missionaries, Dr. and Mrs. Soderstrom, who were then at Lakamti to establish a Swedish mission hospital.

Lambie, whose leave fell due in 1922, decided to travel home via Ethiopia. On reaching Goré, where he practiced medicine for a week, he was asked by the local governor to set up a hospital, and the same happened at Addis Ababa where Ras Tafari offered in a 12-acre tract of land at Gulelé just outside the capital. On the missionary's eventual return to the United States, his board recognized the need to extend its activities to Ethiopia, but was unable to provide the necessary funds. Lambie accordinly embarked on a fund-raising lecture tour, in the course of which he received a large donation of US $70,000 from an American sympathizer, Mr. W.S. George.

This entirely unexpected gift came about one evening at the end of a lecture by Lambie in a small Ohio town, when he was approached by a prosperous-looking man who asked, "What is it that you are in most need of out there?" "A hospital," replied the missionary unhesitatingly. "What would be the cost of the building?" was the next question. "Fifty thousand dollars would build and equip it," said Dr. Lambie carelessly, supposing that his questioner was animated merely by curiosity. "Good," was the surprising answer. "I will send you my cheque for fifty thousand in the morning. And just bear in mind that if that isn't enough there's more where that comes from." It appeared, Lambie later learned, "that years before, the donor, then a lad in his early teens, had been seriously injured while stealing a ride in a freight train. Lying pinned beneath the wreckage he had vowed that some day, should he survive, he would build a hospital in memory of his mother."

Lambie in this way was enabled to found the Ras Tafari Makonnen Hospital at Gulelë which opened in May 1923. It had between 50 and 75 beds. It was equipped, according to Fan C. Dunckley, with "the most modern medical applicances and apparatus," and cared for 1,400 inpatients and 10,000 outpatients a year. Powell, an American traveler who stayed in the hospital compound, related:

> From dawn to dark an unending procession of Abyssinians, rich and poor, nobles and commoners, afoot and astride of gaily caparisoned mules, filled beneath our windows to the dispensary. . . . Thanks to the unremitting and unselfish work of the missionaries American prestige is higher than that of any other nation.

The second missionary institution, the Empress Zawditu Memorial Hospital at Felwaha, specialized in maternity. Established by the Ethiopian government in 1934, it was entrusted to the American Seventh Day Adventist Mission and had 50 beds. It was directed by Dr. Stuart Bergsma, assisted by Dr. Nicola and two nurses and charged inpatients 5 Ethiopian dollars a day, though the poor were treated free of charge.

The third missionary hospital, founded by the Italian Catholic Mission in 1935, was also situated at Gulelé. Though officially called the Hayla Sellasé, most people referred to it as the Italian Hospital. It was run by Dr. Bora, a fascist party leader, who was assisted by Dr. Miglio, and possessed, according to Farago, "the most beautiful building in the land." It was equipped with diathermy and ultraviolet equipment as well as a lift, the first in the capital. The establishment was widely suspected, however, of having been built mainly with Italian propagandistic intent. An Ethiopian minister was quoted by Farago as declaring that the institution was "only an advertisement."

The founding of the above institutions substantially increased the number of hospital beds in the capital and hence the public's familiarty with hospital treatment. Mrs. Dunckley, who spent eight years in the city, suggests that this process was gradual. It took "considerable time," she recalled, before she could persuade any of her servants to consent to being sent to hospital when they were ill, for they were all under the impression that people were sent there "only to die." However, after two or three cases from her compound had been successfully treated by the American hospital, there was no more objection.

The Leprosarium at Aqaqi

Missionaries were also responsible for the country's second leprosarium, the Hayla Sellasé Leprosarium at Aqaqi, just outside the capital, which was set up by the Sudan Interior Mission in 1934. This institution, which was financed by the American Society for Assistance to Lepers, was run by the Canadians Dr. and Mrs. Ralph Hooper, with the assistance of 12 nurses and cared for 200 to 300 lepers, some of whom lived on the premises while others came only for treatment. "Many" patients, Lambie claimed, were successful treated. "All," he added, "had Jesus Christ preached to them, and the definite conversions have been not a few."

Government and Municipal Clinics

The Ethiopian government established a Veterinary Clinic in 1927, and a small Municipality clinic was set up in the early 1930s. Supervised by a French physician, Dr. Martinie, it had five beds. There were also plans for a municipal VD clinic to be staffed by two doctors and 12 nurses, which, on account of the Italian invasion, were never implemented.

Private Clinics

A number of private clinics were also set up in the late 1920s or early 1930s. Dr. H. Ambert, a physician from the Caucasus who had studied in Paris and Bordeaux, established a gynecology and midwifery clinic in 1927, and a year or so later two other French-trained doctors, Jacques Bekiar from Paris and M.S. Mikaelian, an Armenian graduate of Montpellier, opened clinics specializing in gynecology, venereal diseases, and skin compliants. Madame Olga Seniavine, a Russian, founded a clinic for women and children in 1932; at about the same time, Dr. Bruns from Berlin set up a general clinic, and Dr. Rieger of Frankfurt established one for internal diseases, equipped with installations for electric massage and light treatment. A veterinary clinic run by an Armenian, Dr. Kaimak, also dated from about this time.

Such establishments encountered many difficulties. Dr. Näglesbach, in an article in the local journal *Aethiopien Korrespondenz*, noted that private practices in Addis Ababa were not lucrative because the "poor could not and the rich did not wish" to pay for medical services. The public, moreover, was often unable to judge a doctor's qualifications. There were physicians in Addis Ababa, Farago claimed, who had assisted famous medical men in Europe, but could not "get on" in Ethiopia, while there were others who, although unqualified, were "doing well" because they advertized themselves skillfully and winked at treatments that no doctor with a conscience would allow. He cited the example of a young doctor who had worked in one of the largest hospitals in Germany before being driven out by the Nazis. He had come to Ethiopia because he knew that "the people suffered from terrible ophthalmic diseases." At first he had had plenty of work to do, and had treated from 30 to 50 patients daily, but they "suddenly stopped coming." Even his regular patients disappeared. Before long he discovered the reason: a rival practitioner, who was not qualified and had lost many of his patients to him, had started a campaign saying: "This Hakim says on his plate that he is an oculist. What kind of doctor is that if he only cares for the eye. Come to me! I can treat all parts of your body."

The Institut Séro-Vaccinogène

To support the developing health program, the Ethiopian government granted a 20-year charter on July 24, 1924, for the establishment of an Institut Séro-Vaccinogène, which operated as a share company with joint Ethiopian and Italian capital. The organization had a five-year monopoly and was committed to produce 20,000 smallpox inoculations, as well as serum against rinderpest, and antistaphylococcic, antistreptococcic, and antigonorrheic injections. The establishment, which had an Italian director, Dr. Provenzale, was equipped with modern installations and a busy laboratory, which, according to Zervos, undertook analyses for malaria, syphilis, and other complaints.

There were also plans, at the time of the Italian invasion, for the Ministry of the Interior to run a public analysis laboratory.

The Public Health Budget

The above developments led to a steady rise in government expenditure on health, which, according to Zervos, by 1933 was estimated at 550,000 Ethiopian dollars.

The Expanding Medical Profession and the Founding of a Medical Association

The number of doctors—and dentists—grew significantly after World War I, and justified the establishment of an Ethiopian Medical Association in 1927. In the following year it was reported in *Aethiopien Korrespondenz* that there were 25 physicians in the capital.

One of the foremost among this small but expanding medical profession was Dr. Jacob Zervos, a Greek, who served as Hayla Sellasé's personal physician. Closely attached to the monarch for 20 years, he was described by De Monfreid in 1933 as a person of influence who was flattered and courted by the Greeks, but was regarded with jealously by other foreigners. Also associated with the court for a time was Dr. Germain of the French legation, who had insisted—without avail—that Empress Zawditu should cease fasting during her last fatal illness. Other prominent physicians included the hospital directors: the Swede Dr. Hanner of the Bét Sayda, the Frenchman Dr. Martinie of the Menilek, the Americans Dr. Lambie of the Tafari Makonnen and Dr. Bergsma of the Zawditu, and the Italian Dr. Bora of the Hayla Sellasé. There was also a German, Dr. Kurt Ewert, who headed the Ministry of the Interior's Public Heath Office, and two Greeks, Dr. George Kioussis, in charge of the Municipal Clinic, and Major G. Argyropoulos, physician to the army.

Dr. Martin, alias Hakim Warqnah, was still the only fully trained Ethiopian physician. Having left the country at the time of Menilek's death in 1913, he returned in 1919 after 28 years' service with the British government and was from then onwards entirely at the disposal of the Ethiopian government, but served as a provincial governor and later as a diplomat rather than as a doctor.

Dentistry

The number of dentists also increased during these years and, according to Zervos, had reached over a half-dozen by 1935. The doyen of this dental corps was Dr. Caracatsanis, a Greek who was court dentist to Empress Zawditu. His colleagues, or competitors, included the Armenian Dr. Emm Terzian and his son Dr. Andronil Terzian (who had studied in France and had his own clinic) and two other Armenians, Dr. Joseph Davidian and his son Dr. Edward Davidian, as well as a Greek, Dr. Nic Nicolaides.

Another dentist whose history was particularly interesting was Madame Alexandra Dabbert, a Russian aristocrat who arrived in Dire Dawa in 1923, almost destitute. She related, in a personal communication to the present writer, that she was obliged to start work before the arrival of her dentist's chair, but managed with an ordinary chair and some pedal equipment which she had brought with her hand luggage. Some time later she was informed that her cases had arrived and went to the customs to collect them, but when the box was opened she saw that her dentist's chair was entirely broken. "On seeing this disaster," she wrote, "I burst into tears. . . . The insurance would pay nothing as the cases had been insured CIF only as far as the port of disembarkation . . . it was a tragedy." Matters, however, soon improved. It was not long before she obtained many good clients, including the director of the railway company, M. Hetz, who arranged for her chair to be repaired in the company's workshops, and she was officially appointed dentist to the railway in April 1924. At this time, and later in Addis Ababa, she had an average of six to ten patients a day. A large proportion of them were new clients, for she tried to finish a case in one or two sessions rather than fill her waiting room by making them come many times. Ninety per cent of her patients were Europeans, and only 10 per cent Ethiopian. She explained this primarily by the fact that the latter had "excellent teeth," but also because her prices "though reasonable," were "too expensive for most of the population."

After Madame Dabbert's move to Addis Ababa she was appointed dentist to Hayla Sellasé's family in 1932. She recalled that she would ride on horseback to the palace to treat the royal children and would be accompanied by her faithful aide Habta Masqal, also mounted, who carried a small suitcase full of dental appliances, and another servant who bore her heavy pedal equipment. On at least one occasion, however, Empress Manan and her two children, Tsahay and Makonnen, visited her in her own establishment. Dr. Zervos had told her that it was traditional, when treating the ruler's family, first to try the medicine on at least two memebers of their suite. For this reason, she recalled, when giving a solution to the crown prince, she first put it on her own tongue, which seemed to please his attendants. Recalling her other clients she said that the poor made grateful patients. One such was "a little expecting mother, in the last days of her pregnancy, who came with a swollen cheek and asked me to cure her. I do not remember exactly what she paid, it was one or two thalers; I extracted the tooth despite the tumefaction, and she left. Exactly two days later, however, she returned with a small packet—some ten eggs . . . a present with which to thank me. The baby had already been born . . . and the little lady was pretty and happy." The rich, on the other hand, were less appreciative and had the "bad habit" of expecting to be cured free of charge because they knew her socially. To defend herself against demands for free professional attention, she employed a "good and respectable servant" whose duty it was to collect her fees. He would be informed how much each extraction, filling, and so forth would cost, and it was his task to obtain payment—without which she would not so much as touch the tooth. Describing a typical situation, she related that she might be visited by a small provincial chief who had come to the capital on business, accompanied by many servants riding mules, armed with rifles and wearing striking black burnooses bordered with red leather. Despite this retinue, he might well declare that he had no money with him at that time but would surely send the amount requested on the following day. She would then refuse to undertake the work. Her servant would propose that the client leave some object, such as a rifle or a leather cartridge belt with perhaps 40 cartridges, as a pledge of future payment. The servant was always careful to ensure that such goods corresponded with or exceeded the value of the operation to be undertaken. Only when these matters had been concluded to mutual satisfaction would the work begin.

Pharmacies

The number of pharmacies increased significantly in the 1920s and 1930s. The country's first chemist shop, which had been closed when its owner, Dr. Mérab, left to fight the Germans, reopened after his return in February, 1922, and continued in business until his final departure in 1929.

Zahn's pharmacy, the second to be established, also underwent several vicissitudes. It was run by its founder, Hakim Zahn, until 1925, when he fell in love with the daughter of Herr Goetz, a German plantation owner at Adami Tullu, south of the capital, moved to a farm with the lady, and handed over his shop to a fellow German, Dr. Ewert. Zahn, however, left the farm in 1927 because of a conflict with the local population and returned to his pharmacy.

Throughout his long years as a chemist, Zahn encountered many competitors. Three other shops, he recalled, were set up around 1923, one run by a Swiss, another by two White Russians who had come via Egypt, and the third by the strongest competitor of all, a British concern operated by the Abyssinian Trading Company, with two doctors and a couple of pharmacists. The British shop, however, did not remain in business long, for it was "so well done up with mirrors, glass shelves and nickel fittings, that the ordinary Abyssinian did not even dare to enter it." The populace therefore remained faithful to Zahn, while "the British pharmacy was nearly always empty, and was soon liquidated." The two other pharmacies were also abandoned before long, the Swiss returning to his native country and the Russians to Egypt.

Later, more serious competition arose from several Greeks and Armenians, who, Zahn claimed, had neither diplomas nor proper training. "These simple garlic eating people," he sneered, "thought they could catch up with me. They all established themselves near to me. One even opened a shop directly next to mine. This was too much for me!" He protested to the municipality that it was absurd that all the pharmacies should be clustered together, and declared that all that was lacking was for the rival pharmacist to sit on his roof! The competitor soon gave up, but not long afterwards several others established themselves in the area, further demonstrating the growing demand for imported medicine.

At least half a dozen successful chemist's shops were opened after 1925. They included three owned by Armenians (K. Arabian's Pharmacie Principale established in 1925, N. Broussalian's Pharmacie Normale in 1926, and S. Latfian's Pharmacie Impériale in 1932), and three by Greeks (the Pharmacie Greco-Ethiopienne by G. Athanassiades in 1927, the Pharmacie Ethiopienne by D. Zagorides in 1928, and the Droguerie d'Ethiopie by D. Caravidas in 1933).

Zahn's trade also expanded substantially over the years. His principal customers had at first been members of the foreign missions, and it was "many years," Farago claimed, before a significant number of Ethiopians visited his establishment. By the early 1930s, however, they came "from far and wide to consult the popular Hakim Zahn." On one occasion two ragged figures arrived from Tegré, three weeks' journey away. The leader announced that he wanted to see Hakim Zahn. The chemist went forward, and the traveler made a low bow and asked the German to laugh. Zahn, uncomprehending, complied. The man, obviously relieved, then described his complaint. The pharmacist subsequently asked why he had been told to laugh, and the man readily explained: "I heard in my village that you, Hakim, had a gold tooth, and I wanted to convince myself that you were the wise Hakim Zahn before I could confide in you." After receiving the medicine, however, the travelers sat down and refused to pay for the medicine. Their spokesman declared, "We have got the money" (which he showed), but they did not want to pay until they were sure that the medicine was effective. They therefore remained seated "for hours on end," and "only paid when they were satisfied with results." Most of the clients, Farago reported, had "the same complaint—tape worm," for which Zahn sold about 14 tons of *kosso* a year.

Notwithstanding his growing Ethiopian clientele, Zahn also catered to the European community (who were encouraged to enter through a special door) and, according to Farago, used the shop in the critical months before the Italian occupation as a kind of "news agency" which they visited "at least twice a day," bringing their own news and exchanging reports of others.

Provincial Hospitals and Clinics: Harar and Dire Dawa

The medically best-equipped towns were Harar and Dire Dawa. Ras Makonnen's old hospital at Harar—which cost the French taxpayer 60,000 francs a year—was run by a Frenchman, Dr. Joula, assisted by two French Roman Catholic sisters, and treated some 300 patients free of charge every day. The hospital was situated, De Monfreid recalled, in a "magnificent garden" on a site which dominated the city and had its own motor for the production of electricity for light and ice.

Harar also had a Swedish Mission hospital, established in this period. Equipped with 40 beds, it was run by Dr. and Mrs. Agie, and later by Dr. Artoun

Jonson, with the help of Hungarian physician Dr. Franz Pedar and two nurses. Pedar, who had studied at the Rockefeller Foundation for Medical Research in New York, where he had specialized in tropical diseases and diseases of the blood, was quoted on the eve of the Italian invasion as declaring:

> These Abyssinians need me. They are ravaged by terrible diseases and I am not exaggerating when I say that ninety per cent of the population are either syphilitic, or suffering from infectious diseases of the eye. They are not difficult to cure and I have proved that they respond at once to Salvarsan spraying. . . . But we have no Salvarsan, and the Government has no funds . . . the mission is suffering from the economic crisis like everyone else.

The old leprosarium at Harar was also still in service and cared for about a hundred patients. It was run by Father Charles and Dr. Jean Feron, who arrived in 1930. Dr. Feron later stated that he had tried all known treatments—arsenic, mercury, salts of gold and bismouth—but, though these had at first worked with efficacy, they later failed and he had been obliged to change the cure. However, with chaulmoogras oil supplemented by "a series of sudden attacks" with different metals—particularly copper—in salts or in colloidal form, he had "succeeded in inducing an almost complete return to health." Such medicines, however, were "expensive" and therefore he could "only treat isolated cases" with them. Chaulmoogras oil, in particular, was "very expensive," and "large quantities" were required. Steer, who inspected the leprosarium at the time of the Italian war, therefore described the mission's work as "an uphill struggle," the more so as uncured lepers found the exhibiting of their sores a source of income. He nevertheless felt that Feron's lepers, who dwelt peacefully in their own huts and received money to prepare their own food, were "happy couples" and lived to the same age as anyone else.

Dire Dawa was likewise medically relatively well provided. The railway company operated a small hospital for its staff directed by the Frenchman Dr. Renault, assisted by a pharmacist. There was also a municpal clinic run by the Greek pathologist-surgeon Dr. Paspatis with the help of several Ethiopian nurses, a private clinic owned by a certain Dr. Goldstucker, a dental clinic, and a pharmacy attached to the railway hospital. There also were several foreign doctors, mostly Frenchmen, as well as a Lebanese.

Other Provincial Centers

Several other hospitals—most of them run by missionaries—and a number of clinics were established in other provincial centers. Dabra Tabor had a government hospital; Laqamti a 40-bed Swedish mission hospital run by Dr. and Mrs. Soderstrom; Dambidolo, the Jean Orr Memorial Hospital operated by the United Presbyterian American Mission; and Dasé, a small one-man Seventh Day Adventist Mission hospital. There was also an Italian government hospital at Gondar and a mission hospital in Arussi for plantation workers.

Other hospitals were in construction by the Seventh Day Adventists at Dabra Marqos and by Canadian missionaries in Walamo.

Government or mission clinics were to be found in several other provincial centers. At Goré there were two clinics, one operated by the Ethiopian government and the other by the United Presbyterian Mission. The former was directed by an Italian, Dr. Lanzoni, and later by a Greek, Dr. Nikitas Zervos, who also ran a pharmacy. The mission clinic was under the direction of two Americans, Dr. and Mrs. Virgil F. Dougherty, assisted for a time by a surgeon, Dr. Näglesbach. Lanzoni, who had formerly served in Eritrea but had left after having been accused of being an antifascist, reported that at Goré syphilis was

> widespread in a startling manner among the better class, the poor, the townsfolk, and the country-folk. I have not yet encountered a family exempt from this infection. Syphilis cases come to the dispensary and readily ask for intravenous injections without bothering about medical advice. They are satisfied with four injections . . . the treatment which the American mission has been carrying out for some time.

Tapeworm and other helminths, he recalled, were also prevalent and some 1,000 doses of taenicide were dispensed monthly.

There were likewise government clinics at Jijiga, run by a Swede, Dr. Agie; at Asba Tafari, entrusted to an Indian doctor; and in Sidamo, where there was a Hungarian Dr. Saska, as well as a private veterinary clinic belonging to a Greek called Houloussou.

Foreign missions also operated several clinics and dispensaries. At Aira, the German Hermannsburger mission had a clinic run by Dr. Luders, assisted by a sister; at Soddu, the Sudan Interior Mission had a dispensary managed by a nurse, Miss Ruth Bray; and in Bagémder, the mission to the Falashas had a dispensary under the care of a sister.

Provincial Doctors

There were a number of other physicians in the provinces, mostly in the service of governors. In Gojjam, Ras Imru employed a Greek, Dr. Vassiliou, and in Balé, Dejazmach Nassibu another Greek, Dr. Vassilikiotis, while in Jimma, Abba Jiffar made use of a certain Dr. Goggne.

Such activities introduced foreign treatment to an increasing section of the population. Christine Sandford, who ran a dispensary for many years at her estate at Mullu, north-west of the capital, commented that she saw a gradual but steady expansion in the use of imported medicines, though she attached even greater importance to popularizing "elementary rules of hygiene and cleanliness," particularly among the women and children of the peasantry. Describing her own work, she recalled:

> For over ten years the distribution of medicines, disinfectants, and dressings worked many apparent miracles in the countryside within a twenty-mile radius. . . .

Memories were long when help had been given, and steadily the right soil in which to plant the seeds of education in hygiene and elementary first aid was being prepared in many districts.

Smallpox Control

The struggle against smallpox was intensified during this period by the expanding of vaccination services. Shortly after World War I, the Phelps Stokes mission reported that vaccination was "gaining ground," while a decade or so later Rey noted that it was popularly "recognised and appreciated." The local Institut Séro-Vaccinogène, which was established in 1924, initiated a "vast propaganda," Zervos reported, with the result that over 25,000 vaccinations were carried out in Shawa and Harar in the half decade prior to 1930, when financial difficulties resulting from the world slump led to some curtailment of activity. He nevertheless estimated that 50,000 inoculations had been given by 1935. Vaccination was in full swing at the Bét Sayda Hospital, one of the main inoculation centers, when Farago inspected it at the beginning of the war, and reported:

> There was a crowd outside the large zinc building that served as the out-patients' clinic. There were about a hundred Shankala children from Beni Shangul [who] had travelled for fourteen days to be inoculated. . . . They had arrived naked, just as they lived at home, but in the town they had put on coarse sacking. . . . The nurses inoculated them one after the other, with great skill, and immediately they had been treated they set out again for home.

"This scene" he thought, "was symbolic of the new Abysinnia," for the hundred children were "only the start: the next day hundreds more would arrive."

A plan for compulsory vaccination was put forward by one of the foreign physicians, Dr. Näglesbach, but was never implemented.

Control of Rabies

Modern-style rabies inoculation gained great popularity in Addis Ababa after the completion of the railway from Jibuti. In the period before the serum was locally available, persons bitten by rabitic dogs would take (if they could afford it) the three day train journey to the coast, after which they would sail up the Red Sea to be inoculated either at Cairo or Alexandria. Three of four Europeans, Mérab stated, usually did this every year. The necessary serum, however, began to be produced in Addis Ababa in 1927, and its manufacture by the Italians in Eritrea started at about the same time. Inoculations in the Ethiopian capital, according to Mrs. Dunckley, were first given by an Armenian veterinary surgeon, but later by other practitioners as well.

Medical Education

The first Ethiopian students to go abroad for medical studies left during this period. The first to become qualified since Hakim Warqnah was Dr. Melaku

Bayen, who studied in India and subsequently in the United States where he attended Muskigum Missionary College, Ohio State University, and later Howard University, where he received his degree of medicine just prior to the Italian invasion. He duly returned home, but later went into exile in the United States where he edited a newspaper, the *Voice of Ethiopia*, which rallied Negro support for the Ethiopian cause. Other medical students included Hizgias Finas, a Falasha who studied in Italy but died before returning home, Binega Tesfa Mariam, who also studied in Italy, and Getahun Tassama who attended the American University in Beirut. The only student of dentistry was another Falasha, Abraham Abera, who studied in Austria and France, but also died before returning to his native land. Two veterinary students also studied abroad at this period: Alam Warq Beyene, who studied in England, and Ingida Yohannes who attended the American University of Beirut and later New York University.

The first steps in modern medical education within the country itself were taken towards the end of this period. A school for medical auxiliaries was established at the Menilek School in 1935, under the direction of the Greek Major Argyropoulos, assisted by the director of the Hayla Sellasé I Lycée, Professor Malhamé. Twenty students, who had completed seventh grade, were enrolled for a two-year course that included anatomy, microbiology, and analysis, in addition to mathematics and chemistry. It was planned that graduates would be attached to the army or serve in the provinces, but teaching was brought to an end by the Italian invasion. A scheme was also drawn up by Dr. Melly for a medical school, but this likewise was deferred because of the war.

The Ethiopian Women's Work Association and the Red Cross Society

The threatened Italian invasion led to the establishment in 1935 of two new institutions: the Ethiopian Women's Work Association and the Ethiopian Red Cross Society. The former, which was set up largely on the initiative of Princess Tsahay and an official of the British Save the Children Fund, had an influential committee, largely composed of the wives of prominent government officials. Its patron was Empress Manan, and its committee comprised Madame Berhané Marcos, vice-president; Madame Belachew, secretary; and the Rev. A.F. Mathews and Ato Belachew, treasurers. The founding members included the emperor's kinswoman Princess Yesash Warq and the wives of several prominent officials: Madame Zeleke Agedaw, Madame Walda Maryam, Madame Georges Herouy, Madame Ayalé Gabré, Madame Tasfay Tegagn, Madame Sirak Heruy, and Madame Tadessa Meshasha. Although this was the country's first women's organization, it members equipped the first ambulance unit sent to the north and provided all the bandages and dressings for the southern unit. The organization subsequently opened a clinic in Addis Ababa that functioned until the arrival of the Italians.

The Ethiopian Red Cross Society had 200 founder members. Its committee, which was nominated by the Women's Work Association, included Wayzaro Sharanesh, president; Wayzaro Martha, secretary; and Wayzaro Wallata Emanuél, treasurer. The society raised 32,650 Ethiopian dollars by private collection, to which the government later added a further 200,000.

Legislation

Modern medical legislation began in Ethiopia in 1930, when the first attempt was made to put the medical and allied professions on a sound legal footing. Laws were enacted to supervise the professions of doctor, dentist, pharmacist, midwife, and veterinarian, as well as to control pharmacies and the sale of poisons and to render illegal the sale of adulterated or undesirable footstuffs. Such questions were made the responsibility of the Ministry of the Interior, which established a Public Health Bureau. It was entrusted with the supervision of hospitals and clinics; the registration of midwives, doctors, pharmacists, and veterinarians; and regulation of the import and use of poisons, narcotics, and stupefactives. The office was under the direction of Dr. K. Ewert and a committee composed of the Minister of the Interior, as president, and the following members: Dr. Jacob Zervos, Dr. Hanner, Major Argyropoulos, Dr. Ewert (who did most of the work), and the ministry's secretary-general Ayala Sebhat.

The most important law, which regulated the work of the doctor, dentist, pharmacist, midwife, and veterinarian, was issued on July 18, 1930. It specified that no one could exercise these professions, or run a pharmacy, without a relevant diploma. As a temporary measure, however, and subject to special authorization, doctors were allowed to operate pharmacies, and authorized nurses were permitted to treat patients in provinces which lacked any qualified physician. Midwives were prohibited from prescribing medicines or using obstetric instruments and in difficult cases were expected to call a doctor. Pharmacists were forbidden from dispensing medicaments without prescription from a qualified physician or veterinarian. Grocers and other traders were prohibited from selling medicines other than castor oil or sulphate of magnesium.

The law placed the medical and allied professions under the supervision of the Ministry of the Interior and specified that doctors, dentists, pharmacists, midwives, and veterinarians had to shown their diplomas to that ministry within three months to receive official authorization to practice. The ministry was to keep a register of practitioners, and persons failing to register were liable to a fine of from 20 to 2,000 Ethiopian dollars, depending on the gravity of the case—though foreigners could elect as an alternative to receive penalties commensurate with those in their own country.

The law also enacted strict regulations for pharmacies. It specified that they had to have four rooms, and be supplied with all necessary equipment and furniture, as well as a pharmacopeia. All chemical products, drugs, and the like had to be classified, and stored according to their proper stipulations. Stupefactives and poisons had to be locked in a special cupboard. Pharmacists were obliged to declare the number and quality of their personnel and indicate on all prescriptions the name of the pharmacy, the composition of the medicine, directions for its use, its price, and the date when it was sold. Labels on medicaments for external use had to be written on red paper, and all medicines prescribed for Ethiopians had to carry written inscriptions in Amharic. Pharmacists were prohibited from exercising the medical art except in urgent cases, or where a doctor could not be found. If a physician prescribed more than the maximum dose, the pharmacist was expected to reduce the dose unless the doctor confirmed it in writing.

Pharmacists were obliged to remain open at night and on Sundays on a rota basis. All weights, balances, and measures were to be controlled by an Inspector of Pharmacies. The Ministry of the Interior was given the right of inspection to ensure the execution of the law. Vaccines and serums had to be sold before their expiration date and smallpox vaccine within 90 days of its arrival. Tincture of digitalis had to be prepared by the pharmacists themselves and not be imported from abroad. Any contravention of these regulations rended a pharmacist liable to a fine of from 5 to 5,000 Ethiopian dollars, and the ministry had the power to withdraw the right to practice from anyone who broke the law repeatedly.

Another law stipulated that druggists had to be in possession of an assistant pharmacist's diploma or to have passed a special examination after the completion of an apprenticeship of at least three years.

A further law regulated the sale and possession of poisons, which had to be kept in special locked cupboards bearing the sign "POISON;" the same applied to stupefactives, and lists of both types of agents were published.

Finally legislation was enacted to control the preparation and sale of foodstuffs and drinks, both alcoholic and nonalcoholic. The law specified the required composition of flour, butter, fat, oil, mead, beer, pepper and various other spices, honey, salt, sugar, gelatin, cheese, sausages, preserves, sweets, syrups, bread, pastries and chocolates, as well as the age of "fresh eggs" (which could not be more than fourteen days old). Adulteration or imitation of foodstuffs was prohibited, and provision was made for the inspection of shops, storage places, and markets "at any time between dawn and sunset" as well as for the imposition of fines, of from 1 to 1,000 Ethiopian dollars.

Sanitation

Despite such reforms, sanitary conditions in Addis Ababa, as elsewhere, were still poor. "Many" of the capital's wells, Rey reported, were exhausted every dry season, when "great difficulties" were encountered in obtaining water. A few wells, however, operated all year round, and their owners would allow their friends to send servants to collect water from them.

The supply of water for the citizens as a whole was far from "adequate", however, as Christine Sandford asserted, and the poor were often extremely short of water. They were dependent on "the few wells on the outskirts of town," and "many dozens of women" were "to be seen at nearly every hour of the day," Rey stated, "patiently awaiting their turn to fill up their large water-pots by means of a mug, for drinking and cooking purposes."

The Felwaha baths on the other hand constituted a valuable source of healthy warm water for Addis Ababa's more fortunate citizens. Many of the wealthy, particularly among the foreign community, would employ groups of four Guragé porters to go down to the springs with four large tins which they would fill and bring back. The water on arrival would still be so hot as to require the admixture of half as much cold water. A *tanika* (or four-gallon tin) of hot water could be purchased, according to a Swedish resident, General Virgin, for one *bésa* (or 1/32nd of an Ethiopian dollar), and its transportation for a kilometer would cost a further two *bésa*s. Thus it was cheaper, according to the American traveler MacCreagh, to employ Guragés to carry water from Felwaha than to heat it by fire.

Most people in Addis Ababa, as in the countryside, however relied heavily on the often impure water from streams and rivers. Humans and livestock often drank from the same supply, and, Herzbruch stated, dead animals were frequently allowed to remain in the water, for the public disliked carrying off such corpses.

In the absence of piped water the bulk of the population had perforce to wash their clothes, as in the old days, in the city's less than abundant water courses. The river beds, which were largely narrow clefts between the rocks, were often occupied in the morning, Rosita Forbes related, by people who were "engaged in washing themselves, their clothes, or their household effects," with the result that "the boulders were shiny with soap, the water foamed with it, and snow-white chammas drying in the sun contrasted with the figures of their owners, glistening after a vigorous scrubbing." This picture is confirmed by Mérab, who recalled that every day several hundred people could be seen washing their clothes in any of the city's three main rivers.

Scavenging in Addis Ababa, as in other towns, was carried out almost entirely by hyenas, assisted by pi-dogs and vultures. Large numbers of hyenas came up from the river beds each night to clear the town. The pi-dogs, though also useful as scavengers, tended to multiply unduly. The city authorities therefore waged a constant war to control their numbers, and, usually after the rains, took steps to poison them off. The result was that, as British resident Fan C. Dunckley recalled, for days afterwards their bloated carcasses, surrounded by a "curtain of flies," could be seen lying about the streets waiting to be collected.

Addis Ababa also suffered throughout this time from the absence of any adequate drainage system. This became increasingly serious as the population grew and the settlement became denser. Inevitably, as Rey noted, cesspools in the more crowded areas were dug in close proximity to drinking wells.

Another unsanitary aspect of the capital resulted from the dearth of public latrines and the absence of any tradition of their use. Citizens relieved themselves, Rey observed, outside the huts or in the roads at any place or at any time nature urged. At least one large communal latrine, however, was in existence—near the city's main hotel, the Etegé, where the British journalist Harmsworth saw it in 1936. It was visited all day long by "a steady procession of clients," sometimes consisting of a whole family together, while "several attendants with shovels waited hopefully for tips."

A further unhygienic feature of the city in its early days was the windowless butchers' stalls, which, as Mrs. Dunckley recalled, were completely open to the flies. The latter, Mérab confirmed, were very numerous in the dry season. There were also many mice, which, according to the German observer Schrenzel, were to be found in every house.

Addis Ababa, moreover, often was excessively dusty because the streets and squares were neither paved nor washed and might, on holidays and marketdays, be trampled over, Mérab says, by 5,000 or 10,000 people at a time. Eye diseases, perhaps for that reason, were common, particularly in the dry season when as many as a quarter of his clients had conjunctivitis.

Thus conditions in the capital all in all were far from healthy and may well have actually been deteriorating. That at least was the opinion of Christine Sandford, a not unperceptive observer, who declared that the prevalence of smallpox, venereal diseases, typhus, trachoma, and leprosy "increased" as a result of the "rapid growth of the city's population."

XIX

The Italian Fascist Invasion and Occupation

Preparations for fascist Italy's seizure of Ethiopia, the ensuing invasion of 1935–1936, and the occupation of 1936-1940 had major medical consequences.

Eritrea

The Italian colony of Eritrea prior to Mussolini's decision to invade was endowed with but rudimentary medical facilities. General Emilio De Bono, the fascist commissioner for the colony, noted that in 1934 it had "only two hospitals": the Regina Elena at the capital, Asmara, and the Umberto I at the port of Massawa. The former he described as a "good" institution, but the latter as only a "very modest establishment," entirely lacking in the equipment required in a tropical country. According to the Italian author Battaglini, these hospitals together had no more than 300 beds. "In this matter of hospitals, as in every other department," De Bono complained, "lack of available funds . . . had made it impossible to do things that could usefully have been done."

Plans for the invasion caused De Bono to turn his attention to the "essential question" of military hospitals, for it was estimated that 10,000 hospital beds would be required. Accordingly, steps were taken to enlarge the Asmara and Massawa hospitals as well as to establish a number of temporary hospitals elsewhere. This was achieved by the construction of huts and barracks, including temporary Docker houses erected by German workers, and by requisitioning existing buildings. New military hospitals were built at Nefasit, Decamere, May Edaga and May Habar, while the Principe di Piedmonte school at Asmara and the munitions depot at Ghinda both were converted for hospital use. Throughout Eritrea, De Bono noted, "all the local school premises were soon being transformed into hospitals."

The result was that by the outbreak of hostilities, according to Battaglini, the colony was provided with no less than 10,000 military and 5,000 civilian hospital beds—fifty times more than it had had only a year earlier. Provision was also made for the more sanitary operation of brothels. The Italian administration nevertheless faced many difficulties, and Italian road workers often were acutely short of doctors and medicines, including such elementary items as quinine, bismuth and antitetanus serum. Such shortages, Battaglini recalled, were one of De Bono's "major preoccupations" and the cause of strong complaints by General A. Caffo and others.

War Preparations in Ethiopia

Meanwhile, the threatened invasion, as we have seen, led in Ethiopia to the founding in 1935 of the Ethiopian branch of the Red Cross and to the Ethiopian Women's Work Association, a voluntary society established mainly to supply bandages and medical comforts to the troops. For the most part, however, as in former times, the Ethiopian soldiers went into battle with only the most rudimentary medical facilities. As Colonel Argyropoulos, a Greek physician in the Ethiopian army, observed, an Ethiopian army medical service did not "exist at all" and the Ethiopian forces were virtually "without any doctors, without any nurses and without even bandages."

The Invasion

After the outbreak of fighting on October 3, 1935, Red Cross missions arrived in Ethiopia from Sweden, Britain, Egypt, Holland, Norway, and Finland. All, according to Marcel Junod, a Red Cross official, were "first-class and well-equipped." The Sudan Interior Mission also dispatched staff to care for the Ethiopian troops.

These missions, however, soon were deliberately bombed by the Italian air force, apparently in an attempt to bring all Ethiopian and Red Cross activity to an end. The Red Cross hospital at Adwa was attacked on October 25 and the American Red Cross hospital at Dasé on December 6. Targets bombed between December 15 and 31 included the Ethiopian Red Cross ambulance at Negelli, and Swedish Red Cross ambulance at Malka Didaka and the Egyptian Red Cross hospital at Bulalé. Systematic bombing continued into the New Year with attacks on Ethiopian Red Cross ambulances at Dagabur, Waldeya, and Maqalé; on Egyptian Red Cross ambulances or units at Harar, Jigjiga, and Bulalé; on British Red Cross units at Waldeya, Qorem, and Chelga; on a Swedish Red Cross ambulance at Ilyan Serar; on a Finnish Red Cross ambulance at Jigjiga; and on Ethiopian Red Cross planes at Dasé and Qorem.

The bombing of the British Red Cross unit was described by its commandant John Melly, who stated that Italian airplanes dropped about 40 bombs and that as a result the sterilisation and operating tent were wrecked. . . . Five other tents were totally destroyed and a quantity of medical stores and equipment. One lorry was totally smashed, another rendered useless. . . . The 46 ft. square Red Cross flag had a direct hit. There can be no possible question of doubt as to the absolute deliberation of the attack. Practically all the tents and lorries are also clearly marked with Red Crosses.

Faced with this onslaught, in which Dr. Hylander of the Swedish Red Cross was wounded, the International Red Cross Society in Geneva decided that it was impossible to continue with ambulance work. Most foreign medical missions accordingly were withdrawn.

The British Red Cross ambulance retreating from the north duly reached Addis Ababa, where it received Hayla Sellasé's permission to take over the Empress Manan Girls' School as a temporary hospital. With the help of Lady Barton, wife of the British Minister, the conversion was effected in a day, and the hospital, which was operated by nine Englishmen and an Austrian, remained in operation until the arrival of the Italians on May 5, 1936.

Italian Military Medicine

The Italians meanwhile had been devoting considerable attention to the medical needs of their army. Aldo Castellani, a fascist practitioner in London's Harley Street, who had become director of medical services for the invading armies, at first faced considerable difficulties. He was obliged to appeal personally to Mussolini's wife, Rachele. She noted in her diary that, "finding himself unable to secure the despatch of certain men he considered indispensable through the normal bureaucratic channels, he came to enlist my help. I put him in touch with Mussolini, and the necessary action was taken forthwith." Castellani subsequently drew up an enthusiastic account of medical operations under his direction. He stated that this was the first time that such a large number of "white troops" had been "transported to a tropical zone" and that the thought of 500,000 young white soldiers fighting caused "serious misgivings to many experts," as it had become "almost an axiom that to prevent heavy losses from sickness in colonial wars, the bulk of the troops employed should be native troops." Il Duce, however, had not been deterred by such arguments, but "realised immediately the enormous importance of medical preparation and organisation" and "paid the same attention to it as to purely military preparations." As a result, "requests regarding medical personnel and hospitals were immediately acceded to and often doubled. . . . Enormous supplies of quinine and other essential drugs, disinfectants, sera, vaccines were dispatched. . . . as well as hospital, X-ray and laboratory equipment of every kind, and mountains of cotton, wool, gauze and bandages." "I can testify," Castellani concluded, "that on more than one occasion the dispatch of medical and sanitary material took precedence over the dispatch of munitions and war material."

The Italian army in East Africa was equipped with base and field hospitals, each base hospital being provided with a bacterial laboratory and X-ray department, 55 small portable hospitals that could be transported on mules, 13 surgical units, 15 motorized X-ray laboratories, 11 dental motor ambulances, four institutes for chemical and bacteriological research, 12 disinfecting and six disinfection stations, 139 large water sterilizers, and four medical depots. The Italian navy likewise had 20 hospitals and infirmaries and eight hospital ships, and the air force 22 infirmaries. All in all, the Italian forces had no less than 2,484 doctors, 188 pharmacy officers, 384 nurses (one of them the crown princess of Italy), 200 nuns, and 16,139 hospital attendants and male nurses.

Steps were also taken to protect Italian health in other ways. The troops, according to the fascist writer Pisani, were inspected weekly for venereal disease, received "large distributions" of antivenereal medicine, and were subjected to propaganda on the dangers of sexual infection. Each soldier also received three tablets a day of quinine sulphate or bihydrochloride as a prophylactic against malaria. Prominent fascist officers, among them General Graziani and Starace, the secretary of the Fascist party, set the example by swallowing a tablet at every meal, while the soldiers frequently were paraded and one in 10 or 20 made to pass urine, which was tested to ascertain whether the quinine had in fact been taken. To minimize risks of dysentery, efforts were also made to ensure a supply of pure water. "Practically all the officers," Castellani stated, "drank mineral waters—such as S. Pellegrino and Fiuggi— bottled in Italy—and shipped to Africa in enormous amounts." The water for the troops was "obtained from rivers and wells," and "purified by boiling or by some method of chlorination." Soldiers were recommended to wash their hands with a 2% solution of lysol or lysoform after visiting the latrine, and before eating their meals. They were provided with flannel belts to prevent abdominal chills and resultant dysentery and received a lemon a day against scurvy. Extensive vaccination against typhoid and cholera was also carried out, as well as propaganda on the dangers of snakes, poisonous insects, polluted water, and various diseases, as stated in the official Italian publication, *Gli Annali dell'Africa Italiana* (hereafter, *Gli Annali*).

As a result of such precautions, the incidence of disease in the invading army was low. Official fascist statistics stated that from the beginning of fighting on October 3, 1935, to Mussolini's proclamation of an Italian empire, on May 9, 1936, there were only 1,241 cases of primary malaria admitted to hospital; 1,093 relapses (with 23 deaths); 453 cases of dysentery (with one death); 458 of typhoid and paratyphoid (with 161 deaths), 30 of heat stroke (with seven deaths), 17 of relapsing fever (with no deaths), five of tetanus (with four deaths), two of tapeworm and one of smallpox (neither of them fatal), and none of typhus, cholera, or scurvy. The total number of white troops dying from disease was only 599. Castellani, who was rewarded with the title of Count of Kismayu and later given the honor of treating Il Duce, claimed that "mortality and morbidity" in the Italian army in Africa was in fact "somewhat less" than among units in Italy and that "the number of deaths from disease" was "much lower than the number killed in battle."

Medical Care during the Occupation

Addis Ababa

After their occupation of Addis Ababa in May 1936, the Italians took over the city's hospitals which in accordance with fascist practice were promptly rechristened, while other buildings were converted for medical use. Most hospitals were reserved for the exclusive use of the white population. Thus, the well-equipped Bét Sayda Hospital was expanded to become the 300- or 400-bed Vittorio Emanuele military hospital for Europeans; the Hayla Sellasé Hospital was given the new name of Principessa de Piedmonte, Italica Gens, and enlarged as a European hospital with 350 beds; and the Zawditu Hospital was reserved for Europeans.

The old Menilek Hospital, by now largely out of date, was extended, renamed the Duca delgi Abruzzi Hospital, and converted into a segregated institution. As the German Nazi woman, Louise Diel, stated, there were "separate sections" for Italians and for "natives." She claimed that the Italian section, which was the largest, had a capacity of 700 beds while the "native" had 500, but apparently even this was an exaggeration, for an Italian municipal report for 1938 stated that the latter in fact had only 150 beds.

The result of these developments was that the Ethiopian population, which before the war had the use of four hospitals, was left with a share in only one.

Meanwhile, two new hospitals, also exclusively for Europeans, came into existence as a result of the conversion of existing premises: the Empress Manan School for Girls, which, no longer needed as an educational establishment, was turned into the 300-bed Regina Elena Military Hospital; and the house of Ras Mulugéta, for former Ethiopian minister of war, was equipped with 250 to 350 beds, to become the Luigi Razza Hospital for Italian workers. The old Italian Consolata mission, which formerly had cared almost exclusively for Ethiopians, was renamed in honor of Graziani's mother, Adelia Clementi Graziani, and designated to serve partly as a pediatric center for Italian children and partly as a clinic for "native" trachoma cases.

Four small clinics and a venereal disease (VD) dispensary, on the other hand, were brought in to service for the "native" population.

The old Sudan Interior Mission leprosarium at Aqaqi meanwhile was taken over by the Italian Consolata mission, but was retained as a leprosarium. It was responsible for about 240 inmates, all of them "natives."

The racial imbalance with respect to medical care was slightly reduced subsequently, in 1938, when the old Tafari Makonnen Hospital, earlier run by Dr. Lambie for the United Presbyterian Church of North America, was reopened with 60 to 80 beds as the Ospedale per Capi e Notabile Indigeni (i.e., Hospital for Native Chiefs and Notables). Not long afterwards, in the autumn of 1938, a new "native hospital," the Hemanuel Ospedale per Indigeni de Tecla Haimanot (or Emanuel Hospital for Natives of Takla Haymanot), with four pavilions and 80 to 120 beds, was established. Both institutions were situated on the west of the city, which had been reserved for the "native population."

Throughout this period, the Italians were greatly worried, as the fascist author Dario Lischi and the publication *Gli Annali* both emphasize, over the risks of infection confronting their personnel in Ethiopia. The fascist viewpoint, as Diel expressed it, was that "only healthy white men" could "undertake successfully the giant task of colonising Italian East Africa." From this it followed that medical facilites were primarily for the benefit of Italians, who were then establishing themselves all over the country, and that preventive medicine was largely designed to prevent them from being contaminated by the "natives." The prevailing attitude is apparent from a popular Italian primer, L. Carella's *Igiene del lavoro nei climi caldi dell'Africa Orientale*, written for Italian workers going out to East Africa. Its author urged the importance of cleanliness, sanitation, and pure drinking water, explained how to make latrines and why it was advisable to avoid pork and alcohol, and declared that though he did "not recommend complete sexual abstinence" the worker should "constantly take the maximum prophylactic precautions" because "sexual diseases represented one of the gravest dangers in Africa."

The need for widespread preventive medicine, primarily in the interests of the European population, was constantly affirmed. A fascist report on the "First Year of the Empire" emphasized the necessity "to protect the health of nationals" (i.e., Italians) from infection by "natives," while a municipal report for Addis Ababa stated that Italians in the city "quickly understood" the "latent danger of infectious diseases" and the need for "effective preventive action." Dr. Giovenco, an Italian medical writer of the time, urged that for "the integrity, purity and dignity of the race" it was essential that "contact with the native element be avoided" and that the "native population" in the vicinity of Italian workers' camps be kept under sanitary control, while another Italian physician, Dr. Mariani, contended that it was necessary to fight against typhus "not only because of the danger which it represented for the natives and nationals of Italian East Africa, but above all because of the danger of importing the virus into the Mother Country."

Preoccupation with preventive medicine led, shortly after the seizure of Addis Ababa, to the establishment of a "service of general disinfection," equipped, as *Gli Annali* noted, with squads of disinfectors. According to a later municipal report, much use was made of lime, creoline, and creosote. Steps were also taken to institute mass propaganda on basic hygiene, which received considerable attention in the otherwise very meager educational textbooks for "natives." Medical information for the "native population," often in undisguisedly racist terms, was likewise distributed. One somewhat patronizing Amharic text declared:

1. The most dangerous enemy of man is the louse because it transmits two serious diseases: typhus and relapsing fever.
2. The man who does not have lice on his body, in his clothes or in his house can be sure of not being contaminated by these two diseases, even if he is in contact with persons affected.
3. Syphilis ruins the victim and his descendants because it is transmitted to children. It is not cured by exorcisms or herbal decoctions, but by injections which only white doctors know how to give.
4. One must not believe one is cured of syphilis because the external manifestations of the disease have disappeared. The spirchaeta remains alive in the liver, brain, bones, and blood, and is killed only if the cure continues for two or three years: otherwise sooner or later new external or internal manifestations will appear.
5. One does not develop gonorrhoea or venereal ulcers if one has contact only with clean women and washes oneself well with soap and water after intercourse.
6. The disease which has had the largest number of victims is smallpox. Only vaccination, effected with vaccine by the Government, can prevent this infection.
7. The cure of diseases is not obtained through the advice of natives because they are incompetent, not having been to the schools and special hospitals which exist only in parts of the world inhabited by whites.
8. To call the white doctor when one is ill means almost always to be cured and to prevent the disease spreading among persons inhabiting the same house.
9. Soap and water for the body and for clothes are the cheapest means of defence against almost all diseases.
10. Women, if they do not want to have trouble when they are pregnant and wish their children to be born alive and healthy, must be treated by the white doctor. If the pregnancy is not normal he will give them advice and medicine.

The racist motive behind Italian policies was frankly stated by Diel, who noted that the "natives" had to undertake "medical treatment" as "a preventive measure for the protection of Italian garrisons, workmen and the ever-growing Italian population."

Other action in the preventive field included the issue of orders for the compulsory reporting of infectious diseases and a mass vaccination scheme that resulted in some 200,000 smallpox inoculations in 1937. Medical work among the "native" population, however, was seriously handicapped by the fascist reign of terror that followed that year's attempt on Graziani's life. The municipal report for 1938 admitted that "despite intense propaganda . . . the native population for the first few months (of 1937) showed itself mistrustful and did not want to know of our medical cures nor of preventive vaccines against contagious diseases." Such fear, however, was later largely overcome, in part by the use of 64 loudspeaker-vans that made medical announcements in thickly-populated areas. The municipal report for 1938 claimed that Italian medicine gradually gained popularity and that 5,900 "natives" were by then attending clinics each month.

Perhaps the greatest progress was in the ophthalmic field. Dr. Paolo Guerra, a notable specialist, claimed that by May 1937 a "regular service" had been established and that evidence collected by it demonstrated that medical facilities were "truly necessary not only for the assistance of the patients, but also to give an idea of the grave dangers to which our compatriots were exposed" by the widespread diffusion of trachoma, which he termed "one of the most serious and contagious" of diseases. It was therefore necessary to take action with "the greatest possible speed" to shield Italians from "this great threat." Seven eye clinics were soon established, namely the Istituto Gulelé, the Missione Cannosiane (with two sections), the Vicenzo and Consolata missions, a section at the Duca degli Abruzzi Hospital, the St. George clinic, and the mendicants' clinic. Provision was made for the free treatment of trachoma and other eye-diseases every Tuesday.

Fear of infection, and particularly of typhus, greatly reinforced fascist racial theories and was an additional motive for the rigid segregation of Europeans and "natives" which took place during the viceregency of the Duke of Aosta. An Addis Ababa order of September 21, 1938, prohibited Italians or other Europeans from entering the Takla Haymanot or New Market area, reserved for "natives." In the following year Dr. Mariani, considering the medical situation in racist terms, urged the need (1) to place the dwellings of "native servants" far from those of their "white" masters; (2) to separate "the white element" from that of the "native" in offices, shops, schools, places of work and prisons; (3) to prevent the "promiscuous" transport of "whites" and "natives" on public or private vehicles and to create exclusive transport services for "natives"; (4) to systematically disinfect and vaccinate "whites" obliged by their work to have frequent contacts with "natives"; and (5) to remove "natives" from large urban centers to the countryside.

Italian concern with public hygiene also led to the establishment in Addis Ababa of a public slaughterhouse and the provision of covered vehicles for the transportation of meat within the city. There was at the same time a drive against the city's previously extensive canine population, which was considered a potential source of rabies. Maria Landi, an Italian nurse who estimated that there were over 15,000 dogs in the capital in 1936, claimed that over 1,500 were eliminated in the first few months of the occupation, while the municipal report for 1938 later reported the killing of "over 2,000." Diel claimed that after an outbreak that summer in which ten cases of rabies were reported, between 4,000 and 5,000 dogs were "destroyed with strychnine" and "the same number a few months later." The latter figure is, however, probably exaggerated, for D'Ignazio, a more reliable observer, stated that a total of only 6,000 dogs perished. The slaughter was undoubtedly considerable, however, for in 1938 the Swedish observer Svensson saw but two dogs, both accompanied by their owners. Many hyenas were likewise killed off on the outskirts of Harar.

Medical research in the capital was carried out at the Bacteriological and Micrography Institute and the Istituto Sieroterapico Milanese, as well as later at a typhus research institute founded on November 24, 1939, after the outbreak of the European war.

Eritrea

In the provinces, as in Addis Ababa, there was considerable inequality in the medical facilities available for Italians and "natives." The greatest concentration of hospitals was in Eritrea, where, as we have seen, many had been established or enlarged in preparation for the war. Asmara, with a population of over 50,000 Italians in 1940, had the best services. Its principal hospital, the Regina Elena, which like almost all Italian medical institutions of this period was segregated, had about 1,500 beds for Europeans. There were also a polyclinic and several small institutions for "natives," namely an eye clinic, which received patients from as far afield as Kassala and Aden; a VD clinic, attached to the Regina Elena, for "native" prostitutes; and nine other clinics, some run by the municipality, others by the Fondo Nazionale Assistenza. The town also had a medical and prophylactic laboratory.

Massawa, the port of entry for Italian troops, had two hospitals, the Umberto I, with 130 beds for Italians and 160 for "natives," and the Royal Marine Hospital, exclusively for Italian naval personnel. There was also an isolation hospital for Italians at nearby Gurgussam, and a 150-bed clinic, attached to the Umberto, for "native" prostitutes.

There were also small hospitals at Adi Caieh, Embatkalla, Agordat and Assab, and VD (or other) clinics at Belesa (which also had a 200-bed isolation camp for "natives"), Coazen, Edaga Berai, Decamere, Adi Ugri, Addi Quala, May Edaga, Ghinda, Saganeti, Senafé, Ad Teclesan, Agordat, Barentu, Ugaro, Scuimagalle, Nocra, Thio, Assab, and Abroborifahe.

Two prophylactic repatriation camps, established to protect the population of metropolitan Italy from infected returnees from Africa, were also in operation: for the military at Nefasit, and for workers at May Habar. Private individuals returning to Italy were similarly under close supervision—for eleven days before their departure—and had to show that they had been vaccinated for typhus within the previous year.

Medical research in Eritrea was mainly concerned with malaria. An institute for the study of the disease was established in Karan and a second was in preparation at the time of the fascist collapse.

Medical educational facilities were almost entirely for Italians. The only training available for "natives" was a six-month course for dressers, which was attended by an average of 30 pupils between 1928 and 1935, and 50 thereafter.

The inequality of medical facilities available to Italians and "natives" was one of the features which most struck later observers. The 1948 Four Power Commission Report on Eritrea, compiled by representatives of Britain, France, the US, and the USSR, noted that the territory had 2,000 hospital beds, of which 1,200 were reserved for an Italian population of 60,000, leaving only 800 beds for a "native" population of over 750,000. Hospitals and dispensaries, as the British officer Trevaskis noted, "mainly served European interests" and were almost invariably "sited in the principal centres" while "few if any" existed in places without substantial Italian communities. The discrepancy in hospital treatment for the two races is also confirmed by fascist statistics, which show for example that there were 6,179 Italian hospitalized patients in 1938 as compared with 5,467 "natives." That the "natives" were not without need of medical attention is evident from the fact that 160,930 received outpatient treatment that year, the corresponding Italian figure being only 23,600.

Harar, Dire Dawa, Gondar and Jimma

The five principal provincial towns of occupied Ethiopia (i.e., Harar, Dire Dawa, Gondar, Dasé, and Jimma) were all relatively well supplied with hospitals and clinics, albeit mainly reserved for the Italian population. Most of the hospitals in these centers dated from the prewar period, but others were established to meet the expanding needs of Italian colonization.

Harar had two hospitals and a leprosarium, all three build before the occupation. Ras Makonnen's hospital, which by then had 200 beds, was retained as an institution for "natives," as was the old Catholic-run leprosarium. On the other hand, the former Swedish Mission Hospital, which was more modern, was requisitioned as an Italian establishment and used for the training of dressers. Several lesser institutions were later established, namely, a polyclinic, a VD clinic, and a VD station for "native" prostitutes, as well as a small medical laboratory.

Dire Dawa had the old railway hospital, with 150 beds, which was designated for Italians, as well as a polyclinic, a small hospital for "natives," a VD clinic, and a VD station for "native" prostitutes.

As for the other provincial centers, Gondar had a 300-bed combined military and civilian hospital for Italians, a polyclinic, a VD station for "native" prostitutes, a workers' clinic with 20 beds, a 50-bed VD clinic, a gynecological clinic, and a medical laboratory; Dasé, a hospital for Italians, a VD station for "native" prostitutes (capable of handling 100 women), an eye clinic, and a malaria laboratory; Jimma, a 450-bed hospital for Italians (opened in 1940), a hospital for "natives," two polyclinics (one for each race), two dispensaries for "natives," and a medical laboratory.

Other institutions in the provinces included a much-publicized 96-bed leprosarium, for "natives," run by a Catholic organization, the Order of Malta, at Selaclaca, 35 kilometers from Aksum, and a malaria research center at Kombolcha.

The diffusion of Italian military and civilian personnel in many centers throughout the country and the dream of massive Italian colonization also led to the establishment of a number of small—and often only temporary— clinics and dispensaries, attached to local Italian commissariats and set up for Italian road-workers then in the country. In the Dasé area in 1937, for example, there were a 32-bed clinic in Kombolcha and 113 roadside clinics (each with between 12 and 20 beds) in addition to 74 small dispensaries.

These institutions were primarily for Italians and therefore were of little relevance to the "native" population. The medical facilities available to that population actually declined in some provinces as a result of fighting and disturbed social conditions, as well as because of the expulsion of Protestant missionaries, who previously had been one of the principal sources of medical attention in remote areas. Such missionaries were systematically driven from the country. One of the most famous, the Swedish Dr. Harold Nystrom, was expelled by a decree of September 3, 1937. After the expropriation of the American mission hospital in Addis Ababa, a British consular report revealingly observed, "Although no reasons are given, it is thought that the Mission's close associations with the Ethiopians has for a long time rankled in the minds of the authorities who are suspicious of any contact between foreigners and Ethiopians."

Venereal Diseases

The principal illness with which the Italians were confronted were venereal diseases, though in the lowlands these were outstripped by malaria and, to a lesser extent, typhus, typhoid, and tuberculosis.

Venereal diseases, which, as we have seen, had long been prevalent in the country, increased in incidence during the occupation, as a result of the growth of prostitution in the main cities and roadside towns, frequented by many Italians. From their first arrival in East Africa, as the American journalist, Herbert Matthews, explained, the Italian troops showed a great desire to "get together with black women," and a subsequent Italian antifascist open letter to Mussolini told of the soldiers "tasting the delights of the soft black flesh" of gracious *sharmutas* (or prostitutes). In Asmara, the first city to witness a large concentration of Italian troops, the "black" and "white" prostitutes, according to the journalist M. Durand, were soon "coining money fast." Despite the subsequent racial laws, extensive use was made of local prostitutes. Doody, a British traveler who visited Eritrea after the liberation, recalled that at the small Italian naval battery post of Umm Es Sahring, there was a *casa* of military *amore*," which was "still abundantly equipped" with "many thousands of packets of what the French call 'English letters', forming a pile which reached half-way to the roof." "Three females," he added, "were officially 'on strength' . . . one good lady was provided to satisfy the demands of the three officers; number two devoted herself exclusively to the five N.C.O.'s; but the third was the one who could really claim to be doing her bit, for she shared her favors among the 60 other ranks." Italian Eritrea, according to the subsequent Four Power Commission report, had 120 licensed prostitutes in 1939, but many more unlicensed, for in that year no less than 100 clandestine ones were arrested.

On crossing the Ethiopian frontier the Italian soldiers also made considerable use of local women. One Bersaglieri officer was quoted by Durand as declaring, "My men are young robust fellows. They must have their women." The result was a considerable diffusion of VD. *Gli Annali*, though a propagandist work, admitted that normal precautions proved "insufficient" to prevent "sad and sometimes tragic consequences," and that in the Hawzén-Adwa-Sheré area, two field hospitals had to be established for the compulsory treatment of local women reported to be infected. All military dependents were obliged to undergo medical inspection three times a week; healthy women were issued with certificates and had to reside in specified houses where they were frequently examined, while medically controlled women in the Adwa–Aksum area were encouraged to make their way to Italian military camps.

In Addis Ababa the first Italian brothel, according to Ladislas Saska, a Hungarian physician, came into existence within two days of the city's capture and before long "a whole street" was converted for this purpose. Diel claimed that efforts were made to keep prostitution "under vigilant supervision" and 1,500 "native" women in the capital were reserved exclusively for Italians, while 47 Italian girls were installed in a special brothel. Street prostitutes, she said, had to be "in possession of an official permit" and were "medically examined three times a week."Such precautions, however, were by no means fully successful: Saska, writing as a practicing physician, relates that venereal diseases soon "ravaged the Italian ranks, and that no medical assistance was sufficient to deal with it". Discussing the medical care available he added:

> In the Italian military hospital, the treatment was of the worst and lowest. Italian soldiers went to the private surgeries of doctors settled in the town before the occupation, but even they had no adequate means to deal with the number of cases of venereal disease. . . . There were 11,000 cases in 15 months . . . venereal disease destroyed more Italian soldiers than the Ethiopian army. I know of cases where Italian soldiers committed suicide when they heard the nature of the disease. I heard the desperate cries of two Italian boys, almost children, who wept bitterly when I told them what had happened to them.

Gli Annali, though designed to place the occupation in the best possible light, also testified to the extent of VD infection, and stated that, in view of the large number of Italians in the capital, anti-VD provisions were more extensive than elsewhere. A 300-bed VD clinic for "native" women and another for Italian prostitutes were attached to the Duca degli Abruzzi Hospital, while the Luigi Razza Hospital for Italian workers had a special VD department. The hospital's authorities recognized that VD constituted "a grave danger," as Milella put it, "for the integrity of the race." Diel admitted that the Italian "campaign against venereal disease" made but "slow progress," and need was so great that in 1939 Pisani reported plans to establish a new 500-bed VD clinic at Entotto.

In Dasé Dr. Mari, the official in charge of VD treatment, reported that after the occupation of the town a "multitude" of "native" prostitutes arrived from all over the region. Two brothels, staffed, respectively, by 20 "native" and 10 "white" women, were thereupon established, according to *Gli Annali*. There was, Mari recorded, "a sudden appearance of venereal diseases," a "frightening propagation . . . among the metropolitan as well as the native population." Gravely concerned about infection among Italians, he complained that, despite the fascist racial decrees, many Italians displayed "unlimited irresponsibility" when it came to "sexual relations with native women." The incidence of disease made it "easy" to deduce "how frequent and dangerous" were "the occasions of infection, above all in the remoter areas, where workers are employed on road-building and soldiers in distance garrisons."

In an effort to control the situation, in September 1936 the authorities at Dasé set up a VD department in the local army hospital, where an average of 80 military and civilian patients—a large proportion of them suffering from syphilis—were admitted. A women's VD dispensary was established at about the same time and received no less than 12,297 visits in the first six months of 1938. "Continuous propaganda," according to Mari, was also carried out to warn both Italians and "natives" of the risks of VD. Prophylactics were widely used. The "white" brothel was installed with hot and cold running water, washing soap, and *protargol*, and its inmates were subjected to medical inspection three times a week. The "native" brothel likewise had its "prophylactic room," with water, soap, towels, and permanganate and protargol solutions, and its manageress had instructions to recruit only prostitutes with valid licenses. As a result of these measures the incidence of disease, Mari claimed, was greatly reduced by 1938.

Prostitution, and VD, was also extensive in other centers. At Mojjo, General Mischi gave strict instructions, according to Poggiali, that soldiers were to apply for permission, and be medically examined, before each visit to the brothel, and *carabinieri* were ordered to verify the customers' documents. At Harar, according to an official report for 1939, about 300 "native" prostitutes were in possession of licenses and subjected to twice-weekly inspections, while in Dire Dawa a "white" brothel was in operation within the first year of the occupation. Lakamti was described by the Italian journalist Poggiali as "famous for its abundance of prostitutes." He stated in his diary that it had been proposed to establish mobile brothels (or "Cars of Love"), to be staffed with

Italian women, for the Italian workers' camps, but this was vetoed by Davide Fossa (the fascist leader in charge of labor) and the Addis Ababa *fascio*, on the grounds that in places where white families had not yet arrived it would be unseemly for the Italian women to be seen for the first time in the form of the prostitute.

The increasing prevalence of VD in the Italian East African empire was emphasized in an official report that stated that from January to October 1936, some 2,323 cases of syphilis were treated in Amhara, 761 in Eritrea, 305 in Harar province, 150 in Galla and Sidama, and 30 in Addis Ababa. The rate of infection was said to have reached its peak in 1937, when no less than 9.75% (i.e., almost one in 10) of Italian soldiers were affected, and the rate in the following year was still 5.05%. The corresponding rates for Italian civilians and "native" troops, though lower, were still considerable, as indicated in the following table.

Percentage of infection by venereal disease (VD).

	Italian Troops		Italian Civilians		Native Troops	
	1937	1938	1937	1938	1937	1938
Primary syphilis	0.94	0.40	0.182	0.168	0.70	0.27
Advanced syphilis	1.70	0.50	0.127	0.115	1.04	0.71
Blennorrhoea	4.06	2.05	0.664	0.418	1.06	0.70
Soft ulcers	3.05	2.10	0.375	0.265	0.90	0.31
Total VD	9.75	5.05	1.348	0.966	3.70	1.99

In an attempt to control the incidence of infection, VD stations for "native" prostitutes, as we have seen, were established at Asmara, Addis Ababa, Harar, Dire Dawa, Dasé, and Gondar. The latter town had in addition a 50-bed VD clinic. Smaller VD clinics—often no more than huts—were set up elsewhere at many places, among them Adi Ugri, Tessenei, Barentu, and Assab in Eritrea; Adwa, Enticho, Aksum, Hawzén, Abbi Addi, Enda Mehané Alam, Addigrat, May Chew, Qoram, and Alomata in Tegré; Waldeya, Lalibala, Dabra Tabor, Dabra Marqos, Lake Haik, Adi Arkay, Debarek, Matamma, Alefa, Danghila, Kombolcha, Batie, Gorgora, Chelga, Derasgé, Warra Ilu, and Mugia in Amhara; Jigjiga, Asba Littorio, and Afem in Harar province; Sciano, Dabra Berhan, Dabra Sina, Holeta, Adi Salem, Ambo, Bishoftu, Mojjo, and Fitché in Shawa; and Jimma, Negelli, Lakamti, Argio, Moyalé, Arero, Yavello, Goré, Bonga, Alghe, Agaro, Wolisso, Huba, Maji, Soddu, and Gardulla in Galla and Sidamo.

Malaria

Malaria, which traditionally was common in the lowlands, led to considerable hospitalization of Italian soldiers and workers and caused the fascist authorities much concern. In the Bari d'Etiopia settlement scheme for Italian workers, for example, 23 settlers fell victim to malaria. Though the altitude of Addis Ababa was well above the level in which the malaria mosquito could live, the disease was responsible for a large proportion of the admissions to the city's hospitals. The Luigi Razza Hospital for Italian workers thus reported that the largest single number of its patients (445 by 1938) were suffering from this complaint, contracted mainly in the area of the Awash or Omo rivers or the Rift Valley lakes. The study of malaria therefore received a high priority in the field of research.

Epidemics

Several epidemics occurred during the occupation, but failed to reach major proportions. A typhus outbreak in Addigrat prison in December 1936, according to *Gli Annali*, spread to Asmara as a result of the transfer of prisoners there. The governor of Eritrea issued a decree for the compulsory inoculation of Italian officials, civil servants, and soldiers in contact with the "native population" as well as of all persons, irrespective of race, who were connected with hotels, restaurants, cafés, drinking houses, cinemas, brothels, or public or private transport. The majority of Italians in the area were inoculated, *Gli Annali* stated, to prevent them from carrying the disease back to Italy on repatriation. These precautions appear to have been successful, for the infection soon died away.

A new outbreak, however, took place in the autumn of 1937, when the disease was reported between Addis Ababa and Dabra Sina, as well as at Fitché and around the Omo river. Fearing that military operations and the movement of population would spread the epidemic, the governor general ordered resolute action to prevent the disease from "endangering the physical integrity" of Italians and "as far as possible to reduce illness among natives." An Addis Ababa health commission likewise advised extending inoculation to all Italians and "initiating inoculation among the native population, the source of the diffusion of infection." The commission recommended that the entire "white population" be given Weigl vaccine, which was "efficacious and not harmful," while the "natives" should receive "the easiest" vaccine to prepare. Dr. Mariani, who also thought in racist categories, later (in 1939) urged the need for continued precautions, including research on the first cases among the "native population" (particularly in crowded areas, work camps, and among the troops), early diagnosis of Italians thought to be contaminated, and the inoculation of all Italians and foreigners "exposed to the dangers of infection." Widespread inoculations were again ordered, and victims of the disease isolated, for, *Gli Annali* reiterated, the authorities sought above all "to preserve Italians from infection" and to prevent those returning to Italy from introducing the disease there. Typhus, though less prevalent, D'Ignazio claimed, than in former times, nevertheless led to numerous cases among the Italian population: 69 in 1937, 251 in 1938, 127 in 1939, 42 in 1940, and 217 in 1941.

Smallpox, which had declined considerably in the early twentieth century but was still endemic, broke out in March 1937 among road-builders from the Sudan, and threatened Gondar and Eritrea. The principal focus of disease between April and July was at Asmara, where 18 Italians and 76 "natives" were registered as infected, and smaller outbreaks were reported in other parts of Eritrea. Mass vaccinations were carried out at places of work, road-blocks, and markets, with the result—*Gli Annali* claimed—that "no European was infected." The epidemic, however, also appeared among the workers constructing the Addis Ababa airport, whereupon the area was isolated and there were extensive vaccinations, after which the disease quickly subsided. D'Ignazio recorded that eight Italians and several hundred "natives" were hospitalized. Mortality among those not vaccinated was said by D'Ignazio to have run at 40% in the case of Italians and 50% in that of "natives."

A meningitis epidemic was also reported at this time in eastern Tegré and around Dasé, but soon petered out, perhaps because of extensive inoculations.

Vaccination

A fairly considerable amount of vaccination took place during the occupation years. Between 1936 and 1938 there were, according to *Gli Annali*, 1,035,640 vaccinations in Eritrea (which then included Tegré), 200,000 in Shawa, 178,586 in Harar province, 133,402 in Amhara, and 117,198 in Galla and Sidamo, as well as 13,500 typhus injections in Shawa. Local production of rabies serum also started in this period, but was limited, D'Ignazio noted, to only 50 or 60 courses of treatment a year.

Sanitary Conditions

Relatively little was done to improve sanitary conditions, which were particularly poor in the larger towns. In Eritrea, for example, Trevaskis noted that municipal cleansing services "only operated in the European quarters" while the "native quarters" had to be "cleansed by the communal efforts of their own inhabitants," or, more often, "left in a condition of increasingly insanitary neglect". Gandar Dower, another British officer arriving in the colony with the forces of liberation in 1941, exclaimed, "Everywhere . . . enteric fevers and dysentery were endemic. . . . Flies were regarded as inevitable natural phenomena." This was perhaps not surprising, for, as Margery Perham, the well-known expert on colonial practice, argued, the Italians were "not predominantly concerned with the interests of the Ethiopians," who therefore benefited only from "the marginal effects" of Italian medical activity.

Part III

Postscript

XX

The Postliberation Period (1941–1973)

Professor Asrat Waldeyes

The Aftermath of the Italian Occupation

The five-year Italian occupation of Ethiopia ended in 1941. Just before the end, the country was a store-house of both military and nonmilitary equipment, machines, and vehicles, as well as of soldiers and civilians whom Italy had invested in her bid for conquest.

When General Cunningham's forces entered Addis Ababa to receive the surrender of the Italians, the Ethiopians cheering along the streets were held in check by armed Italian police and armed Blackshirts. The Ethiopians, however, saw only the end of a brutal occupation with still vivid memories: the indiscriminate slaughter of men, women, and children; the extermination of the foreign-trained and modern-educated population, the liquidation of dignitaries and civil servants; the massacre of religious leaders and clergy of the Ethiopian Orthodox church; the destruction of churches and monasteries; and genocidal attacks and oppression throughout the country.

Following the "liberation," however, contrary to the belief and expectation of the Ethiopian people, the country was run by the British as an occupied territory, with Italians left holding official positions, at least in the early period. The British effort to make Ethiopia a protectorate continued until the signing of the Anglo-Ethiopian agreement of 1944. Soon after the liberation, all valuable equipment, machinery, trucks, and other Italian property were confiscated as war booty and exported. Italian prisoners of war and most Italian professionals also departed, and only 500 were allowed to remain. However, a substantial number of Italian civilians—artisans, technicians,

241

drivers, engineers as well as doctors—stayed behind in Ethiopia of their own choice. They did so largely because the Ethiopian people, despite all they had suffered, did not carry out the retribution many expected. This was in no small measure due to the influence of Emperor Haile Sellassie,* who, on the day of his arrival in Addis Ababa, called upon all Ethiopians to act with compassion towards their former enemies.

After the liberation Ethiopia, with the exception of a few survivors who had been in exile, found itself virtually devoid of trained or modern-educated personnel and extremely short of seasoned government officials and civil servants. In addition, during this period the Ethiopian government began operating with borrowed East African shillings, which remained the currency of the nation for several years. However, in 1944, through skillful international maneuvering and negotiations, Ethiopia succeeded in establishing its full independence and sovereignty over the major part of its territory. In the first decade after the liberation, the priorities of the nation were consolidation of independence, expansion of modern education, the reunion of Eritrea, development for foreign trade, strengthening of defense, economic development, mining exploration, development of air transport, and the development of the banking system. In this scale of priorities health development had a relatively low place.

This extraordinary background of political, social, and economic circumstances should be taken into consideration in any appraisal of the development of health services in the first decade of postliberation Ethiopia.

Milestones in the Development of Health Services

One week after his arrival—and contrary to the wishes of the British military—the emperor established seven ministries and appointed ministers and vice-ministers to administer them. These were the Ministry of Interior, the Ministry of Pen, the Ministry of Foreign Affairs, the Ministry of Commerce and Industry, the Ministry of Justice, the Ministry of Posts, Telegraphs, and Telephones, and the Ministry of Education. When the Ministry of Interior was established, a Department (or unit) of Health was established within it. To head this unit a Britisher, Dr. Campbell, was appointed Director of Medical Services.

In an attempt to regulate public-health matters, in 1942 a Public Health Proclamation[1] was promulgated, giving powers to the Minister of Interior to

---

*Since the personalities and institutions mentioned by Dr. Asrat Waldeyes in this overview of the post–World War II period belong the recent past it has been deemed expedient to refer to them in the English spellings by which they were, and are still, better known. On the other hand in the earlier, more historical chapters Dr. Pankhurst throughout uses a simplified form of the transliteration favored by the Institute of Ethiopian Studies in Addis Ababa. This has inevitably led to some discrepancies in spelling. The late emperor (and sundry institutions called after him) which were spelled Hayla Sellasé in earlier pages thus appear in this chapter as Haile Sellassie.

regulate matters concerning public health. In the same year a Medical Registration Proclamation[2] was issued, prohibiting anyone from practicing medicine, surgery, or dentistry for gain without being licensed by the Director of Medical Services, and obliging the Director of Medical Services to keep a register of all persons licensed under its provisions. The proclamation also established legal procedures in case of illegal conduct and included provisions for the practice of traditional medicine.

A Pharmacists and Druggists Proclamation[3] was promulgated in 1943, limiting the business of pharmacists and druggists to licensed professionals and licensed premises. In 1945 Ato Araya Abebe was appointed Director General of Health to run the Health Department.

In 1947 the Health Department obtained its own premises, the present site of the Ministry of Public Health. The department, though still under the Ministry of Interior, was headed by a Vice-Minister for Health—Ato Abebe Retta. In the same year a Public Health Proclamation[4] was promulgated. It laid down the structure and function of both the central and local administrations with regard to health, which was made the responsibility of the Ministry of Interior. For the care and promotion of public health, the minister was to establish a consultative and advisory body, the General Advisory Board of Health, to express expert views on matters specified in the proclamation, as well as any general aspect of the public health services, either on its own initiative or when specifically requested. This consultative and advisory board was to consist of not less than eleven persons appointed by the minister through notices in the *Negarit Gazeta*. The board had discretion to co-opt as many experts as necessary, and the minister was responsible for issuing special standing orders regulating the procedure of meetings.

The minister, in addition to regular and general consultations with the board, was to refer to it for expert advice on the following matters: (1) public-health policy and special measures for emergencies; (2) public-health legislation; (3) engagement of professional and specialist staff; (4) budgetary estimates; (5) staff training and medical and sanitary education; (6) professional discipline.

In the same proclamation an executive body, the Department of Health, was established. The establishment of this department (soon to become a ministry) and of the General Advisory Board of Health was a milestone in the development of modern medicine in Ethiopia. The board was to play a key role in the development of health-related activities for the next 27 years.

At about this time an advisor to the Health Department was employed. He was Dr. Hylander, a Swede who had worked as a missionary in Ethiopia for many years and had been wounded by an Italian bomb in the Italo-Ethiopian war when he was chief of the Swedish ambulance unit. He became the first chairman of the Advisory Board and remained chief advisor to the ministry for about two decades until he retired.

The Ethiopian Red Cross Society was restablished by the legalization of its charter by Legal Notice No. 99 of 1947.[5] In its charter the society's objectives in times of war and peace were outlined, together with its administrative system and procedures. The society was to be administered by a Board of Directors consisting of a president and 16 voting members, six appointed and ten elected. The appointed members were: a representative of the Ministry of the Interior, a representative of the Ministry of War, a representative of the Ministry of Education, a representative of the Ministry of Finance, a representative of the Ministry of Pen, and a representative of the Department of Public Health.

The Department of Public Health was made the Ministry of Public Health in 1948, and the first minister was Blatta Zewde Belaineh.

In 1948, a Medical Practitioners Registration Proclamation[6] was promulgated. It repealed the Medical Registration Proclamation of 1942 and the Pharmacist and Druggist Proclamation of 1943, as it covered the same areas as both earlier proclamations. In addition it recognized two changes: the existence and authority of the Minister of Public Health, and the function and responsibility of the board for the licensing and disciplining of medical practitioners.

In 1954, the Gondar Public Health College was established. The ministry, whose approach towards rural health was unique for this time, proceeded to build health centers in rural areas in preparation for the health officers and their teams who would soon be graduating from Gondar.

Nineteen fifty-four was also the year when the first Ethiopian doctor* returned to Ethiopia, after successfully completing his education at Edinburgh University. Other Ethiopian doctors returned in the following years, as graduates of the American University of Beirut, of McGill University in Canada, and later still more from various other universities abroad.

As the number of doctors working in Addis Ababa increased and the quality of the medical work improved, professionalism developed, and through the efforts of a few doctors in the capital, the Ethiopian Medical Association was established. It was registered with the Ministry of the Interior in the late 1950s. In 1962 the *Ethiopian Medical Journal* began to be published, and in 1964 the Ethiopian Medical Association launched its first annual medical conference. The association thereafter grew in both stature and in importance.

The first Ethiopian medical specialists in their country's history were two surgeons who had gone to complete their specializations in the UK, and returned to Ethiopia in the early 1960s. Thereafter other Ethiopian doctors began going abroad for specialization, to return years later as specialists in ophthalmology, medicine, pediatrics, obstetrics and gynecology, and other subspecialties.

---

*This was of course Dr. Asrat himself who is also referred to, obliquely, in later pages. Note: R.P.

The School of Pharmacy was established in 1962. The country's first Medical School, which incorporated the School of Pharmacy, came into existence in 1964, and its first graduating class completed courses in 1968.

The Development of Medical Services
The chief aim of medical development during the Italian occupation had been to uphold the interest of the occupying forces and of the white population. Nevertheless, different forms of segregated medical services reached the Ethiopian population. The most important were for the treatment of venereal disease among prostitutes and in brothels. These newly established and profitable institutions were actively supported, and medically controlled venereal disease clinics—called *borcelle*—were established in many towns.

Italian medicine left influences on Ethiopians that lingered for a long time. These included the preference for medicine by injection rather than by the swallowing of pills, refraining from alcoholic drinks or eating spicy foods while on a course of medical treatment, the enthusiasm for strength-giving injections of calcium preparations called *calcio*, and the belief that surgical operations would have a dangerous outcome.

Medical activity immediately after the liberation was based on rudimentary hospital services and a handful of private practices in Addis Ababa, carried out by the few remaining Italians. From 1941 to 1944 there were also a few British doctors, mainly involved in the British military service and administrative work with the Ethiopian medical services.

The main medical priority immediately after the liberation was the maintenance of existing hospital services. For this work the bulk of the medical personnel available were Italians whose credentials were uncertain. The situation was fairly precarious, for the newly established health unit in the Ministry of Interior was in its formative stage, just beginning to strengthen its reign over the administration of existing hospitals and health institutions.

In the postliberation period the few elementary schools that were opened started to teach in English, which became the country's official foreign language. However, because of the presence of Italian doctors, and the proficiency in Italian on the part of the non-Italian supportive staff, Italian maintained a privileged position as the *lingua franca* of hospitals and clinics.

All hospitals were run by the government, except for a few that had previously been operated by missions and had been permitted by the government to remain in operation. Foremost among these was the Empress Zawditu Hospital which was run by the Seventh Day Adventist Mission of America. A building complex erected by the Italians during the occupation as courts for the "indigenous people" was converted into a hospital. It was named St. Paul's Hospital and was totally reserved for the service of the poor.

In 1948 the present Balcha Hospital was completed by the Ethiopian government and was named in memory of Dejazmatch Balcha, a renowned military leader of Emperor Menilek's time who in his old age—during the Italian occupation—became a great patriotic fighter. When the hospital was completed it was given to the Soviet Red Cross and Crescent Society to run. This hospital through the years grew to be popular among both the dignitaries and the humble.

Around this time, the old leprosarium, renamed the Princess Zenebework Hospital, was gradually developed as a center for the treatment, control, and rehabilitation of leprosy. Two decades later, through the invaluable assistance of various external agencies and governments, an excellent center for training in the treatment and research of leprosy was established in the compound of this hospital.

In 1951 another new hospital was built, on premises which the Italians had planned to use as living quarters and a club for their Air Force cadets. This hospital was built as a memorial to Princess Tsehai, who had trained as a nurse in Guy's Hospital and the Hospital for Sick Children in Great Ormond Street, London, and who finally died in Ethiopia during childbirth. The hospital was equipped mainly by money raised in England in her memory. The whole concept of building this hospital, and the persistent campaign to raise the money for its equipment, was brought to fruition by that indefatigable, staunch supporter and true friend of Ethiopia, Miss E. Sylvia Pankhurst. When finally inaugurated, the hospital had four wards, three of which were named in recognition of the services of Sylvia Pankhurst, Colonel Orde Wingate, and Dr. Melly of the 1935–1936 British ambulance unit. With the hospital, the hospital's nursing school was also inaugurated. This hospital became a real center of modern medicine, rendering the most economical and the best medical services in the country. Finally, the hospital became the first teaching hospital for the Faculty of Medicine. This followed its selection by an international committee set up to advise on the establishment of the Medical School.

The health centers and health stations planned in preparation for the services of graduates of the Gondar Public Health College were built first around Gondar and Begemdir and thereafter in the other provinces. Each health center was manned by a health officer (who was the team leader), a community nurse, a sanitarian, and a laboratory technician. Each center was supposed to care for about 50,000 people. Health stations were manned by auxiliaries, who in most cases were dressers with good practical experience. In Begemdir, the college became responsible for the whole province's health services. This forced the college to expand satellite stations for both the treatment of patients and for the training of its students.

A maternity hospital with gynecological services was built in the center of Addis Ababa by the Indian community living in Ethiopia. Known as the Gandhi Memorial Hospital, it was given to the Ethiopian government as the community's contribution to Ethiopia's development effort and rendered an invaluable service to the population of Addis Ababa and the provinces.

In the early 1960s, a children's hospital, the Ethio-Swedish Paediatric Clinic (ESPC), was built, with Swedish aid, in the area adjacent to the Princess Tsehai Hospital. This clinic was made possible by the initiative, endeavors, and convictions of one man—Professor Edgar Manheimmer. With the establishment of the ESPEC, Professor Manheimmer went on to develop mobile units, based at the clinic, to bring both curative and preventive measures to the people. As he became more and more convinced of the value and importance of preventive measures in Ethiopia, he became increasingly involved in projects and educational activities aimed at satisfying these goals. He was instrumental in both the conceptualization and the procurement of the Swedish assistance that built the Ethiopian Nutritional Institute (ENI), adjoining the ESPC.

The new St. Paul's Hospital was built by the Haile Sellassie I Foundation with assistance from the German Lutheran Church. The hospital operated almost exclusively for the poor. It was a large modern hospital with 450 beds and replaced the old St. Paul's Hospital. Some of its departments were used by the Faculty of Medicine as a teaching hospital.

In the early 1940s, the Central Laboratory was in the lower part of Addis Ababa near the Guenet Hotal. Not only the hospitals but also (and especially) the practitioners of the city were dependent on this laboratory, which employed almost all the available technicians. Then in 1951, the Central Laboratory was moved to its present location. It became the Pasteur Laboratory of Ethiopia, directed by the Pasteur Institute of Paris, and was responsible for laboratory services, production of vaccines, and research into communicable diseases.

In the 1950s, building began on a number of hospitals in different parts of the country. The locations selected depended on political or economic considerations in relation to the various provinces. This continued into the 1960s.

In the late 1950s, the Ministry of Public Health for the first time in its history initiated short- and long-term plans. Planning was started by an energetic Minister of Health, but implementation died out after his transfer to another ministry.

To improve the medical services of developing countries, and to enhance the promotion, prevention and treatment of diseases, the World Health Organization (WHO) in this period called for the promotion and expansion of basic health services. Although Ethiopia was already experimenting in this with its own formula, with the assistance of WHO and other agencies more emphasis was now placed on the expansion of basic health services through health centers and health stations linked with existing hospital services. At length the target of one health center per *awraja*, or district, was achieved.[7]

Finally, the fourth five-year plan was formulated in the early 1970s. This plan was unique in that for the first time, development plans of the various ministries were coordinated by a Central Planning Office. These plans were initially to be tried out on selected *awrajas* which were to be given relative administrative autonomy and financial incentive to enable them to accelerate development. For historical reasons, this plan had no chance to be implemented or evaluated.

The responsibility for the administration of health activities in Ethiopia has always been assumed primarily by the government, with a few nongovernmental agencies involved to a modest degree. Accordingly, about 80% of the service-giving centers were owned by the Ethiopian government, the rest mainly by missionaries. After the 1960s, the Haile Sellassie I Foundation expanded its activities in the health sector. In Addis Ababa it ran the Haile Sellasie I Hospital, St. Paul's Hospital, and the Ghandi Memorial Hospital. Missions of various denominations ran hospitals, health centers, and health stations scattered in towns and rural areas. These missions, despite the country's adverse experience with missionaries in the past, were encouraged by the government to work in health activities.

All health institutions in the country were supposed to work under the strict guidance and control of the Ministry of Public Health. The administration of hospitals, health centers, and health stations was in the hands of this ministry. They were answerable to the Provincial Health Department, which in turn was answerable to the ministry and to the provincial governor. Ideally both the Provincial Health Department and the hospitals were headed by doctors who served, respectively, as provincial medical officer and medical director, with administrators assisting them. Because of the shortage of doctors, provincial health departments were sometimes run by a layman with wide experience in the health services. However, the situation improved in the 1960s and provincial health departments by then were administered by professionals. In the early stages, most medical directors were expatriates, but later newly trained young Ethiopian doctors entered this field, and in the care of small hospitals without directors were often made responsible for them.

Health services run by the government were heavily subsidized, for 75% to 95% of the patients were treated either free or virtually free. Because the tariff was very low, even those who paid were in effect also subsidized.

Governmental hospitals, health centers, and health stations received their equipment and supplies of drugs and other materials from a central semiautonomous governmental organization that purchased medical items and distributed them to all centers in the country.

Peripheral health services are assumed to be backed by the next better institution until, by using the vertical referral system, patients reach an institution commensurate with their health problem. This usually did not work for several reasons—the heterogeneity of medical practitioners, the absence in some areas of staged institutions, and more importantly because the patients were free to refer themselves, and therefore went to any institution of their choice, thus short-circuiting many centers. As a result of the heterogeneity of medical practices, and the irregularities that tended to occur—especially with regard to surgery—there developed a system of consultation in which doctors were selected by the Ministry of Public Health and requested to act as consultants by seeing the patient and giving their advice or conclusions in writing to the treating doctor. This arrangement, called "concillium," operated for a long time and usually was ordered for important personages or officials of the government or their relatives.

Eritrea was federated with the motherland in 1952. Health-service institutions in the Italian colony had been rapidly augmented and improved at the time of Italy's preparation to invade Ethiopia. When the British took charge of Eritrea the health administration was modified somewhat, but the system of racial segregation was retained. Hospitals in Eritrea were manned basically by Roman Catholic nuns who were responsible for both nursing and housekeeping. Most of the doctors, except the young ones, were contracted by the British administration to work in the hospital for half the day, in the morning. The rest of the time was their own for private practice. In Asmara this was carried out in private clinics and in three private hospitals. At the time of the federation of Eritrea with the rest of Ethiopia this system prevailed, but the private sector became more open to the indigenous population.

Ethiopian doctors began to be assigned to Eritrea from Addis Ababa by the Ministry of Public Health around 1963. In 1965 the ministry, with a view to combating the scandalous system of private practice then prevailing in Asmara and Massawa, attempted to reorganize the health services of Eritrea to bring them into conformity with those in the rest of Ethiopia. For this purpose a team consisting of the Minister of Public Health, the Minister of State, the chief advisor, and a senior Ethiopian doctor went to Eritrea. The responsibilities of the two doctors in the team were to evaluate the credentials and suitability of each physician, to classify them on the basis of their qualifications and experience, and to determine their salaries, as well as to evaluate all health institutions and submit recommendations with regard to the reorganization of the health services. The physicians, all of whom were Italian, were reorganized and were employed as full-time employees. They were allotted salaries at least three times higher than they had been receiving before. In addition, as a result of political pressure, they were allowed to continue their private practices. Health institutions in various parts of the province were reorganized at the same time, and those requiring structural change or additions were developed in accordance with their new role or function, according to the recommendations. During the period of the federation, the Ethiopian government also built two new hospitals, one in Agordat and the other in Massawa.

Ethiopia's armed forces—army, air force, and navy—during this period each developed its own health services, through the remarkable efforts of individuals responsible for health administration. The army had three hospitals: one in Addis Ababa, one in Harar, and one in Asmara. The air force had a hospital at Debre Zeit, and the navy used the new Massawa hospital. The police force also had its own medical services, with three hospitals—one in Addis Ababa, one in Asmara, and one in Harar. All these military and police services were extended to the families of serving personnel, and thus contributed to the medical coverage of a large section of the population.

Private practice by the few Italian doctors working in the government hospitals flourished in Addis Ababa immediately after the liberation. These practices were remnants of the occupation period, primarily intended for the Italian population. As more doctors from other countries began to join the health services and many Italian practitioners left after World War II, private practice began to dwindle. This happened at the time when, with the coming of new government recruits, the hospital services were getting stronger. Private practice has never been forbidden by law, but doctors under full-time government employment have not been given permission to have private practices, on the grounds of a possible conflict of interest in doing the same kind of work for both the government and themselves. In spite of this negative attitude by the Ministry of Public Health, many national and expatriate doctors indulged in office-clinics, for a short number of hours, outside their working day. In addition a few highly experienced auxiliary personnel conducted private clinics both in Addis Ababa and the provinces, and rendered various specialized services which won them great appreciation from the populace.

Traditional Medicine

The practice of traditional medicine in Ethiopia consists of the use of herbs, spiritual healing, holy water, bone-setting, and minor surgical procedures. These practices vary in their form, procedure, and content according to the local customs, and are very widely practiced. During and after the Italian occupation, the general population, with the exception of the few privileged groups, depended almost entirely on traditional medicine. In 1942, therefore, its practice was protected by law in Proclamation No. 27 of 1942,[2] which related to the registration of medical practitioners. Article 8 stipulated:

> Nothing contained in this Proclamation shall be construed so as to prohibit or prevent the practice of systems of therapeutics according to indigenous methods by persons recognised to be duly trained in such practice.
>
> Provided that nothing in this Article shall be construed to authorise any person to practice any indigenous systems of therapeutics which is dangerous to life.

Proclamation No. 100 of 1948,[6] relating to the registration of medical practitioners, reaffirmed the same principle as that of Proclamation No. 27. On the basis of these proclamations, traditional practitioners did not need to register, but the onus was on them not to use systems of therapeutics that were dangerous to life.

In the 1950s the registration and the granting of licenses to traditional healers started. Practitioners were supposed to submit to the ministry the herbs they used, so that these could be examined by the Central Laboratory to ascertain whether or not they were injurious to health or life. As for various reasons this was difficult to implement, the system was open to abuse and corruption. For this reason one of the ministers of public health, Ato Akalework Habtewold, changed the procedure of licensing by appointing a committee of doctors who were to be responsible for the proper licensing of traditional practitioners. This was to be done through the evaluation of each candidate. The committee also had to gather information which would assist in the study of the issue and submit recommendations to the minister on the future growth and proper development of indigenous medicine. During this period the committee found that information received was unreliable, as the candidates were secretive and the medicines received from them were compounded and therefore—though on the whole essentially harmless— were not recognizable. The committee, having also taken into consideration the experience of some other countries, such as India, made the following recommentations to the minister:

> the establishment of a legalized association of traditional medical practitioners, answerable to the ministry, to be responsible for the evaluation and licensing of practitioners, formulation of standards and code of practice, and punishment for misconduct and malpractice;
> the provision by the ministry of recognized locations or institutions for practitioners in the association;
> the promotion, through the association, of proper observation of clinical results and identification, analysis, and research into the therapeutic value of identified herbs;
> the promotion and encouragement of dialogue and cooperation between practitioners of modern and traditional medicine.

The minister received these ideas with enthusiasm and began to work on their implementation. However, at that time the administrative framework for such implementation was weak, and when he left the ministry the plan was abandoned. The previous procedure of licensing applicants on request therefore continued as before.

Indigenous medicine was carried out essentially on the basis of private practice, that is, of private agreements between consenting parties. The total cost of treatment cannot easily be assessed, but must have been enormous. If added to the government's own expenditure on health, the true dimensions of national expenditure on medical care can be appreciated.

The development of modern medicine has not in any way reduced the volume of traditional medicine practiced. This is because modern curative services have not been able to catch up with their growing demand or the population increase. Moreover, as modern medicine has tended to be increasingly concerned with preventive measures, and the curative services available have become progressively more distant and inefficient, indigenous medicine has become increasingly appreciated because it is at least readily available.

Specific Projects and Other Health Activities

In developing countries it is impossible to meet all health needs. For this reason it has been necessary to develop priorities. Selection of priorities depends not only on the availability of resources and manpower, but also on political and personal considerations, influence of the donor agencies, whims and ambitions of international experts, and above all on worldwide considerations, campaigns, and commitments on health matters. Such factors have had their influence in the introduction of a number of special projects which were developed mainly with the support of external agencies. These and other health-related activities are considered here to portray the nature of their activities.[7]

Malaria was known to be distributed in Ethiopia in areas below 2,000 meters, and its prevalence varied according to place and season. In 1958, there was a massive malaria epidemic in the country that even affected places such as Addis Ababa which were normally considered too high for malaria. During this epidemic all Ethiopian doctors in Addis Ababa were sent to the seriously affected areas to lead teams for the distribution of chloroquine tablets and to provide assistance to the sick. The concern created by this epidemic, and the previous success of pilot projects using DDT spraying initiated under WHO/UNICEF and USAID sponsorship, influenced the establishment in 1959 of the National Malaria Eradication Centre at Nazareth, which started to train paraprofessional personnel. The necessary administrative and technical organizations having been developed and strategies outlined, in 1966; a drive for the eradication of malaria from Ethiopia by 1980 was launched. To house the administrative center of this organization, a central headquarters was built within the compound of the Ministry of Public Health. However, to conform to a later decision of WHO, the objective was changed from eradication to control. The Malaria Control Service used indoor DDT spraying supplemented by drug distribution, and achieved considerable success in areas where malaria was previously of the endemic and epidemic type.

The global program of smallpox eradication started in 1968, but the program did not begin in Ethiopia until 1971. This program was initiated by the Ministry of Public Health with the assistance of WHO. The development of the program was hampered by various factors, mainly difficult communications, the low number of health institutions in some areas, and organizational problems of coordination. In 1973 the program was still in process of implementation.

Leprosy treatment and some measure of antileprosy work had been carried out by foreign missionaries for many years, and in Addis Ababa it was the responsibility of the Princess Zenebework Hospital. In 1956 a Leprosy Control Project was established, aimed at "bringing leprosy treatment as near to the patients' homes as possible and doing active case finding." This was effected through existing health organizations, both governmental and nongovernmental, but in the areas where there were no health facilities antileprosy work was carried out by mobile clinics.

ALERT (the All Africa Leprosy and Rehabilitation Training Centre) was established within the compound of Zenebework Hospital in 1965 by 11 founding members, including the Ministry of Public Health. The activities of ALERT consisted of training, service, and research. Training was provided for all categories of medical and health personnel. Service included hospital activities (inpatient and outpatient), an antileprosy program in the Shoa region, and rehabilitation. Research activities centered on follow-up. Study of relapsing patients and of the immunological status of leprosy patients are a few of the complex and high-powered research projects that were carried out in this institution.

Tuberculosis (TB) is prevalent throughout Ethiopia. A TB Control Programme was officially launched in 1959 with the establishment of a TB Demonstration and Training Centre in Addis Ababa. A little later, TB centers were established in Asmara and Harar. In addition, TB hospitals were set up in Addis Ababa, Asmara and Harar. It was the policy of the TB Control Programme to involve all health institutions in the control program. However, the idea of involving all these institutions in the scheme remained more an aspiration than a practical reality.

A Venereal Disease (VD) Control Project was supposed to have been established in 1955. All that was visible, however, was a VD Clinic in Addis Ababa started by the Italians. It was unfortunate that such an important sector of health was dismally neglected, despite the prominent attention it had received during the Italian occupation (albeit in the Italians' own self-interest).

Another project that was found difficult to maintain was the Trachoma Control Project. Several attempts were made to organize regionwide or nationwide trachoma control projects, but most of these failed. In recent years trachoma control projects involving limited regions of the country have been established with the assistance of the Italian government. This project gathered momentum, and it is hoped that it in the future will attain a substantial measure of success.

The Central Laboratory and Research Institute was established in Addis Ababa in 1951 as the Pasteur Institute. It came into existence as a result of an agreement with the French government, linking it with the Pasteur Institute in Paris. The building that was to house the institute had been erected before the Italian invasion, when it was a mission hospital known as the Lambie Hospital. Soon after the liberation, laboratory work for hospitals and clinics was carried out at premises near Guenet Hotel. This continued for some years until the various hospitals developed basic laboratory services of their own.

In the early 1960s the agreement with the French was abruptly terminated. The laboratory was renamed the Central Laboratory, and the first Ethiopian director was appointed to lead it into new ventures. In 1968 the organization was again renamed, as the Central Laboratory and Research Institute, and designated for laboratory diagnosis and research activities in the field of communicable diseases. The institute, being a seminautonomous body, had financial difficulty in carrying out its intended functions. To supplement its budget, it increasingly involved itself in clinical laboratory work for which it received fees. This development was facilitated by the inadequacy of the hospital laboratories and the absence of laboratory services in the private sector. The Central Laboratory and Research Institute later become predominantly involved in individual medical work.

The institute for many years also operated a veterinary service section which had the capacity to produce antirabies vaccine. This section was also actively involved with rabies control efforts by the Addis Ababa municipality.

In the mid-1960s, the American navy's laboratory base in Egypt, NAMRU II, moved to Addis Ababa as a result of a bilateral agreement and was established within the compound of the institute. The unit was mainly involved in valuable research into communicable diseases of its own choice.

EPHARM, a pharmaceutical manufacturing organization, was established in the early 1960s by an Israeli firm in collaboration with the Ethiopian government. The organization started with great expectations and promise. Discrepancies between hopes and achievements gradually became evident, however, and the Ethiopian government in 1972 established a high-level committee of professionals and administrators to study the workings of the firm and to make recommendations for its future organization. This study was completed and presented to the Council of Ministers in 1973.

Medical Education
The first post–World War II medical education in Ethiopia began in 1947 when the Department of Health, using the available physicians in Addis Ababa and the secondary-school laboratories at Kotebé, started to train pharmacy assistants and dressers. There were 60 students in all. Later a school for laboratory, pharmacy, and X-ray technicians and dressers was opened in Menelik Hospital, which continued to train these professionals. Laboratory technicians were also trained subsequently at the Central Laboratory and at the Gondar Public Health College.

In the 1940s the Ethiopian government began sending students abroad, on the basis of merit, to complete their secondary schooling, and a number elected to study medicine. Later, in the 1950s, students who had completed their secondary education in Ethiopia, were dispatched abroad for medical studies.

The first nursing school was started in 1950 by the Ethiopian Red Cross in the Haile Sellasie I Hospital, with the assistance of Swedish teachers and materials. At first, nurses entered school with only a primary-school education. Thereafter, the Empress Zewditu Hospital, run by the Seventh Day Adventists, started a nursing school. The Princess Tsehai Hospital followed in 1952, and later the new St. Paul's Hospital and the hospital in Asmara. The Gondar Public Health College trained community nurses. Gradually, better-educated students became available for nursing. By 1970, for instance, a registered nurse would be admitted with an 11th-grade-plus education and 3½ years or nursing school training, while a community nurse would have 10th-grade-plus and three years of nursing training. The training of nurses was the classical one in which they served as apprentices, doing full-time nursing as student nurses, supported by classroom education. Early in 1970, the notion gained ground of changing nursing education to a predominantly classroom setting, in which the student nurse was more of a student who received exposure than a worker-student. Since this was such a major change, it was unfortunate that the issue was not seriously debated in the context of Ethiopia's needs, but rather was adopted as a result of pressure from outside experts and the nursing division of the Ministry of Public Health. In Ethiopia, because of the dearth of health professionals, practitioners at every level find that they have more to do than they are trained for, and the need to improvise is a routine necessity. To function properly, therefore, it is necessary not only to have a good education, but also to have ample practical experience. Nurses in Ethiopia, especially in the provinces, have to undertake a variety of responsibilities, often unaided. Assessing how their education will prepare them to perform these tasks should be a major consideration in the evaluation of the future of nursing education.

A plan for the training of specialized nurses—as nurse anaesthetists, to alleviate the shortage of staff as well as to help start a voluntary blood donation scheme—was conceived by the anaesthetist of the Princess Tsehai Memorial Hospital, Dr. R. Ghose, and the Ethiopian surgeon then working with him. To this end a nurse anaesthetist school was started in 1960 with the approval and support of the Ministry of Public Health. Nurses were trained not only in anaesthetics but also in taking and cross-matching blood, to enable them to perform these tasks with a view to starting small blood banks at whatever hospital they might serve. This scheme was a great success and its graduates were the backbone of surgical work in Addis Ababa and the few provinces to which they were assigned. Unfortunately the program had to be discontinued upon the untimely and unfortunate death of Dr. Ghose.

The College of Public Health and Training Centre was established in Gondar in 1954, through the cooperative efforts of the Ethiopian government, WHO, and USAID. Its sponsors conceived it a a unique school, designed to supply the health-care services with middle-level professionals, who were regarded as a short-cut to solving the huge health problems of Ethiopia.

It was envisaged that these middle-level health workers would take an integrated approach—involving curative, preventive, and promotive activities—with the priority on prevention. These professionals were trained to work together as a team, consisting of a health officer (the team leader), a community nurse, and a sanitarian. They were to be assisted by auxiliary and ancilliary personnel. With health centers dispersed all over the country, each team was expected to—and in fact did—look after about 50,000 people in rural areas.

When the University in Addis Ababa became a chartered institution it was made responsible for all higher education. The Gondar Public Health College and Training Centre, accordingly, was taken over by the University in December 1961. As a result of this development major changes occurred in the curriculum of the health officer. The diploma course was replaced by a degree course, for the bachelorship of Science in Public Health, effective as of 1962. This change did not take into account the tasks the health officers were expected to perform or their future career structure. Their training, moreover, became increasingly academic and decreasingly field-work oriented. The upgraded health officer became more a clinician than a public-health man as originally intended, and the new tasks to be performed were not identified. This lack of synchronization between education and the tasks to be performed became a strain on the system of basic health services as previously envisaged.

In the late 1950s, the Ministry of Public Health undertook a preliminary study of the practicability of establishing a medical school in Ethiopia. The government later commissioned, through assistance, a high-powered international committee to study the feasibility of starting a medical school. Because of the absence of intrastructure and the meager number of students available to study medicine, the commission's recommendation was negative. However, because of the eagerness and insistence of the government to establish a medical school, a second international commission devised a scheme which would make it possible to start training. The plan recommended that selected students from the University College of Addis Ababa be sent to the American University of Beirut for preclinical training, and that in the meantime, and before the return of these students, clinical teaching be organized at the Princess Tsehai Memorial Hospital, and that a preclinical teaching facility be established.

The University, which succeeded the University College and was chartered in 1960, took up the task described above and set about implementing it. The available students (at the time only six in number) were sent to Beirut. The University, after organizing the first conference on Medical Education with the full participation of the Ministry of Public Health and experts from WHO's regional office, went on to organize clinical teaching in the Princess Tsehai

Memorial Hospital, and also established the Institute of Medical Sciences at the University Campus at Siddist Kilo. The University was assisted in this work by British teachers recruited on the basis of bilateral agreements. A little later, the government decided to provide for the needs of the Faculty of Medicine by adding premises for the preclinical department to the new medical center being built as a memorial to the Duke of Harar. This enabled the Faculty to teach both preclinical and clinical courses.

The establishment of the Faculty of Medicine was formally approved by the University's Faculty Council in 1964. The University began its medical program in 1965 with the training in clinical subjects of the six students who had returned from Beirut. Soon afterwards, in October 1966, the faculty began complete training with 22 preclinical students. They were mainly drawn from the Faculty of Science and the Gondar Public Health College, but because of the shortage of eligible students in the country a few were also enrolled from among science graduates of foreign universities.

The majority of the teachers in the faculty were from Great Britain, and the curriculum followed the international pattern with modifications to fit Ethiopian circumstances. For this reason, the degree chosen was an M.D. and internship was made an academic requirement.

The Institute of Medical Science, which incorporated the departments of Anatomy, Physiology, Biochemistry, Pharmacology, and Public Health, as well as the medical library and the dean's office, were housed in the main campus of the University until early 1973, when they moved to their new location in the Duke of Harar Memorial Hospital compound. As the Duke of Harar Hospital was not yet opened, most clinical teaching continued to be given in the Princess Tsehai Memorial Hospital and the adjoining Ethio-Swedish Paediatric Clinic, with some additional teaching at St. Paul's Hospital.

The Ministry of Public Health was the main consumer of the faculty's graduates, and the two institutions had little difficulty understanding each other. Faculty staff were always heavily involved in the ministry and responded to the numerous demands it put on them. The faculty, for example, ran an abridged course for health officers, with one year less in the clinical phase.

At one time, the Ministry of Public Health aspired to have competent and respected medical officers of health running all the provincial health services. It was then felt that the best person to occupy the post would be a health officer who had shown competence and had wide experience in the rural area, and who in addition would be medically qualified. WHO, which agreed with the idea, gave the ministry scholarships for five students per year. Following this, and to assist in the fulfillment of the ministry's aspirations, the faculty trained a total of 20 such health officers. However, for legitimate and important reasons, these graduates abandoned their administrative responsibilities and settled into clinical work. These reasons, if honestly and sincerely evaluated, may provide useful lessons for the future development of the health service. In addition in 1973 the Ministry of Public Health, in response to requests from health officers, awarded ten fellowships per year for four years for seasoned officers to return to study medicine in the faculty. This provided an opportunity for able health officers who had done their duty well, but were stagnating, to develop their career potential.

In 1972 the deanship of the faculty, which had earlier been held successively by three Britons, was Ethiopianized, and the number of Ethiopian staff became the majority. To accelerate and augment the Ethiopianization program, links with universities in the United States and the United Kingdom were developed. Under an agreement between New York University (NYU), the Haile Sellassie I Foundation, the Ministry of Public Health, and Haile Sellassie I University, an NYU–Ethiopian medical exchange program was instituted in 1971. Under this scheme, specialists from NYU came for a month at a time to teach and work in their own fields. This soon led, by a historical accident, to an interest in Ethiopia's development on the part of a Mr. Rubin Cohen, whose foundation was a benefactor to NYU. Through the offer of scholarships received from this foundation and other agencies, the faculty sent candidates to the United States—mainly to NYU—for specialization in various fields, including surgery, otolaryngology, ophthalmology, pathology, dermatology, obstetrics and gynecology, internal medicine, and haematology, etc—so that on their return the faculty would be well equipped for the expected yearly increase in student intake. At the same time, places for students to specialize in physiology, pharmacology, and obstetrics and gynecology were found in the United Kingdom, and doctors were sent to study these subjects, except for pharmacology where the arrangement was dislocated on account of the death of the candidate.

The Haile Sellassie I University developed a program of national service, in which students served in the rural area in the field of their studies for one year before commencing their final year. In the case of the Faculty of Medicine, however, the scheme was altered by agreement between the ministry and faculty to make it more profitable for both the student and the country. A special scheme was devised whereby students, after graduating and completing their internment, served as doctors in the rural areas for two years. This scheme applied also to Ethiopian doctors who had graduated abroad. By 1973, the faculty's graduates totaled 62 and, having been tested both in urban and rural settings, proved highly worthy graduates.

The School of Pharmacy was established in 1961 as a unit of the Faculty of Science, with the aim of providing pharmacists for hospital services and retail pharmacies. In 1964 the School of Pharmacy became part of the Faculty of Medicine, but maintained close academic ties with the Faculty of Science. The School's course ran for four years and contributed invaluable services by providing much-needed pharmacists for hospitals, retail pharmacies, and the drug industry, as well as the administration. By 1973 the School had graduated nearly 90 pharmacists.

Appraisal of Administrative and Health Manpower Support

In the early period—between 1941 and 1944—Ethiopia was struggling for its independent existence. Military material, machinery, industrial plants, trucks, and valuable Italian properties were removed to Kenya and neighboring British colonies, which thus benefited materially while Ethiopia was still occupied and bled cruelly. Although the Ethiopian environment was devoid of material facilties, the 500 Italian doctors, engineers, and artisans who freely remained behind became the basis of valuable technical activitiy in the country. Among the doctors there were a few who were highly capable, and by virtue of the friendship and trust that developed between them and Ethiopian high officials they were able to play an influential role besides providing curative services in Addis Ababa.

The British director of medical services, Dr. Campbell, had as his first duty the organization of hospital services, and for this he utilized such Italian doctors as were available within the framework of the British occupation administration. It was within this framework that the public-health guidelines and the proclamation regarding the registration of medical practitioners and pharmacists was promulgated in the name of Ethiopian government.

At the end of 1944, the signing of the second Anglo-Ethiopian agreement eliminated the earlier limitations on Ethiopian independence. Thereafter an Ethiopian director-general, Ato Araya Abebe, was appointed to head the health unit within the Ministry of the Interior. By 1947 the health unit, which became the Department of Health, was headed by a vice-minister, Ato Abebe Retta, who also was heading the institution with the same rank when it became the Ministry of Public Health. The ministry was later run by another vice-minister, Blata Kidane-Mariam Aberra. In 1950, Blata Zewde Belaineh was appointed the first Minister of Public Health, an appointment which signified the increased attention which the ministry was receiving from the government. Subsequent ministers appointed up to 1973 were Blata Mersie-Hazen Wolde Kirkos (acting vice-minister), Dejazmatch Tsehai Inquo-Sellassie, Ato Akalework Habtewold, Ato Getahun Tessema, Ato Abebe Retta, Dejazmatch Asfeha Wolde-Mikael, Dejazmatch Girmatchew Tekle-Hawariat, and, lastly, Ato Ketema Abebe. The appointment of ministers, as opposed to the directors general of earlier times, reflected the ministry's growth. Starting in 1954 as assistant advisor and progressively climbing in rank to minister d'etat was Ato Yohannes Tsighe who served the ministry uninterruptedly until 1973. During this period he played a dominant and determining role in its affairs.

With regard to the rest of the administration, except for a few Eritreans who had experience working with the Italians, the civil servants were all people with traditional education and experience. It was only in the late 1950s that a few Ethiopians with university education in health-related subjects began to join the ministry. Throughout the entire period, not a single Ethiopian physician joined its central administration.

From the start, the ministry's administrative machinery lacked the backing of professionals because of their absence from official posts. The creation of the General Medical Advisory Board nevertheless provided the administration with the necessary professional complement in all activities. In addition, the ministry made extensive use of advisers from international and bilateral agencies. The board consisted of a heterogeneous group of medical practitioners from various backgrounds who infused into it rich and varied experience. On this basis, for some 27 years, the board was the central force influencing public health policy, public-health legislation, the engagement of professional staff, medical training, education, and professional discipline. During this period the board thus rendered invaluable service to the health development of the nation.

Hospitals at the outset were run by a medical director, who was centrally appointed. He was assisted by a hospital administrator who headed the hospital administration and acted as the director's subordinate. Both were answerable to the Ministry of Public Health (if they were in Addis Ababa) or (in the provinces) to the Provincial Health Department which later slowly developed. As medical directors were for the most part expatriates and did not understand Amharic, this in many instances allowed the hospital administrator to take the initiative and in effect be more influential. As Ethiopian doctors began to assume responsibilities as directors of hospitals the situation improved and the hospital administration became more oriented towards hospital needs. This started to happen after 1963.

Medical technicians began to be trained as early as 1947, and their number and variety steadily expanded over the years. There was in addition an important core of practical technicians and dressers who developed proficiency through practical exposure rather than schooling and gave tremendous service though with little recognition. This medical-technical support staff included senior and junior laboratory technicians, X-ray technicians, and pharmacy attendants and dressers (advanced, elementary and practical). These cadres should have been trained in greater numbers to meet the great shortage that existed in nursing care. Advanced dressers were allowed to become druggists with the result that hundreds functioned as drug vendors in the rural areas.

Nursing education, which began as early as 1950, progressed to produce three kinds of nurses: registered nurses, community nurses, and specialized nurses. For a long time expatriate nurses worked in government and mission hospitals in the fields of nursing, teaching, and administration and made a major contribution to the establishment and development of the nursing profession. The schools of nursing operated independently in accordance with the requirements of the Ministry of Public Health, and produced nurses with practical experience, imbued with a spirit of professionalism and competitive loyalty to their schools. During the period under review, about 1,000 nurses[8] were trained. The majority worked in hospitals, the remainder in health centers, health stations, and special projects. Nurses in Ethiopia, irrespective of where they worked, have given invaluable service by extending their work beyond the confines of nursing and thus sharing many of the duties of the doctor. Nurses on the whole have been well-received and appreciated by a public uneducated about their role. On the other hand they are often blamed for the ills and shortcomings of the medical services, and, having taken an oath of service, have often been mistakenly regarded by dignitaries and the well-to-do as having forfeited all their worldly rights, needs, and aspirations.

The supply of nurses has not been commensurate with their demand, and the question could be asked why there was still a shortage of nurses, dressers, and medical technicians in 1973. The reasons were many, but the significant ones were constraints on the expansion of educational facilities and budgetary restrictions on employment.

Graduates of the Gondar Public Health College and training centers were envisaged as being trained to work together, as teams which were supposed to provide a quick answer to the enormous health problems of the nation. This short-cut solution was to be attained by concentration on preventive and promotive health-care activities. If this was the right course for developing countries to adopt, Ethiopia must be reckoned one of the first to take such a course to resolve the health problems of its rural population. This notion was introduced and supported by WHO and USAID and both, therefore, share with the ministry the successes and failures of the scheme.

From 1958 onwards, health-officer teams, first in the Gondar area and later elsewhere, worked in various health centers in the country, and without exception were given a heavy load of curative work. They were, therefore, mainly engaged, and forced by circumstances, to attend more to the individual medical problems of the community than to community-health problems. They did this well, were much appreciated, and earned great respect for their work from the people they served. A community approach at that time was not possible because curative health problems were untouched and the administrative, social, and economic situation was unripe for such activity. So, ten years after the launching of the health centers, an international commission was set up to evaluate the contribution and impact of the health teams. The commission's yardstick was what the latter had done to prevent disease, and on this reckoning they were considered a failure. The assessors, however, did not give much weight to the teams' considerable services in the curative field since this was not the primary objective of the evaluation.

The health officer, on account of his services, soon became an important person in his locality, but, as there was no career structure originally envisaged for him, he had no opportunity either for the improvement of his life or for the betterment of his knowledge. Difficulties encountered in administration, and in obtaining supplies, became a heavy burden. It is therefore understandable that some of the more determined officers began pressuring the ministry. Some left the profession and took up a trade or farming, while others enrolled in the medical school, went abroad on scholarship to take a public health degree, or entered the regional or central administration. By the end of the period there were about 30 health officers[9] with master's degrees in public health, most of them engaged in administration.

In the late 1960s there was a trend, both in the Faculty of Medicne and the Ministry of Public Health, urging the need for a specially abridged course suitable for health officers, to enable them to become doctors in a shorter than normal time, and thereby to keep this able and competent group within the profession. Unfortunately, shortage of teachers in the faculty was a major difficulty preventing the adoption of such a scheme, which would have involved teaching two bodies of students simultaneously.

The doctors who worked in Ethiopia were of different nationalities, capabilities, and attitudes. In the early period most were Italians, and many Ethiopian patients and auxiliary workers knew enough Italian for this language to be used as a medium of communication in the hospitals. As the number of Italian doctors dwindled and those of other nationalities entered the profession, English became the language of medical communication, teaching, and training. Accordingly, every doctor, before being allowed to practice was obliged to produce certification that he or she was able to speak English. The only place where this rule was waived was the Balcha hospital, where all the doctors and nurses were from the Soviet Union and used an efficient system of translation in Amharic and English to enable them to interact with both the patients and outside organizations.

The first Ethiopian doctor trained abroad returned in 1954. At that time it was the practice for all returning students to be taken to the emperor by the Minister of Education, who would brief them on the education and proposed assignment of the returnee. During the audience, the student before taking his leave normally received advice, directions, and words of encouragement. After this he would go to the ministry or department to which he had been assigned by the Ministry of Pen (in the early period) or the Ministry of Education (later on). The first trained doctor, after first visiting all the hospitals and health-related activities in Addis Ababa, was assigned to work in the Princess Tsehai Hospital.

Thereafter Ethiopian graduates from abroad started to trickle back, and began working in the Menelik Hospital and the Haile Sellassie I Hospital. The increasing number of these Ethiopian doctors, and their increasing involvement in the committee work of the ministry, had a positive impact on its work as well as on the professional activity of the Addis Ababa hospitals. The public's appreciation of the profession was also enhanced. By the early 1960s, Ethiopian doctors had become involved in hospital administration by becoming medical directors, and in 1972 the deanship of the medical school was given to an Ethiopian doctor.

The number of doctors working in Ethiopia in 1973 was about 370.[7] The great majority were expatriates who worked mainly in the cities. Of these doctors, 65% to 70% worked in Addis Ababa, Asmara, or Harar. Ninety percent of the expatriates were specialists, and the greater number were surgeons, followed by gynecologists, then internists, and a small number of other specialists.

There has been criticism, both within Ethiopia and from international organizations, of the scarcity of Ethiopian doctors working in rural areas, the exception being newly trained doctors doing their national service. The situation is not unique to Ethiopia, but rather a fact of life. If a nation believes in the value of doctors and goes to great pains and expense to train them, they must be placed in circumstances in which they can work efficiently and give the society proper service. For doctors to be assigned to a situation in which they are unsupported and can do very little only achieves the glorification of a statistical presence, for in the process of time they merely destroy themselves and are of little value either to themselves or to society. Therefore it is important to consider the factors required to obtain the maximum benefit from doctors working in rural areas: job satisfaction, family and educational considerations, challenges of service, and, above all, medical and administrative support.

In the mid-1950s, doctors began meeting in small groups to discuss their medical problems and experiences, and they later decided to establish a medical association as a forum for exchanging ideas related to their work. To this end an executive committee was elected to draft a constitution and explore procedures to legalize the association. The president elected was a highly respected expatriate Italian, and the secretary was the first Ethiopian doctor returnee. The secretary, together with Ethiopian legal experts in the Ministry of Justice, had the constitution drafted in English and translated into Amharic. After this it was approved by the few members of the association and accepted by the government. The association was then recognized, and registered with the Ministry of Interior.

The *Ethiopian Medical Journal* was launched in 1962 as the official quarterly publication of the Ethiopian Medical Association. Its aim was the advancement and dissemination of knowledge pertaining to medicine in Ethiopia and other developing countries. This journal had many teething and growing problems, but through the efforts of the successive boards of editors, managed to overcome most of them and succeeded in producing the stipulated number of issues per year.

The first annual conference of the Ethiopian Medical Association was launched in 1964 to provide a forum for doctors wishing to make scientific presentations and to exchange views on their medical work. These conferences have since then been held annually, and have grown in professional stature and importance. Burning and controversial issues have been selected for panel discussion, and it has become the custom for a known man of science to read a scientific paper as a theme of the conference.

Conclusion

The above outline of the development of medical activity in the postliberation period from 1941 to 1973 is based mainly on first-hand knowledge, and on information gathered by the author as one of the participants in the health activity of the time. There is, therefore, no pretension that this account is based on research, or guarantee that it may not include minor errors of detail.

In 1974 Ethiopia underwent a revolution unprecedented in its long history, which has resulted in a radical transformation of political, economic, and social circumstances. A component of the intended change is the health sector, which was one of the major issues of the revolution. In addition the World Health Organization has had an inspired vision, and decided in 1977 that the main target of all governments and of WHO in the coming decades is to be the attainment by all citizens of the world of a level of health that will permit them to lead a socially and economically productive life by the year 2000. Ethiopia, as a signatory to this agreement, is fully committed to this goal.

References

1. *Negarit Gazeta* 26 (1942):5–6.
2. *Negarit Gazeta* 27 (1942):6–7.
3. *Negarit Gazeta* 34 (1943):38–39.
4. *Negarit Gazeta* 91 (1947):66–68.
5. *Negarit Gazeta* (Legal notice) 99 (1947):7–9.
6. *Negarit Gazeta* 100 (1948):1–3.
7. *Comprehensive Health Service Directory.* Addis Ababa: Planning and Programming Bureau, Ministry of Health, 1968 EC (1976 G), pp. 8–10.
8. *Ibid.*
9. *Ibid.*

Bibliographic Note

This work is based on a series of studies by the author that have appeared in specialized journals over the last three decades. It has thus been deemed expedient not to burden the text with extensive footnotes. Most of the sources and quotations cited can readily be traced by consulting Dr. Pankhurst's earlier writings cited below.

Chapter I. Introduction: Some Factors Affecting Health

"Some Factors Influencing the Health of Traditional Ethiopia," *Journal of Ethiopian Studies* 4.1(1966):31-70.

"Some Factors Depressing the Standard of Living of Peasants in Traditional Ethiopia," *Journal of Ethiopian Studies* 4.2(1966):45-98.

"The Effects of War in Ethiopian History," *Ethiopia Observer* 7(1963):143-164.

Chapter II. Early Unidentified Epidemics

"The Earliest History of Famine and Pestilence in Ethiopia," *Ethiopian Medical Journal* 11(1973):233-236.

"The History of Famine and Pestilence in Ethiopia prior to the Founding of Gondär," *Journal of Ethiopian Studies* 10.2(1972):37-64.

"Diseases and Medicine" (chap. 18) in *An Introduction to the Economic History of Ethiopia*, 238-240. London: Sidgwick and Jackson, 1961.

"Le piaghi d'Etiopia," *Kos* 6(1984):33-48.

"Legendary Accounts of Medieval Famines and Plagues" (chap. 1), "Famine and Pestilence from the Fifteenth to the Early Seventeenth Century" (chap. 2), and "Outbreaks of the Gondarine Period and Early Nineteenth Century" (chap. 3) in *The History of Famine and Epidemics prior to the Twentieth Century*, 9-56. Addis Ababa: Relief and Rehabilitation Commission, 1985.

Chapter III. Smallpox and Variolation
"The History and Traditional Treatment of Smallpox in Ethiopia," *Medical History* 9(1965):343–355.

Chapter IV. The **Naftagna fangal**
"The History of Cholera in Ethiopia," *Medical History* 12(1968):262–269.

Chapter V. Typhus: Military and Civilian Outbreaks
"Some Notes for the History of Typhus in Ethiopia," *Medical History* 20(1976):384–393.

Chapter VI. Influenza: The **Hedar basheta**
"A Historical Note on Influenza in Ethiopia," *Medical History* 21(1977): 195–200.

"The Hedar Baseta of 1918," *Journal of Ethiopian Studies* 13,2(1975): 103–131.

"The Great Ethiopian Influenza Epidemic of 1918 (Ye Hidar Beshita)," *Ethiopian Medical Journal*, 27(1989):235–42.

Chapter VII. Syphilis
Economic History of Ethiopia 1800–1935, 627–628. Addis Ababa: Haile Sellassie University Press, 1968.

"An Historical Note on Ethiopian Terminology for Syphilis," *Afrika und Übersee* 59(1975–1975):65–69.

"Old-Time Ethiopian Cures for Syphilis, Seventeenth to Twentieth Centuries," *Journal of the History of Medicine and Allied Sciences* 30(1975): 199–216.

Chapter VIII. Leprosy and Leper Mendicants
"The History of Leprosy in Ethiopia to 1935," *Medical History* 28(1984): 57–72.

Chapter IX. Rabies
"The History and Traditional Treatment of Rabies in Ethiopia," *Medical History* 14(1970):378–389.

Chapter X. Tapeworm and Taenicides
Economic History of Ethiopia, 631–632.

"The Traditional Taenicides of Ethiopia," *Journal of the History of Medicine and Allied Sciences* 24(1969):323–334.

"Remedius Prutky's 18th Century Account of Ethiopian Taenicides and other Medical Treatment," *Ethiopian Medical Journal* 19(1972):3–6.

"Europe's Discovery of the Ethiopian Taenicide—*Kosso*," *Medical History* 23(1979):297–313.

"Ethiopian Taenicides in their East African Context," *Ethiopian Journal of African Studies*, 3.1(1983):49-54.

Chapter XI. Traditional Medicine and Surgery
"An Historical Examination of Traditional Medicine and Surgery," *Ethiopian Medical Journal* 3(1965):151-172.

Chapter XII. Thermal Baths
"The Thermal Baths of Traditional Ethiopia," *Journal of the History of Medicine and Allied Sciences* 41(1986):308-318.

Chapter XIII. Wesheba *or Steam Baths*
"Old-Time Ethiopian Cures for Syphilis," 207-213.

Chapter XIV. The Coming of the First Foreign Medical Practitioners
"The Beginnings of Modern Medicine in Ethiopia," *Ethiopia Observer* 9(1965):114-116.
"The Medical Activities in Eighteenth Century Ethiopia of James Bruce the Explorer," *Medizin historisches Journal* 17(1982):256-276.

Chapter XV. Foreign Medicine in the Early Nineteenth Century
"The Beginnings of Modern Medicine in Ethiopia," 116-120.

Chapter XVI. Developments During the Reigns of Téwodros and Yohannes
"The Beginnings of Modern Medicine in Ethiopia," 120-123.

Chapter XVII. Menilek's Era of Innovation
"The Beginnings of Modern Medicine in Ethiopia," 129-139.
"The Great Ethiopian Famine of 1888-1892: A New Assessment," *Journal of the History of Medicine and Allied Sciences* 21(1966):95-124, 271-294.
The History of Famine and Epidemics, 57-120.
"Early 20th century Ethiopian Noblemen's Requests for Medical Attention," *N.E.A. Journal of Research on North East Africa* 1.3(1982):183-187.
"The History of Prostitution in Ethiopia," *Journal of Ethiopian Studies*, 12.2(1974):159-78.

Chapter XVIII. The Tafari Makonnen-Hayla Sellasée Period
"The Beginnings of Modern Medicine in Ethiopia," 139-160.

Chapter XIX. The Italian Fascist Invasion and Occupation
"The Medical History of Ethiopia during the Italian fascist Invasion and Occupation (1935-1941)," *Ethiopia Observer* 16(1973):108-117.

Index

Ethiopian names which appear throughout most of this volume have been been transliterated on the basis of a simplified version of the system favoured by the Institute of Ethiopian Studies. However, there are three categories of exceptions: 1) names of persons of the present or recent past who prefer, or preferred, to be known—or are better known—by other spellings; 2) places which acquired prominence during the Italian occupation of Eritrea, and are therefore more widely known by Italian transliterations; and 3) names mentioned in Professor Asrat Waldayes' postscript whose own system of transliteration is to be found in the final section of the book. Cross-references have been added where necessary to avoid confusion.